Compliments of
The Black-Zandveld Lecture
in the History of Medicine
and
The Department of Humanities
December 2003

Physician and Philosopher

The Philosophical Foundation of Medicine:
Essays by Dr. Edmund Pellegrino

Physician and Philosopher

The Philosophical Foundation of Medicine:
Essays by Dr. Edmund Pellegrino

Foreword by Daniel P. Sulmasy, OFM, MD, PhD

CARDEN JENNINGS
PUBLISHING

Printed in the United States of America

ISBN 1-891524-09-7

Carden Jennings Publishing Co., Ltd.
375 Greenbrier Drive, Suite 100
Charlottesville, VA 22901
www.cjp.com

CONTENTS

PREFACE ix

ACKNOWLEDGMENTS xv

FOREWORD by Daniel P. Sulmasy, OFM, MD, PhD xvii

SECTION I **TOWARD A PHILOSOPHY OF MEDICINE** 1

Chapter One *What the Philosophy of Medicine Is* 3

Chapter Two *Toward a Reconstruction of Medical Morality: The Primacy of the Act of Profession and the Fact of Illness* 18

Chapter Three *Philosophy of Medicine: Problematic and Potential* 37

Chapter Four *The Goals and Ends of Medicine: How Are They to be Defined?* 56

Chapter Five *The Relationship of Theory and Praxis in the Philosophy and Ethics of Medicine* 66

Chapter Six *Being Ill and Being Healed: Some Reflections on the Grounding of Medical Morality* 72

Chapter Seven *The Healing Relationship: The Architectonics of Clinical Medicine* 80

SECTION II **OTHER PHILOSOPHICAL AND ETHICAL ISSUES CONFRONTING THE MEDICAL PROFESSION** 97

Chapter Eight *The Virtuous Physician, and the Ethics of Medicine* 99

Chapter Nine *Toward a Virtue-Based Normative Ethics for the Health Profession* 113

Chapter Ten *The Anatomy of Clinical Judgments: Some Notes on Right Reason and Right Action* 130

SECTION III THE NATURE OF AND EDUCATION FOR HUMANE CLINICAL PRACTICE AND HUMANE CLINICAL RESEARCH 151

Chapter Eleven *Educating the Humanist Physician: An Ancient Ideal Reconsidered* 153

Chapter Twelve *The Caring Ethic: The Relation of Physician to Patient* 166

Chapter Thirteen *The Book of Job* 179

Chapter Fourteen *Beneficience, Scientific Autonomy, and Self-Interest: Ethical Dilemmas in Clinical Research* 191

SECTION IV HEALTH PROFESSIONALS AS MORAL AGENTS 203

Chapter Fifteen *The Medical Profession as a Moral Community* 205

Chapter Sixteen *Hospitals as Moral Agents* 214

Chapter Seventeen *State University of New York at Stony Brook Health Sciences Center* 223

Chapter Eighteen *Academic Health Centers and the Medical Marketplace: A Faustian Compact Examined* 263

Chapter Nineteen *Access to Health Care: The Ethical Imperative Beyond Insurance* 277

REFERENCES 285

PREFACE

This book represents a unique way to explore the many sides of the professional life of a person who is becoming increasingly recognized as an extraordinary, humane, polymathic, and highly productive human being living amongst us. Some persons enter our collective consciousness by virtue of a burst of visible activity, while others seem to enter gradually into our awareness over a more prolonged period. Edmund D. Pellegrino is in the latter category, but even there he is different from many other great persons of extraordinary talent and achievement, in that Dr. Pellegrino has excelled again and again in several fields by doing a variety of things and playing a variety of roles over the length of his extended professional career.

We, the editors and conceivers of this project, came to the conclusion that this man's entire prolific career as a philosopher deserved more focused attention in depth and breadth. Thus the Association of Academic Health Centers commissioned a paper by Professor Daniel Sulmasy, asking for a critical analysis (written for the non-philosopher) of the main corpus of Dr. Pellegrino's writings in philosophy and ethics. Dr. Sulmasy, a physician and a distinguished medical ethicist himself, got his doctorate under the tutelage of Pellegrino. Sulmasy agreed to evaluate Pellegrino's career and publications as a philosopher and was asked to evaluate those works from the point of view of the professional philosopher as well as from the point of view of their overall meaning to the profession of medicine. Physicians for many years have regarded Edmund Pellegrino as one of the leading medical philosophers, ethicists, and teachers of human values within the family of medicine, but the legitimate question can be raised as to how his work is assessed by professional philosophers. Dr. Sulmasy did not disappoint us as you will discover when you read his essay, published as a centerpiece of this book. Not only has Dr. Sulmasy provided a careful analysis of Pellegrino's philosophy of medicine, but he has given readers a clear and concise review of the competing conceptual frameworks that have evolved since the dawning of the modern era of medical ethics, which Pellegrino did so much to bring about in the 1960s and 1970s.

Our intention had been to publish a recent reflection by Ed Pellegrino on the current state of affairs in the world of medical practice and education along with the Sulmasy piece in order to make a useful contribution to the literature, as well as to connect medicine more completely with philosophy in honoring Dr. Pellegrino and his career; he has long been known to argue that medicine and philosophy are all of a piece. However, we soon concluded that this approach might be only half a loaf, because Pellegrino, in his eighty plus years, has been outstanding in more than as a practitioner and teacher of the practice of medicine and as a working academic in the field of philosophy and ethics.

We soon began to consider the many ways that we have known of him. At a national and international level, we have known Pellegrino as a leading academic physician/researcher, as chairman of the department of medicine at the University of Kentucky, and then as dean of medicine at the State University of New York at Stony Brook (SUNY Stony Brook). We have known of him further as a leading proponent in the 60's and 70's of the health care team, of respecting the roles of other health professionals on the team and of recognizing the concept of shifting captaincy of the team; this led him to leadership positions of entire health science centers (SUNY Stony Brook and the University of Tennessee), one of which (Stony Brook) he designed with the team concept in mind. He also has led two health care delivery organizations with great distinction, one community-based (Hunterdon Medical Center, Flemington, New Jersey) and the other a more traditional teaching hospital setting (Yale/New Haven Medical Center, Inc.).

Throughout all of these many leadership experiences, Pellegrino sustained his own clinical efforts as at least a part-time clinician, maintained a laboratory investigating the biochemistry of calcium metabolism and its relationship to certain diseases, and became increasingly active in the field of philosophy, particularly as it related to medicine and health. He was at the same time an innovator, being a central figure, if not the central figure, in the founding of the Society of Health and Human Values, the *Journal of Medicine and Philosophy*, and the resurgence of human values and ethics as legitimate subjects of teaching and research in medical and other health professional schools. How could he have done all these things well?

Perhaps the confluence of all these sets of intertwining activities, when joined to Dr. Pellegrino's serious and lifelong commitment to his religious faith, created the circumstances that led to his being appointed the first (and thus far the only) non-clerical president in the hundred-plus year history of the Catholic University of America, a position he held with great distinction for five years. One of the major reasons why this elevation to a prominent position so closely aligned with the Church itself did not reduce Dr. Pellegrino's effectiveness with health professionals across the board, with and without any particular religious faith, was his analysis of the doctor-patient interaction, which spoke to a meeting of two separate moral agents, the patient and the doctor. That is, the patient has important rights including a right to know what is going on and might be going on with her/his treatments, but the doctor also has rights, including a right not to carry out interventions that are unacceptable within her/his moral code.

Most recently, Pellegrino took a leadership position in Georgetown University's efforts to establish and develop centers for Health Ethics and for Clinical Ethics. As a full-time philosopher (albeit he remained clinically active) these past several years, his work with graduate students and his productivity as a thinker in these areas has proliferated and prospered to a level that might make some people envious. In fact, some thirty years ago, when he had achieved growing national recognition as a physician, a researcher, an educator, and an administrator, we recall the sotto voce criticisms sometimes leveled at his research and educational ideas by more hard-core, traditional medical scientists along the lines of, "He's a jack of all trades and master of none! He's dabbling and hasn't paid his dues sufficiently in any one of these various areas for us to take him seriously."

Most others, who noticed the multi-tiered productivity of this person, expressed wonderment at the variety of his accomplishments and the clarity and conciseness of his lectures and talks. Clearly, here was an exceptional teacher as well as one who excelled in many other areas.

As the explosion of biomedical science spawned a proliferation of medical specialties in the latter half of the twentieth century, the modern academic profession, which had patterned itself after William Osler, began to wonder, with the rapid demand for medical science research in medical schools, whether it was possible any longer to combine in one person the "triple threat" excellence in clinical practice, in teaching, and in research. More and more physicians in academic medicine and in private practice were and are asking, "Where have so many of the triple-threaters gone?"

Clearly, Pellegrino has excelled in all three aspects that make up the "triple threat" in academic medicine (practice, research, and teaching). In addition, Pellegrino, along with a handful of other high-profile physician leaders of the twentieth century, initiated and administered major organizational enterprises, and has become a "thought leader" for the entire profession.

In the latter regard, however, Pellegrino stands alone amongst other great physician "thought leaders," in that he has spent more of his time than any of the rest in serious work within the fields of medical ethics and philosophy. Thus Pellegrino is not only a triple threat, but he has been a potent contributor in five areas, when you add "thought leader" and "institutional leader" to the mix.

There is, in fact, a sixth area of excellence that Pellegrino shares with a subset of his twentieth-century peers among the great physician geniuses of modern times. Colleagues, students, and patients have noted the human excellence Pellegrino has demonstrated through the quality of his personal life, his character, and his inexorable humane-ness. We are not in a position to sensibly comment further on this dimension, except to note that many of the great modern physicians would surely say that everything else in their lives flows from this personal dimension.

Thus, we came to the conclusion that we would supplement the Sulmasy paper by carefully selecting, from among Pellegrino's more than 500 publications, examples of his best and most significant written contributions illustrative of several of these various "lives" of his. Through this collection, interested readers can explore for themselves the many facets of Edmund Pellegrino and answer for themselves the question about whether his multiple positions and functions are really separate and unconnected dabblings or whether they are all of a piece, linked at their core to the various aspects of what Pellegrino might hope to have become, i.e., the complete physician.

We posit a unity in his professional life, rather than a dispersion of talents and efforts in a variety of unrelated activities; and, as such, we celebrate, through this book, his contributions thus far as part of an integrated life covering many sectors and qualifying him as a humane, complete physician and teacher, highly productive philosopher, and institutional leader, of a stature that puts him in a class with only a few others past and present. Perhaps even more important, rather than attempting a biography of this exceptional person, we provide here a selection of his own writings, chosen with his involvement, which should allow readers to make their own significant scan of this man's extraordinary career.

Roger J. Bulger, MD
The Association of Academic Health Centers

John P. McGovern, MD
The McGovern Foundation

ACKNOWLEDGMENTS

While it is difficult to acknowledge every individual who has had an impact on the publication of this book, we wish to thank the following organizations, institutions, and individuals for their generosity, collective wisdom and collaborative support: the Board and leadership of the Association of Academic Health Centers, the McGovern Foundation for making it financially possible, Daniel P. Sulmasy, OFM, MD, PhD, for an inspiring introduction, Ken Massey and Debbie Bretches for persistence and excellence in design and production, and the long list of professional publishing companies who generously shared their previously published work for use in this well-rounded project.

David B. Ern
Carden Jennings Publishing Co., Ltd.

Roger J. Bulger, MD
The Association of Academic Health Centers

FOREWORD

The Essentialist Medical Ethics of Edmund Pellegrino: Analysis and Critique

Daniel P. Sulmasy, OFM, MD, PhD
The John J. Conley Department of Ethics,
Saint Vincent's Hospital and Medical Center, New York, NY
and The Bioethics Institute of New York Medical College, Valhalla, NY

It is a dangerous rhetorical device to compare the work of a living author with that of a luminary from the past. The comparison can sometimes inadvertently make the living author look very small. But when the comparison is genuinely apt, it can be a mistake not to note it. And so, in reflecting on the work of Edmund Pellegrino, I do not think it hyperbolic to compare his work with some of the medical giants of the past whose names are familiar to many of us. I believe these comparisons are apt, and it would be a mistake not to note them. Pellegrino and his predecessors of earlier ages practiced and taught medicine, even as they became well known outside their field. Pellegrino, as have his predecessors, has given us scientific medical works as well as treatises reflecting on the practice of medicine and its place in the world. To read their works is to discover keen intellects and an amazingly wide range of interests and reading. All were medical leaders, who trained and influenced several generations of physicians. Such leaders have affected the course of medical education significantly, not only by the results of their research and experience, but by writing about medical education and by using their leadership positions to help usher in the reforms about which they wrote.

But like any comparison, there are also differences amongst the individuals in any such group. I would assert that Pellegrino's writings on the nature of the medical enterprise, its moral underpinnings, and its place in the wider world are actually more incisive, systematic, and rigorous than anything his medical predecessors have written. What others did for the scientific aspects of medicine, Pellegrino has done for the humanistic aspects of medicine.

In preparing the present paper, one of the most remarkable discoveries I made was how fresh Pellegrino's writings from the 1960s and 1970s sound. Many seem only truer at the present than they were when he first wrote them. For instance, he was writing about the importance of computers in the work of physicians in 1965,[1] about the need for physician re-certification, about balancing population-based medicine with the care of individual patients and about the care of the underserved in 1973,[1] about the affective aspects of medical education in 1974,[1] and about "institutional ethics" in 1977.[1]

MEDICAL ETHICS AND PHYSICIANS' "DISCRETIONARY SPACE"

Pellegrino also put his diagnostic finger on a serious and persisting anomaly in the relationship between medicine and society that he has called the problem of "the discretionary space" of the practitioner.[1] We are still convulsively grappling with this issue today and will be for the foreseeable future. What he means by this is that every society must decide what sort of latitude it will give to its professionals – if one will, how much decisional autonomy professionals should have. Multiple forces have recently combined to move society to place limits on physicians' discretionary space – changing social mores, the explosion of technology, health care inflation, physicians' own abuse of power and lack of self-policing, to name a few.[2] Some of the contraction in physicians' discretionary space that has occurred over recent decades, however unpleasant, has been a morally necessary response to historical circumstances. By contrast, some has been morally unnecessary, or even misguided. Yet, Pellegrino also notes that at the same time that society is busy limiting physicians' discretionary space, we have witnessed a contradictory tendency of society to expand the physician's discretionary space by increasingly medicalizing aspects of life once thought outside the domain of medicine, e.g., poor school performance, firearms in the home, automobile safety, human rights abuses, and death itself.[1] Pellegrino knew this twenty-five years ago. His insight only grows truer every day. One of the great and overriding issues society now faces with respect to medical ethics is the question of how to bring practitioners' discretionary space into a morally appropriate equilibrium in the face of profound social change.

It has been in the midst of such turbulent times that Pellegrino has written most of his work. As he himself has stated,

> Ethics comes into existence, properly speaking, when morality itself becomes problematic, when the validity of beliefs about what is right and good comes into question, or when a conflict between opposing moral systems or obligations must be resolved.[3]

Such are the times in which we live. Morality itself has never been less certain or more contested. The discretionary space of physicians is in constant flux. This is precisely why medical ethics, defined as the systematic, critical, reasoned evaluation and justification of right and wrong, good and evil in medicine, and the critical evaluation of the kinds of persons physicians should be, is so vitally important at this moment in the history of medicine. As Pellegrino put it, "We have had 2,500 years of medical morality, but only 30 years of medical ethics."[4] Pellegrino has not only written about medical ethics in this period. He has served as one of the prime forces sensing the need for medical ethics and ushering in the era of formal, critical reasoning about medical morality – the era of medical ethics.

The range of Pellegrino's writings and the sheer volume (as of Sept. 30, 2000 — 18 books, 51 scientific papers, and 519 papers in the medical humanities) makes an account, analysis, and critique of his contributions a daunting task. And to help to put this achievement into perspective, it is also impressive to note that Pellegrino actually wrote most of these himself. He did not have a cadre of research fellows writing scientific papers on which he is listed as senior author without having done much of the actual research or writing.

I have read many but certainly not all of his papers and books. To help focus the task of presenting an analysis and critique of his contributions in medical ethics, I therefore decided to concentrate on his books. Since these often contain reworked versions of the papers he considers his most significant, such a filter seems appropriate. These are the papers he most wants to present to us.

In my view (which I do not think would be contested by most scholars in the field) the four most important of these books are: *Humanism and the Physician* (1979), *A Philosophical Basis of Medical Practice* (1981), *For the Patient's Good* (1988), and *The Virtues in Medical Practice* (1993). The latter three were co-authored with his longtime collaborator and friend, David Thomasma. These three books contain the core of his philosophical project in medical ethics. They are certainly not the last word, however. Even as I write, he and Thomasma are actively engaged in revisiting, refining, and elaborating upon the work they undertook in *A Philosophical Basis of Medical Practice* in a new book. This promises to be a work of great significance.

The ideas in these four books run throughout much of Pellegrino's work. They help to situate his philosophical project not only in the context of the social changes discussed above, but also with respect to competing voices in the hotly contested field of medical ethics. When right and wrong are no longer taken for granted, a myriad of commentators have stepped forward to offer their views. Some are familiar; some are obscure. Where does Pellegrino's ethical thinking fit within this broad field?

THE CURRENT STATE OF AFFAIRS IN MEDICAL ETHICS

A wide range of theories of medical ethics have been proposed over the last thirty years since the era of formal medical ethics began. Of these, four have had the most substantial influence. To put Pellegrino's work into perspective, I will briefly discuss these, and then mention several other theories before offering a broad critique of all of them in a manner I will attribute to Pellegrino. This survey and critique will help to show how radically Pellegrino's approach differs from all of these other theories of medical ethics, and provide a springboard for explaining what his approach might have to offer.

1. Principlism: The most commonly taught approach to medical ethics today is known as "principlism." This approach attempts to bypass the fact of radical disagreement about the nature of morality to find common elements at the level of principles that could be agreed to by all persons regardless of their underlying theories of ethics. Beauchamp and Childress,[5] who first introduced the familiar four principles of autonomy, beneficence, non-maleficence, and justice best exemplify this approach. The tension that is evident in moral dilemmas in medicine is often aptly described as a clash between these principles, as when a Jehovah's Witness may autonomously refuse a transfusion that a physician beneficently thinks is indicated. Recourse to these principles often illuminates the right course of action in cases. While very popular, this approach has been criticized as unhelpful because it leaves the resolution of the dilemma of conflicting principles in specific cases to intuition. It has also been described as providing a checklist of moral concerns in specific cases, but not, properly speaking, a guide to action.
2. Contractualism: The theory underlying most legal approaches to ethics is one popularized by Robert Veatch.[6] In the tradition of Locke and Rousseau, he avers that there is no medicine without the consent of the treated. He describes a "triple-contract." Society in general has a contract with each human being who is a member of that society. Medicine as a profession also has a contract with all the members of society, prescribing duties and limits on power. Finally, each individual patient engages in a contract with each individual physician for each medical encounter. Social policy is the ground of the ethics of the first contract. Health policy is the ground of the ethics of the second contract. And informed consent for any and every medical action is the ground of the ethics of the third contract. This theory has been criticized as paying insufficient attention to the reality of the situation of patients, who are often in no position to negotiate "contracts." It has also been criticized as painting too dark and untrusting picture of the character of human beings. But it is, to a great extent, precisely how the laws of a democracy like the USA, based on contractual political philosophy, actually work.
3. Casuistry: Another approach to medical ethics that has attracted a wide following is the casuistic approach of Albert Jonsen.[7,8] Casuistry is a case-based approach to ethics. Since clinicians deal primarily with cases, this approach has great appeal among physicians and nurses. In the form promulgated by Jonsen, casuistry is unmoored from any particular moral theory, and thus holds an attraction for a morally pluralistic society. And for those predisposed to distrust approaches to ethics based upon deductive logic, casuistry offers an alternative — a way to reason about present cases based upon their analogy to paradigmatic cases from the past. In the casuistic approach, one need not apply abstract principles to particular cases. Once a certain morally problematic case has been resolved to everyone's satisfaction, one need only decide whether the case at hand is sufficiently similar to that paradigm case that it ought to be settled in a similar manner. This approach has also been criti-

cized. At the very least, critics would say, casuists are relying upon the principle that "similars should be treated similarly," and so it is really not free of principles. Critics have also expressed concerns that a line of cases that is not hemmed in by firm moral rules may eventually lead to ethically troubling conclusions. Still, this remains a very popular approach and at the very least, elements of casuistry are a major part of what ethics committees all over the world do on a regular basis.

4. Liberalism: Another very important approach to medical ethics is the application of liberal political and moral theory to medical situations. These approaches place a great deal of emphasis on concepts such as human rights and personal autonomy. A major proponent of this liberal approach to medical ethics is Dan Brock.[9] This approach suggests that beyond a basic commitment to liberty and equality, very little of a substantive moral nature can be settled in a truly democratic society. Such a society must promote liberty and equality in everything, including health care. One cannot ever hope to impose a particular substantive view of the good life on the whole population. Thus, the answers to contested questions such as the morality of abortion or euthanasia cannot be given by ethical theory. Each person must be free to make such decisions by his or her own lights. On the other hand, society has an obligation to provide equality of access, and so individual autonomy may be curtailed in order to promote equality. Such an approach can be criticized as having contradicted itself – by promoting liberty and equality it is already declaring a particular substantive theory of the good. Liberal approaches also fail to specify how one balances liberty with equality. But despite criticism, this approach to medical ethics is enormously popular in Western culture, suffused everywhere by liberal political theory.
5. Other Approaches: The superficiality of this incredibly brief survey of the major theories of medical ethics must be acknowledged. But one must also acknowledge that the breadth of medical ethics is even wider than the theories discussed thus far. The plethora of approaches includes many others. Care-based ethics, emphasizing the paradigmatic moral relationships of dependence and vulnerability, often associated with the moral reasoning of women has become popular.[10,11] Feminist theories of medical ethics have also appeared.[12,13] Narrative approaches, based upon the primacy of personal history and stories, criticize all forms of reasoning about ethics as abstract.[14] A form of clinical pragmatism based upon the philosophy of Dewey and James has been proposed.[15] Utilitarianism has strong adherents who base their bioethics upon this theory.[16] Deontologists, basing their approaches upon rules and duties, have also proposed theories of medical ethics.[17] Libertarians, prioritizing freedom over equality, have proposed theories of medical ethics.[18] And while very few ethicists still actively propose situation ethics,[19] this approach, in fact, still has many quiet adherents "in the trenches."

This is the state of medical ethics today. The first 2,500 years of Western medical history, characterized by a lack of ethical theory, have now given way to an era characterized by an excess of ethical theory. The fragmentation of contemporary philosophical ethics has now been foisted upon medicine. Every contested theory of general ethics has been applied to medical ethics. Even the list above is not exhaustive. Religious theories also abound. Some postmodern interpretations would even suggest that this ethical cacophony is precisely where the dream of ethics based upon reason must inevitably lead, because all of ethics is merely a screen behind which raw struggles for power and domination are being waged.

PELLEGRINO'S CONSTRUCTIVE ALTERNATIVE

Where does Pellegrino's approach fit in the midst of this seeming ethical chaos? Pellegrino offers both a critique and a constructive alternative. His approach offers both a way of explaining why we seem so lost and a suggested route out of the dark forest.

Even if Pellegrino has not specifically enunciated it, one can infer his critique of these other theories from the alternative he proposes. This critique is simple. First, every attempt to specify a theory of ethics that is devoid of substantive content regarding concrete moral problems is doomed to failure for one of two reasons. Either it will end up specifying some sort of content subrosa (such as making liberty a substantive moral good in itself rather than a procedural, formally necessary condition for moral action), or it will be of such a broad or vague nature that it is of little help. Of the theories discussed above, only Culver and Gert's theory avoids this by plainly proposing a set of substantive, concrete moral goods. But even so, this theory, like all the others, can be subjected to the second critique. Namely, every one of these theories is "applied" ethics. It is the application of some general moral theory or approach to medical situations. Each, as it were, "imposes" ethics on medicine from above. They do not first attempt to understand medicine. They first attempt to understand ethics, and they apply this abstract understanding to concrete clinical situations. Such an approach may be wrong-headed from the start.

What Pellegrino proposes (in my view uniquely) over and against all these other theorists, is a "bottom-up" as opposed to a "top-down" approach to medical ethics. Rather than pulling one or another ready-made but highly contentious general theory of ethics off the shelf and applying it to the practice of medicine, Pellegrino suggests that perhaps one should start by looking at medicine first and then build a theory of medical ethics from the ground up. One way out of the moral cacophony in medical ethics that may preserve actual normative content would be to try to understand medicine qua medicine first, and then to try to figure out what moral obligations flow from a clearer understanding of medical praxis. In other words, medical ethics should be part of the philosophy of medicine, not the application of moral philosophy to the problems of medicine. This is the approach Pellegrino has championed for several decades.

The basic assumptions of this "essentialist" approach may be characterized as follows:

1. Medicine has a fundamental, knowable nature – an essential core.
2. Through the philosophy of medicine, one can come to an understanding of the nature of medicine and its purposes.

3. From this understanding, one may derive a set of moral expectations of those who practice medicine, and define a morally correct relationship between a society and its medical professionals.

I will spend the rest of this paper explaining this approach in more detail, examining its implications, and offering a critique.

PELLEGRINO'S ESSENTIALIST FOUNDATION

As Thomasma has explicitly put it, Pellegrino first and foremost has engaged in a struggle to find a genuine foundation for medical ethics.[3] Much contemporary ethical theorizing has abandoned the notion that this is possible, preferring instead to say that ethics is either merely the expression of emotions, a thinly disguised power struggle, or a more or less stable consensus reflective of a particular time and place. Pellegrino, by contrast, thinks that there are ethical rules that transcend space and time, that they can be known, and that they are at least *ut in pluribus* true. Just as MacIntyre suggested that particular human practices have defined ends that specify the good for that practice in an objective way,[21] Pellegrino has long contended that medicine is a human practice with a particular nature and objective ends. To silence the cacophony of disparate voices in medical ethics, Pellegrino, the reflective practicing internist, turned to the practice of medicine to find a foundation for his medical ethics.

Those writing before him within the medical profession have made some feeble attempts to develop their own ethical systems. But these, he notes, have not withstood careful scrutiny.[2] Codes of medical ethics have been asserted since the time of Hippocrates, but never justified or given a foundation. Arguments about the nature of medicine (for instance, whether it is a science, an art, or applied science) have long been contested and may be irresolvable. But what Pellegrino finds inescapable is the reality of the relationship between the individual practitioner and his or her patient. His "starting point"[2] is the clinical encounter – "matters of fact rooted in human experience."[2] It is there that he has located the foundation for medical ethics.

Perhaps the seminal paper in his career was originally published in 1979 and later included in *A Philosophical Basis of Medical Practice* as the linchpin chapter, entitled "A Philosophical Reconstruction of Medical Morality."[2] Here he lays out what he believes are timeless, universal, and irrefutably true characteristics of the practice of medicine upon which a theory of medical ethics can be constructed. He calls these the fact of illness, the act of profession, and the act of medicine. While these are, in turn, based upon earlier work in the philosophy of medicine, these concepts are the essential elements of his philosophy of medical morality.

THE FACT OF ILLNESS

Pellegrino contends that the human phenomenon of illness is profound and unique. The primary assault is upon the unity of body and self that constitutes the person. It affects every other possible expression of human freedom. Life and health condition all other freedoms, and the limitations on personal autonomy imposed by illness are therefore ontologically prior to other human freedoms. And, as such, the degree of vulnerability is greater in illness than in almost any other human situation.[2] He calls this state "wounded humanity."[1]

THE ACT OF PROFESSION

Pellegrino next notes that those who possess the specialized knowledge and skill to help those who are ill literally "profess" that they will use their skills for the benefit of the sick by accepting their diplomas and swearing oaths to do so after actually graduating. This pledge is re-articulated each time a patient enters a room and a physician, wearing the symbols of this public profession, asks, "How may I help you?"[2]

THE ACT OF MEDICINE

Pellegrino uses the phrase "act of medicine" to designate what it is that the physician and patient actually do together in the clinical encounter. This is why the philosophy of medicine is so critical to his medical ethics. He calls the clinical encounter "an event" characterized by "mutual intentionality."[2] The act of medicine is first and foremost a relationship. Its goal is the well-being of the patient. The clinician practices his or her craft by exercising judgment, involving both scientific knowledge and practical wisdom. The defining limits of this craft are that it is practiced through, with, and in the human body. Morality arises out of the link between scientific knowledge about human bodies and the care of individual human persons.[2] The physician must answer three questions: What can be wrong? What can be done? And what should be done? The latter is necessarily a moral question.[2]

Medicine, for Pellegrino, is "an activity whose essence appears to lie in the clinical event, which requires that scientific and other knowledge be particularized."[1] All moral obligations flow from the existential situation of the patient (the fact of illness), the moral purposes and commitment of health care professionals (the act of profession), and the relationship between a clinician and a patient based upon a shared intention to seek healing for the patient (the act of medicine). The aim of the clinical event is "a right and good healing act for this patient."[1,2] Medicine is thus an inherently moral activity.

THE PATIENT'S GOOD

Profound moral obligations arise from the essence of medicine, so understood.[2] The predicament of the patient requires trust, which in turn requires trustworthiness of the clinician. The act of profession requires competence, or it is a lie. The shared intention to seek healing for the patient requires a degree of altruism — that the clinician be willing to forgo some degree of self-interest for the sake of the patient. The radical inequality between the healer and the sick person requires patient involvement in decision making to help restore the "wounded humanity" of the patient. Pellegrino and Thomasma call this model of the physician-patient relationship, "beneficence-in-trust."[20]

This means that respect for patient autonomy, far from being a separate and competing principle of medical ethics, becomes an integral aspect of beneficence. For Pellegrino, the act of medicine demands that the good of the patient be the primary focus of the medical event, but this good is manifold and can be specified at four distinct levels.[20]

These levels are the biomedical good, the good as the patient has chosen it, the good of the patient as a person, and the patient's designation of the ultimate good. These levels of good are arranged hierarchically. This gives his system an advantage over principlism in that the Pellegrino system gives substantive advice about resolving moral conflicts, not merely leaving everything to intuition. The biomedical good of the patient is only a limited good. It is humanly good only if it serves the good of the patient at all the other levels. Thus, a physician pledged to act for the good of the patient may know what can be wrong and what can be done for a patient with gangrene of the left lower extremity. And he or she may know what ought to be done from the limited viewpoint of the biomedical good of the patient. However, this does not mean that he or she knows what ought to be done, until, as an integral aspect of the relationship that constitutes the central event of medicine, an understanding of the role of amputation in the overall good of the patient at all four levels has been mutually understood. Thus, if the patient knowingly and deliberatively after being fully informed says, "I do not think that this amputation serves me, for who I am, at this stage in my life," it would be a violation of the physician's pledge to work for the good of the patient to perform the amputation. Likewise, if the patient were to say, "As a Christian Scientist, my concept of the highest good precludes me from undergoing the amputation," the mere fact that it serves the biomedical good of the patient is not sufficient moral warrant to proceed.

It is clear, from this, that Pellegrino is committed to the belief that no system of ethics, let alone a system of medical ethics, can proceed without some sort of understanding of what it is to be human – a philosophical anthropology.[1] For decades, Pellegrino has been impressed by the centrality of questions about the nature of humanity itself and the inseparability of an answer to such questions from a genuine philosophy of medicine and medical ethics. Since at least 1966, in his writings about medicine in the modern world, he has sensed the importance of Augustine's question, "What am I that I have become a problem to myself?"[1] In his view, the poverty of other approaches to medical ethics is their attempt to avoid this question altogether. At the same time, of course, the controversy about Pellegrino's approach is that he does attempt to answer the question, at least in a limited way, based upon an exploration of the meaning of the clinical event. He firmly holds that genuine medical ethics is only possible if it is based upon such an essentialist foundation. This foundation requires a commitment to an understanding of the essence of medicine, which in turn requires a commitment to an understanding of the essence of being human. Yet, he expounds a somewhat limited form of essentialism, based not upon a complete philosophical understanding of the human but an understanding of the human as patient and of the form of human agency known as medicine. He believes that careful reflection, even in a morally pluralistic society, will allow persons of good will to come to a shared understanding of these limited elements of human essence through reasoned reflection on the central event of medicine – the clinical encounter.

MEDICAL DUTIES AND VIRTUES

Specific morally required medical duties follow from this conception of the nature of medicine. If medicine, as a praxis, is to achieve the kind of whole-person healing that any reasonable human being and any reasonable clinician would expect from the encounter, then not just any decision, any way of communicating, any way of acting, will be consistent with this goal. Whatever is consistent with this goal, as it is carefully explicated and placed within the boundaries of a complete philosophy of medicine, is morally praiseworthy. Whatever is inconsistent with this goal or strays outside a proper understanding of the nature of medicine, as he has expounded it, merits moral blame. This leads to multiple concrete conclusions about what physicians are and are not allowed to do, and about the limits society may properly place upon the discretionary space of clinicians. It also leads to a set of concrete duties for patients, and a delineation of the limits that may be placed upon their autonomy as well. Thus, for instance, the stands that Pellegrino has taken regarding such controversial issues as truth-telling, physician-assisted suicide, the morality of financial incentives for physicians to limit patient access to clinical services, and the duty of society to provide healthcare to its members all flow from Pellegrino's carefully laid foundations. In other words, they depend upon knowing what medicine is.

It is sometimes thought that Pellegrino's system is so oriented to the service of the individual patient that it amounts to a complete catering to the whims of patients. But this is not true. Patient duties also follow from the foundations Pellegrino lays out. These include duties of veracity, probity, tolerance, and trust.[20] The patient must also recognize the clinician as an individual moral agent, and respect the consciences of those who serve in the health care system. In addition, because the patient is a citizen, the patient must also abide by whatever limits society has placed upon the discretionary space of the physician.

VIRTUE

I did not mention virtue as a competing conception of medical ethics because Pellegrino's work is often (correctly) associated with virtue theory. Virtue theory, concerned as it is with the character of agents, has enjoyed a resurgence in moral philosophy in recent decades, especially since the publication of Alasdair MacIntyre's *After Virtue*.[21] The book was highly critical of all moral philosophy written since the time of the Enlightenment. MacIntyre argued that for several centuries, ethics has been concerned only with action – the outcomes of actions or the duties of moral agents to perform or not perform certain actions. Ancient philosophical ethics, however, was primarily concerned with character, not action. MacIntyre argued cogently that character still counts. Many in the field of medical ethics picked up on this quickly. They were in search of what was missing from medical ethics education for medical students, who could be taught how to pass a test in ethics but did not thereby seem to become good doctors.

Virtue plays an important role in Pellegrino's system of medical ethics. He has an affinity for ancient thought that made virtue theory congenial. Virtue theory also interdigitates well with a system of teleological ethics like Pellegrino's, concerned with progress towards an ideal goal. Pellegrino appears to adopt an Aristotelian definition of virtue, although in most places he refers to virtue as a "concept" with multiple facets rather than supplying a precise definition. Thus, he approvingly cites the

Aristotelian concept of virtue as "a habitual predisposition to act well," but rejects Aristotle's doctrine of virtue as the mean between extremes.[22] He cites multiple other historical definitions of virtue, but writes, "A set of common themes seems discernible in these many definitions. Virtue implies a character trait, an internal predisposition habitually to seek moral perfection, to live one's life in accord with the moral law, and to attain a balance between noble intention and just action."[20]

Virtue rounds out the system of medical ethics that Pellegrino has proposed. The goal of being the perfect physician is impossible to attain. As Hippocrates once put it, "Life is short and the art is long."[23] Yet, a good physician is always striving to be better. Medicine, in fact, for Pellegrino, demands a higher standard of moral behavior and calls those who have professed this way of life to the pursuit of virtue as part of a new moral community.[22] Specifying the duties of physicians merely defines the moral floor below which no physician should be allowed to fall. Beyond this is the wide-open space of virtue – genuine excellence in the practice of medicine. A major concern of Pellegrino's is the good physician – the one who can be trusted to do what is right, even when no one is looking; the one who goes beyond mere duty; the one who does the right thing for the right reasons and with the right attitudes, motives and emotions; the one who can serve as a role model and teach by example. In sum, he wants to define what makes "the physician's physician" just so. Virtue theory therefore has a prominent role to play in his system.

Pellegrino specifies some of these virtues. They lay out the routes by which physicians can grow in their habitual predisposition to excellence in achieving the "right and good healing act for this patient." These include phronesis ("practical wisdom"), fidelity to trust, compassion, justice, fortitude, temperance, integrity, and self-effacement.[22]

One of the major virtues of a good physician is phronesis. Dan Davis has written an excellent examination of the place of phronesis in the thought of Edmund Pellegrino.[26] Davis shows how Pellegrino's concern with the act of medicine leads him to place significant emphasis on what Aquinas called *recta ratio agibilium* or "right reasoning about action."[2,22] But however significant this emphasis, however "cardinal" a virtue phronesis might be for physicians in Pellegrino's schema, Davis goes a bit too far in assigning it absolute centrality. As I have shown, Pellegrino's schema is more complex than that. As Pellegrino himself states, "Medicine, then, is all three – science, art, and virtue synergistically and integrally united in the clinician's daily activities."[2] Phronesis is a cardinal virtue, but not the central virtue. Virtue has a prominent role to play in Pellegrino's ethics, but his is not a pure ethics of virtue.

Therefore, when those who think that in attacking virtue theory in medical ethics they are attacking Pellegrino[24,25] really manage no more than a glancing blow. Pellegrino himself notes the deficiencies of pure virtue theory and states, "A virtue-based ethics is difficult to defend as the sole basis for normative judgments."[20] Far from promoting a pure virtue ethics, Pellegrino consistently looks for links between virtues, principles, and duties.[22] The role of virtue in Pellegrino's system of medical ethics is more subtle, complex, and circumscribed than either his proponents or his detractors are sometimes prepared to admit.

CRITIQUE

In a nutshell, Pellegrino's system of medical ethics is a foundationalist system that is based upon an essentialist understanding of medicine. He locates this essence in the clinical encounter, believing that certain elements of that encounter are timeless and irrefutably true. From an analysis of the critical elements of this encounter, he is able to specify moral duties for physicians and patients. These duties delineate the moral floor. He then elaborates a theory of medical virtue to help specify the traits of character that predispose individual practitioners towards excellence in healing. Any and all specific judgments of morality in medicine flow from this structure.

Like any proposed theory of medical ethics, Pellegrino's does not meet with universal approbation, however.

First, some have suggested that his attempt to develop a full-fledged philosophy of medicine is very incomplete, and therefore the ethics that flows from it is not sufficiently well established to be universally accepted (van Leeuwen and Kisma 1993). Despite the breadth of his reading, especially in classical philosophy, Thomism, and neo-Scholasticism, Pellegrino is not actually trained as a philosopher, and so some professional philosophers find that his arguments fail to take account of more contemporary philosophical techniques and critiques. Some are unconvinced that his "ground" is irrefutably established. Sometimes the steps he takes from the essence of the clinical encounter to the concrete moral conclusions are not clearly explicated. In other words, just how does he deduce all of those concrete conclusions about the morality of medical practice from the fact of illness, the act of profession, and the act of medicine? The answers are not always clear.

A related concern is that at times the books seem to read like catalogues of one sentence-long throwaway lines about what famous philosophers have said or might be thought to have said about particular issues in the philosophy of medicine and medical ethics rather than careful explications of these positions accompanied by solid arguments to refute them or to show how they support Pellegrino's position. In fairness, since most of his books are co-authored with Thomasma, it is often difficult to tease out exactly whose voice is whose in these writings. But the dominant voice in these books appears to be that of Pellegrino, and certainly both authors must be held accountable for the style of writing and argument throughout the whole book.

Another related concern is voiced by those who think that there is no such thing as an independent philosophy of medicine. These critics would place medicine under the umbrella of philosophy of science. Still other critics doubt that it is reasonable to develop a special philosophical theory of ethics for every single kind of human endeavor. They would make medical ethics applied ethics. They ask why should medicine be so special that it needs its own ethical theory? As a *reductio ad absurdam*, one might ask whether there is also a need for a philosophy of policing and police ethics, or a philosophy of ballet and ballet ethics?

Third, Pellegrino's system has been attacked as narrow. His emphasis on the clinical event seems to place a significant amount of medical activity completely outside the ambit of his philosophical concerns. His description of the "fact of illness" really does not seem to apply to preventive medicine or to public health. Perhaps a consumer model is more appropriate for these encounters. And if so, what does this say about the timeless and fundamental nature of the philosophical system he is proposing? Further, many have argued that Pellegrino has overemphasized the relationship between clinician and patient. They would argue that this view is no longer viable in the present historical and economic environment. This narrow focus, they argue, pays insufficient attention to the common good and the needs of the wider society.

Fourth, Pellegrino's system has been attacked as chauvinistic. His emphasis is on physicians, and by extension, other health care professionals. While he orients the moral duties of health care professionals towards the good of the patient, still his system of ethics does not seem so much concerned with the patient as with the beliefs, attitudes, emotions, and actions of the health care professionals. Thus, to some observers, it can seem elitist.

Fifth, some consider Pellegrino's views overly idealistic. These critics say that he has proposed a system that presumes too much of physicians. They argue that physicians cannot be expected to have a higher standard of moral behavior than anyone else does. They believe it is unrealistic to assume that this is possible, and potentially dangerous to patients to presume that physicians will act according to these professional ideals.

Finally, his views have been attacked as based upon an outmoded view of philosophy. These philosophical critics contend that essentialism is long dead, along with those classical and Scholastic philosophers who espoused it. They argue that there are no actual essences for anything. There is no essence of an atom, no essence of a human being, and certainly no unchanging essence of any human practice. Some of these critics are foundationalists of a logical positivist stripe, who contend that nothing exists that is not empirically verifiable, and that ethics is nothing more than the expression of emotion. Others are anti-foundationalists who accept the existence of the non-empirically verifiable, but suggest that moral (and perhaps other) standards are arrived at intersubjectively by consensus or coherence with other beliefs. On this view, such notions as what medicine is, or what it requires morally, are changeable concepts that can be "invented" according to the needs of a given society at a given place in time.

This list of criticisms, while not exhaustive, serves to demonstrate where Pellegrino's views fit within the ongoing debate about medical ethics. Space limitations preclude a point-by-point analysis of the merits and flaws of these criticisms. But they are part of the active and ongoing debate in which Pellegrino continues as an active participant. While I will leave it to him to respond to these critiques himself, I cannot help but note that in spite of all these criticisms, the core event that he describes as the essence of medicine retains a powerful appeal, especially for clinicians and those who have been seriously ill. Likewise, the system of ethics he has elaborated seems to capture and explain the previously unarticulated intuitions of many centuries of medico-moral thinking. Pellegrino's system cannot be easily dismissed.

CONCLUSION

Pellegrino's contributions to medical ethics have been seminal. Even his most ardent critics readily acknowledge him as one of the fathers of the field. He was writing about humanism and medicine decades before it was popular. Through his founding of the Society of Health and Human Values and the *Journal of Medicine and Philosophy*, he helped to create the field of medical ethics. Through his influence as a medical educator, dean, university president, and academic medical center president, he helped to make medical ethics and medical humanities a standard part of the curriculum in medical schools and residency training programs. His system of ethics continues to have great appeal. It is unique. There are any number of principlists, any number of pragmatists, and any number of utilitarians writing in medical ethics. But there is only one Pellegrino. Time will tell whether his views will have the staying power to perdure into the twenty-first century or beyond. Whether or not this will happen, ironically, will probably depend in large measure on what happens to the discretionary space of physicians in the next century – a problem he himself has so aptly described.

I

Toward a Philosophy of Medicine

The reader who has read Daniel Sulmasy's interpretive introduction before delving into the Pellegrino essays themselves will be rewarded by watching the pieces fall into place over three decades. It should be clear that Dr. Pellegrino was writing credible philosophy even as he served in a series of other "day jobs."

CHAPTER ONE

WHAT THE PHILOSOPHY OF MEDICINE IS

> *I will now turn to medicine, the subject of the present treatise, and set forth the exposition of it. First I will define what I conceive medicine to be.*[1]
>
> *... The philosopher is under obligation to study the nature of philosophy, itself...*[2]

INTRODUCTION

Philosophical reflections about matters medical are as old as medicine and philosophy. In every era, critical thinkers, both in medicine and philosophy, have sought levels of understanding about medicine and its practice not attainable within the purview of the methodology of medicine itself. Only recently, however, has a debate arisen about whether or not there is, or can be, a legitimate field of inquiry called the philosophy *of* medicine. If there is such a field, in what does it consist? Can it be distinguished from the philosophy of science? What is its relationship to the emergent field of bioethics? Does any practical consequence follow from these distinctions?

I will set forth my current personal response to these questions based on my interest in this field as presented in my own work as well as my collaborative work with Dr. David Thomasma.[3,4,5] I will divide my responses into two parts. Part I deals with these perspectives on the present state of the question "Is there a philosophy of medicine, and, if so, in what does it consist?" Part II compares, contrasts, and distinguishes four models for conducting philosophical inquiry into medicine, i.e., philosophy *and* medicine, philosophy *in* medicine, medical philosophy, and philosophy *of* medicine.

I shall argue, *contra* Caplan,[6] that there is a defensible and legitimate field of philosophical inquiry that can be termed properly the philosophy of medicine, that it can be distinguished from other forms of philosophical reflection about medicine, and that the distinctions are of more than heuristic value. In doing so, I shall expand on a set of distinctions I proposed more than twenty years ago, but which are even more cogent now than they were then.[7]

STATE OF THE QUESTION: THREE PERSPECTIVES—NEGATIVE, EXPANSIVE, AND SPECIFIC

The history of philosophical reflections about medicine is long, complex, and parlous. I cannot possibly do justice to its historical development nor to the many versions in which it has appeared in the past and the present. Fortunately, there are several fulsome reviews of that history in the ancient and modern worlds, to which the reader may refer.[8,9,10,11,12] These reviews speak to the long duration of the dialogues between medicine and philosophy, the several forms they may take, and the range of topics that may fall within—and between—the domains of each discipline. While I will not repeat that history, I will draw upon it selectively to illustrate some of the distinctions and definitions I hope to make.

What is evident in that history is the apparent inevitability of the dialogue for both positive and negative reasons.[13] On the positive side, there is the fact the preoccupations of medicine with humanity's complex and urgent problems—like life, death, suffering and disease—could hardly escape the inquiry of critical minds in any era. On the negative side, there is the obvious conflict of methodologies, the observational, empirical and experimental bent of medicine colliding with the analytical, speculative and abstract deliberations of philosophy. Attractions and repulsions notwithstanding, neither physicians nor philosophers could in fact desist from puzzling over such universal human experiences as the nature of illness and healing, the ethics of the professed healer, or the relationship of those phenomena to prevailing philosophical schools of thought.

Until recently, however, these reflections rarely met the criteria for formal, systematic, orderly analysis required to qualify them as a legitimate branch or sub-branch of philosophy. Today, however, physicians and philosophers have begun to speak seriously of the possibility of the philosophy *of* medicine as a field of inquiry, either to affirm or deny it. Today's interest in what Engelhardt and Erde have termed "a newly emerging field of philosophical study"[14] has several sources.

First, is the mutuality of interest in the subject matter of medicine to which I have already referred. In every era, there were physicians who wanted to understand the phenomena they observed and the nature of the art they were practicing. In every era there were philosophers fascinated by the need for a deeper understanding of the phenomena than medicine could afford. To achieve these ends, the critical trans-medical perspective of philosophy has always seemed essential.

A second reason for the current interest in philosophy of medicine is the tremendous emphasis in the last twenty-five years on medical ethics and bioethics. As successive theories of medical ethics have surfaced, it has become apparent that there is need for a grounding for ethics in something beyond principles, virtues, casuistry, care, hermeneutics, etc. The first step in this grounding would have to be the articulation of a theory and philosophy of medicine. Such a theory is necessary if we are to put the competing ethical theories into some proper relationship to each other and resolve some of the contradictions between and among them. In short, we need to move from medical ethics or bioethics to a more comprehensive moral philosophy of medicine and the health professions.

A third factor fostering interest in a philosophy of medicine is the turn of Existential, Hermeneutic, Phenomenological, and Post-Modern approaches to ethics and philosophy. These philosophical perspectives are more open to lived experiences of patient and physician and to the particularities of moral choice, suffering, dying, finitude and compassion. These are phenomena of great interest to philosophers who seek to comprehend them in more concrete ways than is congenial in the analytical mode still dominant in contemporary Anglo-American philosophy. These are also the same phenomena physicians and patients confront experientially every day. Critical reflections on these lived experiences lead naturally to the kind of fundamental and comprehensive grasp that could qualify as philosophy of medicine. To be sure, a post-modern philosophy of medicine would reject ideologies, emancipatory narratives, and absolutism in favor of a diversity of language and concept. But it still would be a philosophy *of* medicine.

Currently, in response to these forces, three general positions are held regarding the nature and existence of the philosophy of medicine. For convenience of discussion, I will label these the negative, the broad, and the narrow positions.

The *negative* viewpoint is that of Arthur Caplan who contends that there is at present no legitimate field of inquiry that warrants designation as philosophy of medicine.[15] Engelhardt and Erde,[16] Engelhardt and Schaffner,[17] and Engelhardt and Wildes,[18] on the other hand, recognize a very broad field of inquiry under the rubric of philosophy of medicine. Last is the narrower view of David Thomasma and myself, who hold to a more specific definition of a field we identify as philosophy *of* medicine *qua* medicine.[19,20,21] In our work, we go further and ground our philosophy of medicine in a theory of the healing relationship. Alfred Tauber builds a philosophy of medicine on the philosophy of Levinas.[22] Different combinations and versions of these three perspectives can be found in the issues of the *Journal of Medicine and Philosophy* and *Theoretical Medicine*, in the long series *Philosophy and Medicine*, and in recent books which have included philosophy of medicine in their titles. All qualify as philosophical reflection broadly speaking, but not all qualify as philosophy *of* medicine. They form a spectrum of philosophical reflections on the matter of medicine, and it is within this spectrum that I wish to locate philosophy of medicine as a distinguishable region of inquiry.

The Negative View: Philosophy of Medicine as Non-Existent

Caplan's line of argument is as follows: He sets forth the criteria he deems essential to define a legitimate field of inquiry. Then, he shows what he believes to be the failure of current definitions to meet those criteria. Caplan's own criteria include key books, articles, special journals, and a distinctive set of problems. He admits that, on further specifying his definition of the philosophy and medicine and the criteria that would give it intellectual stature, he concludes, regretfully, that there is no such field.

Caplan's evidence against the existence of a field of inquiry is as follows: First, he says, there is no agreement upon definition. He then offers his own definition which he then proceeds to show is not met by any of the current fields of study. Caplan says philosophy of medicine is not to be equated with bioethics which is normative, while philosophy of medicine should be metaphysical or epistemological. He likewise rejects identification of philosophy of medicine with humanities in medicine, health care policy, or medical aesthetics. He holds it as evidence against existence of philosophy of medicine that there is not enough "...debate, anguish, posturing and mutual recrimination."[23]

Caplan offers his definition of philosophy of medicine as "...the study of the epistemological, metaphysical, and methodological dimensions of medicine: therapeutic and experimental; diagnostic, therapeutic, (*sic*) and palliative."[24] But, if this were in fact the case, he argues, philosophy or medicine would deal with "key problems" in the philosophy of science and thus be a subdiscipline of the philosophy of science—not a distinct discipline. Caplan's position is similar to that taken by Jerome Shaffer twenty years ago in the first volume of the Engelhardt and Spicker Series entitled *Philosophy and Medicine*[25] when the debates began, at least in the United States. It also accords well with the span of topics proposed by Sadegh-Zadeh and Lindahl as the domain of the philosophy of medicine which was the focus of the journal *Metamedicine*, later renamed *Theoretical Medicine*.[26,27]

Caplan admits the existence of a large literature and several organizations identified with philosophy of medicine. He even admits the possibility that there might be a "field" of inquiry but it is not one now because it is not part of a broader field, has no recognizable canon of books and no distinctive set of problems. Caplan laments the non-existence of the philosophy of medicine since he thinks a philosophy of medicine would be important as a foundation for bioethics, for the philosophy of applied science, and for certain special problems in genetics and similar fields.

The Broad View: Engelhardt Et Alia

Caplan's line of argument against the existence of the philosophy of medicine is circuitous, ambivalent, and based largely on simple assertion. Engelhardt and Erde, and Engelhardt and Schaffner are much more definitive in their assessment of the evidence for the existence of the philosophy of medicine. They define philosophy of medicine, not too differently than Caplan, as "...encompassing those issues in epistemology, axiology, logic, methodology and metaphysics generated by and related to medicine."[28] However, they specify several broad areas of inquiry they see as distinctive to the philosophy of medicine such as models of medicine, concepts of health and disease, the logic of diagnosis, prognosis, clinical trials, artificial intelligence, disease causation, etc. Engelhardt and his co-authors support their contention by a substantial bibliography of work drawn from many eras and countries, covering an extraordinarily wide range of topics at the juncture of medicine and philosophy. It is difficult to see how Caplan could dismiss such an extensive body of work as not constituting a field of inquiry.

The Engelhardt and Erde, and Engelhardt and Schaffner, definitions of philosophy of medicine are close to Caplan's. But, contra Caplan, their review supports the criteria for a "field," given the great range and number of books and articles they cite that deal with philosophy of medicine. For their part, however, they have cast their net too widely. Many of the works they cite are at the margin of their own definition. Some, however, are now so often cited as to constitute a beginning "canon." The Engelhardt, Erde, Schaffner, and Wildes definition embraces every conceivable intersection between philosophy, medicine, and physical and social science. While such studies are important, such a broad definition, which embraces such a wide spectrum of studies, dilutes the specificity of philosophy of medicine and weakens the identification of a definitive set of problems. Yet, this specificity is precisely what needs to be examined more closely if we are to determine whether an independent philosophy of medicine does, indeed, exist.

Much of what Engelhardt, Schaffner, and Erde cite as work in the philosophy *of* medicine could qualify, just as Caplan suspects, as the philosophy *of* science or biology or as sub-branches of extant fields of philosophical inquiry like metaphysics, epistemology, or axiology, or, in my terms, as philosophy in medicine. This would not diminish the importance of the questions studied. But it does obscure the outlines of a philosophy of medicine, a field whose focus would be more narrowly on the precepts, presuppositions, concepts, and values peculiar to medicine as medicine and not simply as examples of problems already pursued in science or philosophy.

It is interesting, and somewhat puzzling as well, that the philosophies *of* many disciplines other than medicine are recognized as legitimate fields of inquiry. The most recently published *Dictionary of Philosophy*,[29] for example, has no entry under "philosophy of medicine." Neither does the currently available but outdated *Encyclopedia of Philosophy*.[30] Yet both reference works have entries for philosophy of biology, economics, education, language, law, literature, logic, mathematics, mind, religion, psychology, science, and social science. Each of those philosophy of "…" articles speaks of the concepts, methods, theories, presuppositions, and justifications fundamental to the discipline in question. Thus, for every discipline, except medicine, a narrow, specific field of philosophical inquiry is recognized that deals with the "what is" question and the problems "internal" to the discipline but not susceptible to resolution by the method of the discipline itself.

Engelhardt and Schaffner's article embraces the whole range of philosophical reflection on medicine. Some of their citations would be classified as philosophy of science, much as philosophy *in* medicine or philosophy *and* medicine, and some as medical philosophy. To some extent, this is also the case with Van der Steen, who identifies philosophy of medicine with (a) questions "left over" from science, (b) normative questions, and (c) methodological questions.[31] Other authors also take the broad or expansive view of philosophy of medicine, [32,33] In the remainder of this paper, I shall attempt to define the various regions of philosophy of medicine more clearly, particularly that region of the spectrum I believe to be distinguishable as the philosophy *of* medicine.

FOUR MODES OF PHILOSOPHICAL REFLECTION ON MEDICINE

In this section, I wish to compare, contrast, and distinguish these four regions in the spectrum of philosophical inquiry into medical matters. I shall not distinguish between different philosophical methodologies, e.g., Anglo-American, Analytic, Classical, Medieval, Phenomenological, Post-Modern, or Hermeneutical systems of thought. Any, or all, of those schools of philosophical thought can be applied to medicine or can examine problems specific to its own enterprise as it exists in the context of medicine. What is significant in defining the field of philosophy of medicine is not the school of philosophical thought but the end and purpose for which that philosophy is applied to medical topics.

Philisophy and Medicine

In this mode of philosophizing, philosophy and medicine each retains its identity and enters as a distinct discipline into independent and autonomous dialogue with the other. The subject of that dialogue is variable. It can be an effort at identification or at comparing and contrasting the way each discipline studies the phenomena peculiar to medicine. It can define similarities and differences in subject matter, method or mutual influences of one on the other. In the Hippocratic writings, for example, the two treatises, "The Art"[34] and "Ancient Medicine,"[35] are devoted to establishing the independence of the method of medicine from that of philosophy. The Hippocratic authors affirm the importance of observation of individual cases and reasoning based in empirical evidence. They repudiate speculation and particularly speculation as practiced by certain philosophers and philosopher-physicians.

Socrates and Plato, for example, frequently used medicine as an example of a techné practiced within ethical constraints.[36] Plato, at one point, went so far as to liken the physician who was also a philosopher to a god. Galen, who practiced both medicine and philosophy, took this identity relationship seriously in his own work. On the other hand, in the Symposium, Plato chides the physician, Eryximachus, for his technicism, for his attempt to explain all human existence through his art.[37] Elsewhere, he has Nicias say that physicians should not presume to go beyond knowledge of the nature of health and disease.[38] Here, Plato clearly seems to disapprove of medicine extending its reach into philosophical problems.

Medicine, for its part, was equally ambivalent about philosophy. In the Hellenic Period, physicians and physician philosophers drew heavily on the teachings of the major philosophical schools—The Academy, the Peripatetic, and the Stoa—for their theories of disease and healing.[39,40,41] Each of the major schools of medicine—Methodists, Dogmatists and Empiricists—adopted and adapted the philosophical doctrines of the major schools of Greek philosophy. In a similar way, in later centuries, Stahl's theory of vitalism drew on the philosophy of Leibniz, while mechanistic theories of medicine drew on Descartes and J. O. de la Mettrie. Lester King provides a detailed account of how seventeenth- and eighteenth-century philosophical systems drew upon theories of medicine, especially for their metaphysical and logical content.[42]

This reliance on philosophy for theoretical understanding was a reversal of the stance of the Hippocratic School which had been explicit in distancing itself from philosophy. Thomas Sydenham and other eighteenth century "Hippocratic" physicians repeated this rejection of philosophy:

> In writing the history of a disease, every philosophical hypothesis whatsoever, that has previously occupied the mind of the author should be in abeyance. This being done, the clear and natural phenomena of the disease should be notes—these and these only.[43]

To the contrary, others in later antiquity and the early Christian periods made medicine and philosophy identical with each other. Varro (BCE 116-27), for one, included medicine as one of the several liberal arts[44] and Cassiodorus (490-585) and Ennodius (473-521) identified *philosophus* and *medicus* as one and the same.[45] This intermingling became stronger in the later sixteenth and in the seventeenth centuries when the growing influence of physical and experimental science on medicine became widely manifest. Discovery of the telescope and microscope opened up new ways of observation of nature and the possibility of subjecting philosophical speculations to empirical vertification.[46] On the other hand, these extant observations were often interpreted in terms of newer philosophical systems. The philosophies of Descartes, Leibniz, Malebranche, Bacon and others were closely interwoven with the new visions of reality uncovered by the access the new instruments gave to both the microcosmos and macrocosmos.

In the seventeenth century, the "natural philosophers" and the newer philosophers of science were often interested in medicine as a science as a branch of chemistry; physicians or mathematics. They exchanged ideas and occasionally blows over the proper methodology for investigation of nature. Medicine, because it is both a science and in many senses one of the humanities, occupied a central place in these debates. Later, in the eighteenth century, as experimentation and clinical investigations were introduced into medicine, philosophical interest shifted to questions of nosography, the logic of diagnosis and theories of health and therapeutics as well as logic of statistical inference, and ideas of causality.[47]

In the last twenty-five years, philosophical reflection on medicine has shifted again, this time to medicine as an ethical enterprise.[48] In the 1960's, philosophers were attracted by the need for a more rigorous and sophisticated analysis of the dilemmas of medical progress than medicine itself afforded. Physicians and philosophers drew on principles and concepts developed in the great ethical traditions - the classical, medieval, the Kantian, and the Utilitarian. Most recently, as philosophers explored the practical issues, they also uncovered the need for a more substantial grounding for medical ethics than ethical analysis, problems, dilemmas or cases could provide. As a result inquiry was directed to alternative theories to those based in principles. Ethical theories based in casuistry, philosophies of care, experience, or virtue became prominent. In Europe, more attention was paid than in America, to hermeneutics, phenomenology, narrative and interpersonal relational theories as they were exemplified in medical ethics and practice.[49,50,51]

Equally apparent today is the realization that medical ethics cannot be pursued without a closer inquiry into the moral philosophy *of* medicine.[52,53] Medical ethics requires clarity not just about the ethical concepts on which it depends, but clarity also about the ends and purposes of medicine as well. Healing, caring, suffering, finitude and a variety of other concepts have come to be legitimate objects of philosophical inquiry in their relation to the ends of medicine. As a result, need for mutual understandings of philosophy and medicine, or the science and praxis of medicine, and the healing relationship, have become active fields of research, has become evident.

Philosophy in Medicine

By philosophy *in* medicine, I mean the application of specific, recognized branches of philosophy—e.g., logic, metaphysics, axiology, ethics, aesthetics—to matters medical. This is essentially what Engelhardt and Schaffner would define as philosophy of medicine. Most of their attention is devoted to philosophical study of the scientific foundations of medicine. This is the sense in which most recent review articles and books now interpret philosophy of medicine. Also, on this view, theories of medical knowledge or ethics, for example, drawn from existing theories of epistemology or moral are applied to medical problems, concepts, or experiences.[54,55,56,67] Medical diagnosis, for example, is examined for its logic, and concepts of health and disease are examined for their ontological or epistemological status. In these cases, the starting point is a question of interest to philosophy as such. The concepts, methods, or presuppositions of science generally, or of the social sciences, statistics, logic, etc., are examined as they may be specified in the activities peculiar to medicine.[58]

Wulff et al., for example, draw on phenomenology, hermeneutics, and existentialism as well as on the philosophies of Kierkegaard, Heidegger, and Gadamer to gain insights into the phenomena of medicine.[59] Similarly, Natanson extrapolates the philosophy of Heidegger and *dasein* analysis to the data of classical psychiatry.[60] Sinha looks for insights into the concepts of health and disease and the ontological, axiological, and epistemological problems of medicine in the Asian philosophical tradition.[61,62] In the same spirit, Fleck undertakes the socio-cultural epistemology of medical fact,[63] and Foucault does so with the clinical "gaze" and the birth of the clinic.[64] Another example is Brody's use of Rawls' method of reflective equilibrium to study the placebo effect and the ethics of its use. Other examples of philosophy in medicine would be the treatises on medical logic.[65,66,67] Similarly, exploration of the themes of explanation and reasoning, and probability and normality, have employed philosophical modes of analysis. Current inquiries into the use of Bayesian logic, artificial intelligence, and decision analysis are further examples of philosophy's effect on medicine.

Obviously, philosophy *in* medicine has been, and is, fruitful for both medicine and philosophy. For philosophy, there is the discovery of subjects of intrinsic interest to the enterprise of philosophy itself. For medicine, there is the opening of the subject matter of medicine in ways not contained within the language and method of medicine itself.

The most fruitful example of the power of philosophy in medicine is the principle-based system of Beauchamp and Childress.[68] They have skillfully and wisely taken four principles of "the common morality" as *prima facie* guides to the resolution of practical medical ethical dilemmas. But the success of their system is now questioned because the *prima facie* principles are not grounded in a more general or fundamental moral philosophy.[69] While I believe principles are essential to any viable ethics of medicine, I have tried to ground them in a philosophy of medicine, one derived from the clinical phenomena of medicine itself.[70] In doing do, I hope to show that there is no essential conflict between philosophy *in* medicine and philosophy *of* medicine.

Medical Philosophy

Another category that needs definition is medical philosophy. This is the vaguest and most loosely defined of the current terms. I take it to mean any informal reflection on the practice of medicine—usually by physicians on clinical medicine based in their reflections on their own clinical experiences. Here, we might include "styles" of practice such as: therapeutic enthusiasm, nihilism, or minimalism; diagnostic enthusiasm which leaves no test unused; diagnostic artistry which pursues an elegant form of clinical epluchage, selecting just the right number and kind of tests; then there are those who want to be a friend to the patient; those who, on the contrary, feel a certain "distance" is more conducive to the healing relationship; those who favor formal or informal modes of address or dress, etc. These matters are rarely subjected to formal analysis but are argued as conducive to good or bad care of patients.

There is also a kind of medical philosophy, based in the clinical wisdom of reflective clinicians has always been a source of inspiration and practical knowledge for conscientious clinicians. Among writers in English, one thinks of William Osler[71] and Francis Peabody[72] or Richard Cabot[73,74] and Lewis Thomas.[75] Their works are not philosophical in any formal sense, but in the more informal, traditional sense of the search for wisdom—in their cases, as that wisdom emerges from reflective and meditative cogitation on years of learning by experience. They are examples of practical wisdom, the kind of reflective understanding beyond empiricism of how to practice a craft with perception contained in the Greek notion of *techne*.[76,77]

In contrast to this kind of informal medical philosophy, well-grounded in the received wisdom of experienced clinicians, are the grand theories and systems of medicine that emerged in the late seventeenth and eighteenth centuries.[78,79,80,81] These were attempts to classify, explain, and treat diseases according to mostly fanciful appropriations of quasiphilosophical notions. Some examples use Stahl's animism, John Brown's theory of stimuli, Hoffman's mechanism, Hahnemann's homeopathy as well as vitalism, mesmerism, and many other lesser known theories, all energetically debated. Some of those speculative medical philosophies were directly influenced by philosophical systems, e.g., Descartes' influence on J. O. de la Mettrie, Condillac's on Pinel, or Leibniz's on Hoffman.[82,83]

Descartes' flirtations with medicine illustrate how complex a serious philosopher's reflections on medicine may be. For one thing, Descartes wanted to draw "...rules for medicine... more firm than those which have been attained to present."[84] At the same time, he looked to medicine for a definition of the goals, ends, and purposes of human life and ethics. Finally, he wanted to ground medicine in infallible demonstrations and sought from it to extend his own life and health.[85] Descartes employs philosophy *in* medicine to develop rules for medicine, philosophy *of* medicine to develop the goals of life, and philosophy *and* medicine to mathematize medicine and make it a branch of his philosophy.

With these difficulties as illustrated in Descartes and other works cited above in mind, I will turn now to that portion of the spectrum of reflection I believe properly qualifies as a philosophy of medicine.

Philosophy of Medicine

The philosophy of medicine consists in a critical reflection on the matter of medicine—on the content, method, concepts and presuppositions peculiar to medicine *as medicine.* To this end, philosophy of medicine, of necessity, must transcend the methods of medicine (i.e., the methods of science, clinical observation, and clinical judgement). Its purposes are different than the purposes of medicine *per se.* Philosophy of medicine makes the specific method and matter of medicine the subject of study by the method of philosophy. Philosophy of medicine seeks philosophical knowledge of medicine itself. It seeks to understand what medicine *is* and what sets it apart from other disciplines, and from philosophy itself. It seeks to show what medicine is, as did the Hippocratic physicians in their two treatises on the nature of medicine ("The Art" and "Ancient Medicine").[86,87] This is no trivial task or labor at the obvious. Lain-Entralgo, perhaps the most astute of the Hippocratic commentators, took this question to be among the most profound in the Hippocratic corpus.[88] Lester King had to admit that he abandoned his project of writing a history of eighteenth-century medicine because he could not determine "...what medicine was."[89]

Philosophy of medicine has the same relationship with philosophy as the philosophies of history, art, law, literature, etc., have to those disciplines. In each case, critical reflection seeks something beyond the content of those disciplines, something beyond the methods of inquiry peculiar to each as a discipline. The philosophy of any discipline is a search for ultimacy, for a grasp of the reality of the things studied beyond what is discernible by the discipline studied.

It is impossible to define clearly what constitutes the philosophy of medicine without a definition of medicine itself. Indeed, the controversy about whether the philosophy of medicine is nothing more than the philosophy of science hinges on what we mean by medicine. If medicine is nothing more than a branch of science, i.e., if we equate it with the sciences basic to medicine (e.g., anatomy, physiology, biochemistry), then the philosophy of medicine is, indeed, only the philosophy of science. But if medicine embraces activities beyond those inherent in the pursuit of scientific knowledge, then a philosophy *of* medicine is a separate and separable entity from philosophy of science. Whether medicine is more than science is a question to be answered factually and phenomenologically in one sense, and by philosophy of medicine in another.

Obviously, medicine does rest, in part, on the sciences of human physiology and pathophysiology as well as pharmacology, microbiology, psychology, genetics, etc. Those are the realms of physical, chemical, and biological phenomena observable by the methods of science in studying the functioning and malfunctioning of human organisms. The end and purpose of the sciences basic to medicine is the pursuit of truth, a grasp of the realities of human bodily function and dysfunction to the extent that they are subject to observation, hypothesis formulation, and experimental manipulation. But medicine is more than a search for truth. It is a search for truth determined by a practical end which truth serves, namely health and healing of human beings.

Medicine *qua* medicine comes into existence in the clinical encounter or in public health when the knowledge of the sciences basic to medicine is employed for a specific end, i.e., for the cure, containment, amelioration, or prevention of human illness in individuals or in human societies. Medicine *qua* medicine, therefore, is shaped not just by the ends and purposes of the sciences. Medicine uses scientific knowledge for its own specific ends, which are healing, helping, curing, and preventing illness and disease and promoting health, i.e., the optimum well-functioning of the whole human organism or human society. Pursuing those ends with individual patients and families is the enterprise of clinical medicine; pursuing them with communities and societies is the enterprise of public health or social medicine.

Philosophy *of* medicine as medicine, then, has as its subject matter the problems of clinical and public health medicine that it examines with its own perspective—one different from the perspective of science and even from clinical or public health medicine themselves. Philosophy of medicine seeks to understand the nature and phenomena of the clinical encounter, i.e., the interaction between persons needing help of a specific kind relative to health and other persons who offer to help and are designated by society to help.

Philosophy of medicine is concerned with the phenomena peculiar to the human encounter with health, illness, disease, death, and the desire for prevention and healing. It is rooted in concepts and conceptions like healing, helping, curing, health, illness, disease, care, the good of the patient, and the moral claims of the sick on the well, on society, and on the health professions. Concepts like causality, probability, taxonomy, logic, and mind-body relationships are studied as part of a philosophy of medicine to the extent that there is something in them that is peculiar to the human encounter with bodily and psychological well-being or dysfunction. Philosophy of medicine examines these ideas and phenomena as instantiations in the experiences of individual persons, in the relationships of physicians with patients or with physicians, patients, and society.

Medicine draws upon every discipline important to attaining its *telos*, a right and good healing decision and action for a given individual or society. Medicine uses all, shapes all, and studies pertinent branches of knowledge in terms of its *telos*. Indeed, medicine *qua* medicine comes into existence when it appropriates knowledge and skills, no matter what their origin, in order to further its healing purposes.[90,91]

Thus medicine is not the arithmetic sum of the disciplines on which it draws—whether they are the humanities or the social, physical, or biological sciences. The philosophy of medicine, therefore, is not the sum of the philosophies of science, biology, the social sciences, literature, etc. Its special domain is the way the concepts, presuppositions, and methodologies of the disciplines it draws upon are differently nuanced by the complexities of the human relationships, as well as by the purposes of those relationships peculiar to medicine.

A philosophic study of causality, for example, could be approached in several ways. As a topic in the philosophy of science, it would be necessary to examine the concept in its most general form. This would require abstraction from the differences in the way causality operates in the medical relationship. This would be philosophy *in* medicine or philosophy of science *in* medicine. But if the emphasis were on those things that make causality in illness and disease unique—if such exist—then we would deal with a philosophy of medicine. Here, attention would be directed to the phenomena peculiar to medicine as the particular kind of activity it is. Claude Bernard recognized these differences in nuance in the idea of causality in his epochal work on experimental medicine.[92]

Similarly, a study of Bayesian concepts could be examined as a problem in mathematical logic. However, it would become a problem for the philosophy of medicine when, and if, there were elements of application of Bayesian logic peculiar to the realities of medical observation and decision. Again, the philosophy of psychology would focus on understandings of the nature of the mind-body problem as a general phenomenon of human life. Examined as a question in philosophy of medicine, the focus would be on the uniqueness of the anxiety, dependence, suffering, vulnerability, and exploitability of a sick person seeking help from another person who has the power and the skill to help and heal, as well as to harm. Or, its focus could be the way mind may produce illness and dysfunction of body or body cause emotional and psychic dysfunction.

Any topic examined as part of the philosophy of medicine should start with the realities, phenomena, and data of medicine itself. Such a study would derive from what medicine *is* as a phenomenon of the real world. In its turn, a philosophy of medicine would help to define what medicine is ontologically and morally. This is a narrower view than the more expansive definitions of philosophy *of* medicine, but it is more suited to the depth and levels of understanding and the reach for ultimacy that characterize philosophical reflection when it is directed to medicine as medicine.

The emphasis on medicine's realities and phenomena does not imply that physicians are the best, or the only, philosophers of medicine. For obvious reasons of inadequacy or lack of formal training in philosophy, personal identification with the phenomena as persons or professionals, and an inclination to scientific positivism, physicians may not be qualified at all. They may lack the emotional and intellectual distance that critical analysis of their own enterprises requires. Contrariwise, the putative possession of critical distance by philosophers need not necessarily authenticate them as philosophers of medicine. Philosopher or physician, the person who reflects philosophically on medical matters must respect simultaneously the phenomena of medicine and the canons of valid philosophical inquiry.

At this point, it might be objected that all of this is well and good, but the question remains: is not what I have described simply the sum total of the knowledge and skills pertinent to the sciences basic to medicine? To this I reply that the difference lies in the unifying perspective and integrative aspects of the conceptions of helping and healing that are specific to medicine and not to any of the contributing sciences. But the objection now might be that the microbiologist also seeds healing when she synthesizes an antibiotic for the specific purpose of killing a specific bacterium, virus, or fungus. In doing so, does microbiology become medicine, or the microbiologist a physician?

They do, in a limited sense, in that now microbiology becomes a science basic to medicine and, thus, different from the study, let us say, of bacterial or viral genetics with no therapeutic purpose in view. But, even so, this is not medicine in the fullest sense, since to be medicine the fruits of microbiological science must be integrated into the life of particular patients or societies by and through an interpersonal relationship. Microbiological knowledge is essential to curing an infection but not sufficient to "heal" the patient. Healing requires a much fuller grasp of the patient as a person, of the place of *this* illness in his life at *this* time, and, in the future, of the ethical dimension and inter-relationships between the patient and his environment—the persons, places, jobs, etc., in her life story. None of the sciences of medicine—clinical, basic, epidemiological, etc., even the psychological—fully encompass all these dimensions as they relate to healing and helping. In ways still only vaguely grasped, the interpersonal relationship between healers and patients conditions the healing process not only in "psychological" disorders, but in "physiological" disorders as well. Psyche and soma, soma and psyche, are inseparable in health as in illness, for both individuals and societies. Like individuals, societies have physiologies as well as pathologies. Like individuals, they can be healed and harmed. Both involve a relationship of persons to a specified purpose not contained in science as science.

Medicine must be concerned with the "good" of the patient. As David Thomasma and I have emphasized elsewhere, the patient's good is a compound notion. It is not synonymous with the patient's medical good. Healing means "to make whole again." Therefore, ascertaining and enhancing all four realms of the patient's good are involved in healing - the patient's biomedical good, his own conception of the good for him as an individual, his good as a member of the human species (i.e., the good for humans), and his good as a spiritual being (i.e., the good for the soul).[93,94] The concept of wholeness, together with its asymptotic attainment through relationships between, and among, persons is the specific end of medicine. It is not an end proper to any of the sciences basic to medicine. But without a concept of healing, medicine as such does not exist.

In short, medicine embraces a wide range of physical and social sciences as well as the humanities. Its distinction lies in its organizing principle of healing, in its centering on human inter-relationships, on its reach beyond a simple addition of disparate pieces of information from a wide variety of sources and its need simultaneously to engage the ethical as well as the technical dimensions of illness and healing.

Again, it is important to emphasize that medicine embraces insights from the humanities as well as the physical and social sciences. Healing is an experience as are illness and suffering. Literature, history, philosophy, language, and theology are all full of rich insights into these human experiences and, in this sense, medicine is a "humanistic discipline." But medicine is also distinct from other humanistic disciplines since its specific *telos* is helping and healing. One may use the humanities as one uses the sciences, to assist in healing, but healing is not the defining characteristic of literature, let us say, that it is for medicine in the fullest sense. A philosophy of medicine would relate philosophy, theology, science, etc., to medicine conceptually, but it would not conflate them.

Medicine is also an ethical enterprise since it is aimed at the good of patients not their harm and, therefore, it must discern what is right and good, what *ought* to be done as well as what *can* be done. Medical ethics is also an ethical enterprise since its end is the good of the patient, i.e., what ought to be done as well as what can be done. A philosophy of medicine would concentrate on the ethics "internal" to medicine[95], to those ethical issues arising in the kind of activity medicine is—one based in a healing relationship and one founded in the phenomena of that relationship as well as competence in knowledge and skill appropriate to a healing relationship.[96,97,98,99,100]

Medicine has been called a "science of particular."[101] This is a useful, but not a precise, description. It is useful in placing emphasis on the necessity of taking into account the existential particularities of illness and the requirements for curing, caring, or healing in particular patients. But medicine-*qua*-medicine is also interested in, and capable of, generalized principles, that is to say, of a theory of medicine. The sciences, for their part, are also deeply concerned with particularities. It is out of particular instances and specified experimental or observational conditions that general scientific laws are derived by induction or applied by deduction. In its practice, science draws validity from the richness and reliability of its particulars. Solution chemistry must deal with particulars - temperature, ionic strength, ionization constants, ionic sizes, hydration envelopes, equilibrium conditions, etc. It is as much a science of particulars as medicine. But the theory of solutions must abstract from these particulars to a general set of laws governing all types of solution.

Like a chemical theory of solutions, a philosophy of medicine begins in the particularities, in phenomena determined by the kind of activity medicine is, and the phenomena it must consider in pursuit of its healing purposes for individuals and societies. The practice, the ethics, and the social role of medicine depend on the philosophy of medicine to which we commit ourselves. So, too, do answers to such issues as: the ends of medicine and how and by whom they are determined; the dependence or independence of medical ethics *vis-à-vis* politics, law, or economics; the place of bioethics; the resolution of cross-cultural conflicts in a world society, etc. These are the contributions a philosophy of medicine can make to those who actually use medicine—one of Caplan's criteria for a legitimate field of inquiry.[102] Our responses to this challenge must wait for another time.[103] For the moment, I have confined myself to an attempt to show that philosophy of medicine does indeed exist as a legitimate field of study.

CONCLUSION

Philosophical reflection on matters medical is a very old enterprise. Given the projects of medicine and philosophy, the dialogue between them is inevitable. Four ways in which philosophical reflection may take place are (1) philosophy *and* medicine, (2) philosophy *in* medicine, (3) medical philosophy, and (4) philosophy *of* medicine. Three opinions exist on the nature of philosophy *of* medicine: that it does not exist as valid field of inquiry, that it includes all forms of philosophical reflection, and that it is a definable field of its own, a specific form of philosophical reflection.

I have argued (1) that the philosophy of medicine is a definable field with its own specific perspective on the subject matter of medicine; (2) that its subject matter and *telos* are different in kind from those of the sciences basic to medicine; (3) that the practice of medicine draws upon the physical, biological, and social sciences and humanities, but medicine is not a sub-branch of any of those disciplines. Rather, the disciplines pertinent to medicine become part of medicine when they are used to advance the healing, helping, caring, and curing purposes of the patient-physician and medicine-society relationships. It is the critical, reflective, systematic study of the concepts and presuppositions of the healing encounter between human persons as individuals or societies that is the domain of philosophy of medicine, philosophically considered.

CHAPTER TWO

TOWARD A RECONSTRUCTION OF MEDICAL MORALITY: The Primacy of the Act of Profession and the Fact of Illness

INTRODUCTION

State of the Question

Is a commonly accepted code of professional morality possible in a democratic, morally pluralistic society? Are there philosophically justifiable obligations that bind all who profess medicine, or more generally, all who profess to heal? Can obligations be derived that are prior to, and independent of, the particular positions physicians or patients may take on the specific medical moral dilemmas of the day? In short, is it possible to reconstruct a professional morality more suited to contemporary requirements than the Hippocratic ethic?

These are fast becoming the central questions in medical ethics despite the heavy emphasis thus far on the resolution of specific moral dilemmas. Several factors specific to contemporary life dictate at least equal concern for the more general question of the moral conduct of the physician *qua* physician.

First is the gradual erosion of the acceptance of the traditional sources of medical morality. Fewer physicians subscribe to the religious foundations of medical ethics than before. Fewer still can claim to be faithful to all the injunctions of the Hippocratic Oath and the kind of life it enjoins. The hieratic, magical, and Aesculapean elements that once bound physicians together exist now only as remnants.

Then there is the wide divergence in values and opinions which characterizes the debates about so many moral dilemmas—abortion, euthanasia, the right to medical care, human experimentation, recombinant DNA research, and many more. The divisions among physicians, patients, and public on these issues are sharp enough to preclude the possibility of a commonly acceptable set of normative guidelines.

In addition, all codes to date have been developed *by* the profession, *for* the profession, and without participation of either patients or society. The Codes propagate a unilateral view of professional authority increasingly under question in a participatory democracy. They are inconsistent, too, with the ideas of contract or covenant now gaining significant support as models of the patient-physician relationship.

Also, even the most ancient codes have lacked a philosophically explicit derivation. They have rested largely on applications of existing theological or philosophical moral systems to medicine. The behavior of the good physician as physician has not been formally derived from a theory of medicine or the nature of the patient-physician relationship.

As a result, today codes of professional ethics are less universally accepted, narrower in the obligations they assume, more legalistic and cautious in tone, and more centered on scientific competence than humane considerations. While the special obligations to protect the subjects of human investigation have been recognized, little attention has been paid to the moral agency of patients in the more mundane and more multitudinous daily interactions with physicians. Even scantier notice is given to the physician's social responsibilities and their potential conflicts with his responsibilities to individual patients.

Two alternatives seem open at present: One is to abandon the possibility of a common set of higher moral principles and return to the simpler and less demanding ethics of a craft. This was the model of the early Greek physician; it assures at least the promise of competence, a promise which should survive even in a morally pluralistic society. The other alternative is to seek a philosophical reconstruction of professional ethics, one derived from the natures of medicine and medical acts and their interrelationships in the act of healing.

This essay takes the second alternative and seeks a foundation for medical morality—some irreducible source which can define the moral conduct of the human relationships specific to medical activity. This foundation should be prior to, and compatible with, a fairly wide range of value systems insofar as specific moral dilemmas are concerned. It should also be susceptible to expansion, enrichment, and illumination by additional obligations derived from theologically or humanistically based value systems. In short, this essay seeks a basis for professional ethics which defines the normative guidelines which must, of necessity, bind all who profess to heal.

While medicine and the physician will be used as the illustrations, the principles we derive are intrinsic to the professional activity of all health professionals—nurses, dentists, optometrists, allied health workers, psychologists, social workers, pharmacists, and podiatrists. Indeed, they could form the basis for a single common code of ethics for all the "healing" professions.

My inquiry will advance in three stages. First, the traditional sources for professional morality are examined and found wanting; then a philosophical basis for professional ethics is proposed based on the relationships of the act of profession, the act of medicine, and the fact of illness; finally, the obligations which derive from these relationships are outlined briefly.

Sources of Medical Morality

All codes of medical ethics reflect certain implicit philosophical assumptions: about the nature of medicine, the patient-physician relationship, and the good life. These assumptions dictate what is right conduct for both the physician and the patient. They give rise, therefore, to at least three constantly interacting levels of moral decision: what is right conduct for the physician *qua* physician and for the patient *qua* patient, what is right conduct for physician and patient irrespective of their situations as physician or patient, and the conjunction of these two levels in a third—determining right conduct in a specific moral dilemma.

The first level is that of professional morality properly speaking, and is the focus of this essay. The second is more properly the realm of general moral philosophy, and the third comprises the agenda of biomedical ethics as it is usually construed today. All three are closely intermingled in any medical decision or act and are disentangled with difficulty.

The philosophical foundations for each of these levels constitute the sources for the normative expressions of professional codes. Medical morality will differ greatly, depending on whether we view medicine as religion or magic, as craft or profession, science or art, as unique service or contract for a commodity, or as an instrument primarily of solicitude for individuals, or of social purpose. Overlaying these differences are the conceptions of the good life we hold: Aristotelian, Platonic, Stoic, Epicurean, Christian, Jewish, Moslem, socialistic, atheistic, or materialistic, Finally, the whole is modulated by which theory of morals we prefer—deontological, theological, consequentialist or utilitarian, or some combination.

The nuances of this triad of interactions in the historical and philosophical evolution of professional morality are beyond the length and scope of this essay. It is pertinent to my thesis, however, to examine some of their interactions around that most crucial source of professional ethics—the conception of the relationship between patients and physician. Ultimately, our conceptions of medicine, our philosophy of the good life, and our theories of ethics must converge on this point.

The most pervasive and influential conception of patient-physician relationships is the Hippocratic ethic. Under this rubric are subsumed a congeries of rules and practices successively elaborated over the centuries and forming a more or less generally accepted blueprint of medical morality. An examination of this ethic will expose the need for, and the requirements of, a reconstruction of professional morality.

THE HIPPOCRATIC ETHIC AND ITS METAMORPHOSIS

Origins

A fairly consistent image of how the Hippocratic physician regarded his relationship with the patient can be extracted from the *Corpus Hippocraticum,* especially from the "deontological" books (the *Oath, Law, Decorum, Precepts,* and *The Physician*).* The relationship these described was centered in the physician. It was a creation of

* I have drawn heavily for this section on the excellent William Osler Oration in the History of Medicine.[1]

the profession and meant for the profession. The physician, at first a craftsman, and later a more elite personage, had great concern for his corporate and personal reputation. The physician's conduct was as much motivated by the practical matter of economic success as by moral considerations. By virtue of his greater knowledge and skill, the physician was presumed to act as a benevolent authority in both technical and moral matters. He took upon himself the cares of the patient, decided what was "best" and whom he would treat. He was expected to be competent, freely to seek consultation, and to set reasonable fees with some regard for the patient's ability to pay. He was not to harm the patient and was to safeguard confidence. Edelstein has shown that the more austerely moral proscriptions of the oath—those against abortion, surgery, giving of poisons, and the injunction to lead a pure life—were Pythagorean precepts, not by any means uniformly held by all Greek physicians.* Something of the pluralism we experience today must have characterized Greek medical morality.

The "ethical" books are notable for their silence on a number of moral questions involving the physician-patient transaction which are of intense interest today. There is, for example, little mention of the patient's part in the relationship except to urge that he not impose upon the doctor impossible or dangerous treatments which might fail and thus harm the doctor's reputation. "The Art has three factors, the disease, the patient, and the physician. The physician is the servant of the Art. The patient must cooperate with the physician in combating the disease".[4] But the cooperation required of the patient is that of the child or servant following the order of the master. Thus, "If the physician is to help, his relationship to the patient must be that of the person in command to one who obeys".[5]

There is even a sense of the patient as antagonist: "Keep a watch on the faults of the patients, which often make them lie about the taking of things prescribed".[6] For this reason, too, the physician is urged to visit frequently or leave one of his pupils, never a layman, in charge. This assures that failures in treatment will not be held against the physician's reputation. We see here again the recurrent concern about reputation which seems to have obsessed the Hippocratic physician.

Edelstein attributes this partly to the fact that the early Greek physician was a craftsman, and his ethic was that of a good craftsman. By doing the job well, he could best distinguish himself in the public's eye from the charlatan or quack. According to Edelstein, this craftsman's ethic was the foundation for the humanism of the Greek physician. The famous quote, "Where there is love of man, there is love of the Attic precepts," was, in Edelstein's opinion, not a love of mankind in the sense of Stoic, religious, or secular humanism.[7] Rather, it bespoke a friendliness and kindliness essential to gaining the confidence of the patient, and thus to convincing him of the physician's capability to heal. That confidence, as every clinician has always known, is an important element in successful therapy.

In none of this is the patient seen as a partner in the decision, but rather as someone to be protected against the anxiety of too much knowledge. The physician knows

* This superb piece of textual criticism established the provenance of the oath as a Pythagorean document and seems more cogent in every way than W. H. S. Jones's *Philosophy and Medicine in Ancient Greece* (1946).[2,3]

what is best: "Perform all this calmly and adroitly, concealing most things from the patient while you are attending him."[8] "Sometimes reprove sharply and emphatically and sometimes comfort with solicitude and attention, revealing nothing of the patient's future or present condition. For many patients through this cause have taken a turn for the worse."[9] The physician clearly is expected to decide for the patient. "Patients in fact put themselves into the hands of their physician."[10]

If he did not participate in the physician's decisions, the Greek patient was nonetheless expected to know how to pick a good physician. The book called *Affection,* for example, is devoted to instructing the layman so he can make some of these judgments himself. In the book *On Joints,* the physician is enjoined to publish his cases, and admit when his treatments are bad.[11] These injunctions seem at odds with recommendations in other books of the *Corpus.* An interesting feature of the whole *Corpus,* in its therapeutic as well as its moral contents, is that the Hippocratic books often seem to be commentaries on each other, not infrequently giving contradictory opinions on important topics. Yet these differences are almost never dealt with directly or dialectically.

There is little in the *Corpus* to suggest an obligation to obtain the patient's consent—certainly not in the way we understand consent today. Nor is there acknowledgment of the possibility of a conflict in the physician's obligations or of differences with the patient about what might be "good" for him. The Hippocratic image is predominantly that of the benevolent, authoritative, authoritarian, autonomous physician who knows what is best. He assumes moral as well as technical agency for the patient. While the patient is considered in some treatises as essential to healing, his role is passive; his cooperation is obtained by persuasion, not by conscious choice among alternatives.[5]

The moral tone of the *Corpus* ranges from the austerity of the oath to the pragmatic concerns for the reputation of the physician and the profession. An example of the latter is the discussion about whether or not to treat "hopeless" cases (see *On Fractures, On the Art,* and *Decorum*). The *Corpus* is nonetheless a remarkably moral collection, mixing nobility and practicality, concern for the patient with a sharp eye for enhancing one's practice and position in the community.

The Hippocratic books are clearly moral documents, since they espouse a fairly consistent set of beliefs about the right conduct of physicians. They are not, however, strictly speaking, ethical treatises in any formal sense. They do not provide systematic justifications for the obligations they impose; no debates and no dialectic are offered defending or defining the moral principles so freely asserted. The tone is hortatory and not dialectical, moralistic rather than philosophical.

There is, of course, no question that the morality of the *Corpus* was shaped by the Attic and Hellenistic philosophers. The early ethic of the craftsman owes its origins to the notion of medicine as *techne* in Plato and Aristotle. It was later broadened by the conceptions of the good man, and the good life, propounded by the Hellenistic philosophies upon which medicine relied for its theories of disease. Their moral philosophies were imbibed with their cosmologies. The oath was a Pythagorean manifesto; *The Physician* is consistent with Aristotelianism, *Precepts* and *Decorum* with Stoicism, *Law* with Democriteanism. Other books are flavored strongly with Platonism, Skepticism, and Sophism.[12,13]

But the philosophical foundations of the ethics of the *Corpus* consisted in the application of general moral philosophies to medicine rather than development of a moral philosophy specific to medicine. Medical ethics was not grounded in an analysis of the special nature of the medical transaction or of the illness. Plato and Aristotle devoted much attention to the nature of medicine and its relationship to other disciplines, like politics, rhetoric, and poetry. They often used it as a model for practical morality. The implications of their theories of medicine for professional ethics are still in need of fuller explication.*

In the case of Aristotle, Joseph Owens[15] has recently shown that medicine was viewed as the servant of ethics. The physician has a responsibility to heal the bodily ills which impede habituation to the good. He is expected to use his art to make the patient a good man. Again, as Spicker[16] observes, a form of paternalism emerges which can have dangerous implications. What is important for our thesis is that, despite intensive interest in theories of medicine, even Plato and Aristotle did not ground medical ethics in a philosophy of the special human circumstances of the healing relationship.

The oath and the Hippocratic *Corpus* were given the powerful sanction of theology when they were adopted, with some modifications, by Christians, Moslems, and Jews. The obligation to act compassionately on behalf of the sick became mandatory for anyone who believed that all men were brothers created by the same God. Solicitude for the suffering was expected, especially from those whose vocation was healing. With the benediction of religion, the Hippocratic Oath became the universal ethical guide in the West—a status it did not enjoy in the pagan world of its origin.

The oath was therefore the common bond uniting physicians whose religious views might otherwise differ drastically. The religious sources of medical ethics remained powerful to modern times and were especially influential in nineteenth-century America.† Their strength and universal acceptance obscured the need for a philosophically derived system of professional morality, and indeed made it unnecessary.

Only in the twentieth century has that necessity become urgent. The major religions no longer agree on the fundamental questions of life, death, and the purpose of human existence. Adherence to formal religion and acceptance of its authority are declining. Pluralism and relativism have come to dominate moral philosophy. The common bonds that once joined all physicians are now so tenuous that many wonder if any common source of medical morality can exist at all.

To be successful, any contemporary effort to reconstruct a common medical morality must begin at a point prior to the divergencies that characterize medicomoral debates today. It must be grounded in a reality common to physicians as physicians, whatever their other beliefs and values may be. That reality is the special nature of the

* A. E. Jonsen and A. E. Hellegers[14] have analyzed traditional codes in terms of a more general ethical framework.

† Chester Burns[17] shows how the code of professional standards in American medicine in the eighteenth and nineteenth centuries depended explicitly on a Christian code of gentlemanly behavior. Burns further points out that during the eighteenth and nineteenth centuries a philosophical basis for professional ethics was specifically ruled out as "godless" or the result of heathen speculation.

human interactions demanded in the act of healing—a reality experienced by both physicians and patients. To be acceptable such a philosophy must not start with existing philosophies or theologies, but with an analysis of the medical transaction itself.

The Stoic and Later Influences

The first intimations of an explicit philosophical basis for the physician's moral obligations as physician to his patient are found in Scribonius Largus[18], who lived at the time of the Emperor Claudius. In this treatise *On Remedies,* Scribonius holds that the physician incurs the obligation to sympathy, humaneness, and a true love of mankind because it is inherent in the nature of the "profession," the vocation or calling of the doctor. Edelstein[19] traces Scribonius's view back to its origins in Cicero's *De Officiis*[20] and in the second century Stoic philosopher, Panaetius.* Panaetius held that we must be faithful to the role we have assumed in life, and that each profession has its own specific ethics. The physician has assumed a role in life that demands compassion and humaneness. These are the physician's professional virtues. Caring, on this view, is as much a *raison d'etre* of medicine as curing. The same sentiments are expressed by Sarapion in the second century A.D. and by Libanius. The latter's speech to young physicians represents the pagan epitome of the obligations and empathy a physician owes his patients.†

These noble sentiments of Libanius derive from some of the loftier elements of the Stoic philosophy.§ They perpetuate, nonetheless, a theory of the physician-patient relationship based on the duty of the physician to be benevolent, kind, and loving, for that is the role he has voluntarily assumed. We are not told whether that kindliness and love of humanity extends to treating the patient as an independent person with an identity of his own which can be smothered even by a loving but authoritarian physician. In fact, evidence would indicate that the "loving-kindness" is that of a father and not the respectful solicitude of one adult for another. This is, nonetheless, for its times a truly remarkable moral image, considering the inhumanity of so many other sectors of ancient life.

These Stoic influences significantly modified the older Greek notion of the physician as ordinary craftsman. They implied a certain nobility of dedication and a love for mankind which tended to confer a privileged status on the "profession." This privileged status took on a different complexion in Galen's *De Placitis,*£ where the physician

* See Scribonius Largus[21] and Deichgraber[22]. Both are cited by Edelstein[23]. It is Edelstein's interpretation of Scribonius which stimulated my own thoughts about the possibility of an ethics specific to medicine. I have translated the relevant portions for myself and concur with Edelstein's reading.

† Edelstein quotes Libanius's moving speech to the young physician which contains such exhortations as "cultivate love of man," "share in the pain of those who suffer," "consider yourself a partner in the disease." Such sentiments call for a degree of empathy with the patient rarely equaled in any era.[24]

§ The Stoics were the first philosophers to suggest that taking an oath or professing a human service was an earmark of personal integrity and necessarily led one to an acceptance of a code of ethics. In this regard, see Marcus Aurelius.[25]

£ Edelstein refers to Galen on this point.[26]

is accorded special privilege as a Roman citizen, and later in Thomas Percival's ethics, where the emphasis is on the physician as "gentleman" (see Percival 1975). The American Medical Association (AMA code of 1848) and its later emendations reflect this spirit. The idea of privilege, rather than vocation, has all too often predominated in the history of the profession.

The Stoic notions of *humanitas* and *misericordia* were given a spiritual significance with the rise of the great religions in the West. For the Christian, Moslem, and Jew, the physician's "profession" was fundamentally a religious act. He was ordained to care for the sick as brothers under the fatherhood of God. The Hippocratic Oath was consequently cleansed of pagan references. Its Pythogorean prescripts were consistent with religious humanism and were perpetuated in the Christianized oaths of the early Middle Ages, the *Fifty Admonitions to Physicians* of Isaac Israeli, and the Moslem Code of Ishaq al-Ruhami.[27]

In the later Middle Ages and into modern times, the idea of the patient-physician relationship was further transformed by changes in the notion of profession and the nature of medicine. Profession took on an even more explicitly religious meaning, beginning with the later Middle Ages, as the act of public declaration of a cleric who, on entering one of the orders, "declared" his dedication to a life of special service and devotion. Gradually, however, this religious dimension was lost as the elitist and privileged aspects gained ground over the idea of vocation, especially in late-eighteenth-century England. Percival's ethics insisted that the physician be courteous, kind, interested, yet objective; his comportment must be courteous and inspiring of confidence. Compassion and kindness were more a matter of *noblesse oblige* than a direct obligation of being a physician as Scribonius Largus had held.

Equally profound are the influences exerted by changing conceptions of the nature of medicine. Since Descartes, the supposition has grown that medicine is really a science more akin to physics and chemistry than to the arts or crafts. The unprecedented practical and theoretical successes of the experimental method made a strong argument in favor of the scientific model. Professional morality based on this model places primary emphasis on competence, objectivity, the advancement of knowledge, clinical experiment, and certitude—definable end points. The scientific model requires that the patient be seen as an object of observation and measurement. While it need not do so, the scientific model often tends to depreciate the caring and nontechnological aspects of the medical relationship.

One final example of a powerful force shaping professional morality is the Lockeian philosophy of autonomous individuality. Physician and patient, in this view, are seen as free agents, contracting with each other for the delivery of a service. Medicine becomes a commodity like other commodities, and a legalistic spirit invades the relationship of the professional with his patient, who even begins to be called a "client." In the contractual model, kindness and compassion become matters of enlightened self-interest. They are essential ingredients for a constructive negotiation of contract terms and fulfillment. They do not require the love of humanity Scribonius Largus thought was so unique to the act of medical profession.

Contemporary Medical Morality

Many other construals of medicine could be mentioned—medicine as an instrument of social and political policy, as in the Soviet states; or medicine as the means of social justice, as in the activist movement in our own country; or medicine as the guarantor of all human happiness. Each construal alters our idea of the patient-physician relationship and its right conduct. What is important to the main line of my argument is that we are heirs to a complex set of modulations and variations on a theme originally formulated as the "Hippocratic" ethic. The way each physician weaves these themes together determines the pattern of his/her personal medical morality. There may be considerable logical incompatibility between individual patterns. Some are more impressed by economic influences, others by the scientific, and others by the hieratic and magical. Some physicians pursue an ideal they know can never be attained fully; others are pragmatic or even political in their interpretation of the privileges of the profession. Some others yearn for a "return" to the simplicity they perceive in the Oath of Hippocrates which takes on for them a quasi-scriptural significance.

Lacking a formalized theory of medicine or philosophically derived notion of the relationship with patients, our society finds it more and more difficult to codify principles of moral behavior for the "good" physician. Witness the serial transformations in the professional code of the AMA from 1848, when it was introduced, to the latest suggestions for revision in 1978.[28] The first document was more specific and more detailed about relationships with patients. The first code was more strongly shaped by Percival's concept of the physician as gentleman, but it did evince a spirit of lofty ideals even if they were unilaterally defined.

In the latest version, the moral statements are much sparser—ten brief paragraphs in all. The language is pragmatic, reserved, and almost legalistic in tone. The emphasis is on scientific competence. It eschews terms which might suggest personal and human commitments* beyond those we expect in a mere contract. Like its predecessors, the current AMA code is created by, and for, the profession. While the preamble states that the code is to aid in relationships with "patients, colleagues, members of allied health professions and the public," there is no evidence of consultation with these groups.

Like the Hippocratic Oath and ethics, the AMA code makes no specific reference to patient consent or conflicts on values and obligations between physician and patient or between physician and healthcare team or hospital. There is no acknowledgment of the specific concerns which have led to the promulgations of patients' bills of rights, of the conflicts between obligations to individuals and to society. Moral responsibilities are not defined in such urgently felt matters as resource allocation, natural death acts, or the humane uses of medical technology.

These observations are not intended as an indictment of the current professional code, but to indicate the need for a more fundamental philosophical foundation than is now available. The profession has carried an honorable and high-minded set of principles from the past into a world which questions some of the very principles on which the ancient model is constructed. Patients today are educated; many live in democratic

* The 1978 revisions omit the following phrases from the current version: "service to humanity," "meriting the confidence of the patient," "rendering a full measure of service and devotion." Also omitted in the seventh paragraph are the phrases "limiting income," "adjusting fees to patients' ability to pay."

societies; they have the legal right to determine the disposition of their bodies; they want to define health in their own terms, or at least assess the worthwhileness of medical advice without necessarily accepting the doctor's concept automatically.

The recent versions of the AMA code are tending more in the direction of the craftsman's ethic which obtained in classical Greek times. The legalistic restraint, while understandable in the climate of litigation which prevails, is disappointing in a profession with such noble traditions. A profession so enmeshed in human concerns as medicine must run some risk in the name of compassion, dedication, and service.

To its credit, the code does not try to give specific answers to, or prescriptions for, all the many vexing medical-moral issues of the day, such as abortion, euthanasia, behavior control, experimentation, organ transplantation, and the like. In this sense, it does qualify as a set of principles directed to the physician-patient relationship. But these principles are not derived from an explicit, formally developed philosophy of the physician-patient relationship. They are subject to the unpredictable vacillations of political, social, and legal events. It is the force of those events which seems to be shaping the evolution of the AMA code, rather than the more permanent demands of the physician's act of profession to a person in need.

The philosophical difficulties exemplified in the past and present history of traditional codes of professional ethics converge, therefore, on the central question of this essay: Is a philosophical basis derivable for professional ethics, one which arises out of the nature of the relationship of doctors with patients and which could serve to reconstruct future codes more suitable to a democratic, educated, morally pluralistic society?

A PHILOSOPHICAL BASIS FOR THE PATIENT-PHYSICIAN INTERACTION

The remainder of this essay attempts to establish a philosophical framework for professional ethics based on three phenomena specific to medicine: the fact of illness, the act of profession, and the act of medicine. The interrelationships of these three phenomena are sufficiently unique to medicine to constitute a specific and unique kind of human relationship which ought to be conducted in certain specific ways to be morally defensible.

The Fact of Illness

Medicine and physicians exist because humans become ill. Illness is a subjective state, one in which a human being detects some change, acute or chronic, in his/her mode of existence based in anxiety about the functions of body or mind. Illness may or may not be associated with demonstrable pathology. What is crucial to being ill is the perception of an altered state of existence, one in which the patient interprets some symptom or sign as an indication that he/she is no longer "healthy," according to the patient's own definition of that fluid and multi-interpretable word.

A person who arrives at the conclusion that he/she is "ill" becomes a patient—one who bears some disability, some deficiency or concern, one who is no longer "whole," one who perceives special limits on his or her accustomed activity.

The person who becomes a patient suffers what is nothing less than an ontological assault. In our usual state we see ourselves identified with our bodies, facing the world and acting on it in essential unity. In illness the body is interposed between us and reality—it impedes our choices and actions and is no longer fully responsive. The body stands opposite to the self. Instead of serving us, we must serve it. It intrudes on our existence rather than enhancing or enriching it. We can no longer use it for transbodily purposes.

With this assault on the ontological unity of body and self, illness erodes the image we have fashioned of ourselves over the years. That image harmonizes our deficiencies and our strong points; we carefully and laboriously protect and refurbish it; we delicately balance it against the external exigencies of human life. Illness forces a reappraisal and that poses a threat to the old image; it opens up all the old anxieties and imposes new ones—often including the real threat of death or drastic alterations in lifestyle.

This ontological assault is aggravated by the loss of most of the freedoms we identify as peculiarly human. The patient is no longer free to make rational choices among alternatives. He lacks the knowledge and the skills necessary to cure himself or gain relief of pain and suffering. In many illnesses, the patient is not even free to reject medicine, as in severe trauma or other overwhelming acute emergencies. Voluntarily or not, the patient is forced to place himself under the power of another person, the health professional, who has the knowledge and the skills which can heal—but also harm. This involuntary need grounds the axiom of vulnerability from which follows the obligations of the physician.*

When a person becomes "ill," he is therefore in an exceptionally vulnerable state, one which severely compromises his customary human freedoms to use his body for transbodily purposes, to make his own decisions, to act for himself, and to accept or reject the services of others. The state of being ill is therefore a state of "wounded humanity," of a person compromised in his fundamental capacity to deal with his vulnerability.

How unique is the state of illness? Is not vulnerability a common condition in many other human situations? After all, the prisoner is deprived of freedom and civil rights; the poor and the socially outcast are constrained even in the most mundane matters of life; none of us is totally "free"; we must all conform to some set of social conventions. But in none of these situations is our capacity to deal with our vulnerability so impaired as in illness. We feel, usually, that we can cope with almost all of the other states of vulnerability if we have our "health." After all, we perceive health as a means toward freedom and other primary values. We ask only to be released from prison, given a job or money, and if we are healthy, we can rebuild our humanity and the integrity of our person. In illness, none of these things will help. Our essential mechanisms for coping with all other existential exigencies are compromised; we face the threat of loss of life itself, or we are suddenly asked to live a life which appears not worth living.

There is, therefore, a special dimension of anguish in illness. That is why healing cannot be classified as a commodity, or as a service on a par with going to a mechanic

* This aspect of illness is underdeveloped in Ramsey's account of the covenant between patient and physician. Illness of the body, by that very fact, determines the need for the relationship. One is not as "free" in the relationship as Ramsey supposes.

to have one's car fixed, to a lawyer for repair of one's legal fences, or even to a teacher for repair of one's defects in knowledge. The teacher-student, lawyer-client, serviceman-customer relationships have some of the elements of the physician-patient relationship. There is in them an inequality of knowledge and skill, and one person seeks assistance from another who professes to provide it. What is different is the unique ontological assault of illness on the body-self unity, and the primacy of the freedom to deal with all other life situations which illness removed. Without denying the analogy with, let us say, the lawyer-client relationship, it would be difficult to argue that the degree of injury to our humanity and the kind of injury we suffer in litigation are identical in their existential consequences to being ill.

The Act of Profession

In the presence of a patient in the peculiar state of vulnerable humanity which is illness, the health professional makes a "profession." He or she "declares aloud" that he has special knowledge and skills, that he can heal, or help, and that he will do so in the patient's interest, not his own. According to the *Oxford English Dictionary,* the etymology of the word "profession"—from the verb *profiteri,* to declare aloud or publicly—is closer to the meaning of the act than more recent formulations. That is what entering a profession means—not simply becoming a member of a defined group with a common education, standards of performance, and a common ethic. These are all secondary conditions of the central act of profession, which is an active, conscious declaration, voluntarily entered into and signifying willingness to assume the obligations necessary to make the declaration authentic.

All health professionals make this act of profession publicly when they accept a degree at graduation, when they take the oath of their profession, and, most important, every time they present themselves to a patient in need who seeks their assistance in healing. They make the act of profession implicitly, but nonetheless undeniably. The expectation is thus induced in the ill person that the declaration will be true and authentic, that the professional's knowledge and skill are genuine, and that the professional's concern for the patient's interests will be truly exercised.

Medicine is, of course, not alone in making an act of profession which invites specific expectations of performance. Lawyers, teachers, and ministers similarly declare a special competence and its use in the interests of those who seek their aid. Their clients also lack something they need. Like the patient, they too are vulnerable to varying degrees. The ethics of each profession rests on the authenticity of its claim—the physician's claim to restore health, the lawyer's to seek justice, the teacher's to redress ignorance, and the minister's to teach the way of salvation.

The act of profession is a promise made to another person, who is in need and therefore existentially vulnerable. The relationship between the professional and those he or she serves is characterized by an inequality in which the professional holds the balance of power. All the usual ethical obligations of making and keeping promises apply, but with a difference—the inequality of power poses special obligations on the person who professes. The professional-client relationship is not simply a contract between equals in which each party can negotiate in his own interest, since one part is not free *not* to negotiate. Medicine, law, teaching, and the ministry do not supply products in the usual legal and commercial sense.

Each profession fulfills the promise inherent in its act of profession by a specific action which identifies that profession. This central act is the vehicle of authenticity and the bridge which joins the need of the one seeking help with the promise of the one professing to help. We can examine that central act only for medicine, though analogous analyses are applicable to other professions.

The Central Act of Medicine

A patient in need who consults a physician wants to know what is wrong, what can be done about it, and what should be done.[29] These three questions, and the subjects of questions which contribute to answering them, taken together constitute the anatomy of clinical judgment previously developed. The final question—what should be done?—is the major focus of the patient's attention and the end toward which the whole process must be directed. It eventuates in a recommended action. While all the other questions leading to it can be reopened, the recommended action is, once taken, irretrievable.

The end of medicine, formally considered, is therefore a right and good healing action taken in the interests of a particular patient. All the science and art of the physician converge on the choice: among the many things that can be done, that which should be done for this person in this particular situation of life. It is a choice of what is right in the sense of what conforms scientifically, logically, and technically to the patient's needs and a choice of what is good, what is "worthwhile" for this patient. The recommended action intermingles technical and moral dimensions which may not always be immediately reconcilable.

This culmination in a right and good healing action is what constitutes medicine *qua* medicine. Diagnosis and therapeutics singly and together serve this end. The physician acts as physician only when he particularizes the conclusions about what is wrong and what can be done in a decision about what ought to be, must be, may be, or should not be done for this patient, here and now.

The patient expects the end of medicine to be an action which is right and good for him. This is the promise he perceives in the act of profession, collectively from organized medicine, and singularly from his personal physician or physicians. It is what he expects also from medical and health organizations—the team, the hospital, or the agency.

The medical act combines technical and moral decision making in a way which makes it a moral enterprise of a special kind. Each medical decision involves the complicated interplay of several value sets—those of the physician, of the patient, and of society. In a pluralistic society, these value sets may differ sharply from each other. The possibilities of conflict in the conception of the good between physician and patient are many. A very special problem in medical decision making is how to resolve these conflicts in a morally defensible way.

For the conflicts of values occur in a relationship of inequality inherent in the vulnerability of the patient, as we have outlined it above. The assault of illness on the usual freedoms of the human being presents an immediate and present danger that the patient's values might be violated or that the physician may confuse technical with moral authority. The patient's moral agency is at risk, and a special obligation of the act of profession is to protect that moral agency while treating the patient.

By virtue of his act of profession, the physician raises specific expectations and thus voluntarily assumes certain specific obligations. It is these obligations, as well as those of the patient to the physician, which we shall examine next.

Obligations Arising from the Special Nature of the Patient-Physician Relationship

The obligations which arise from the construal of the patient-physician relationship outlined here could form the philosophical basis for a professional ethic—one which would bind the physician regardless of the position he might take on any of the specific moral dilemmas of medicine. A cursory examination of these obligations can illustrate the primacy of the acts of profession and medicine taken in the face of the fact of illness.

Let it be clear that no new moral principles need be elaborated. The well-adopted moral principles of truth telling and promise keeping, as well as the principles of non-harm and vulnerability, will suffice, but modulated by those special existential circumstances which define the relationship of one needing to be healed confronting one professing to heal. The same principle would apply by analogy to the lawyer-client, teacher-student, minister-subject relationships, each modified by the specific expectations generated by the act of profession each makes when a patient or client is confronted seeking assistance.

To begin with, the act of medical profession is inauthentic and a lie unless it fulfills the expectation of technical competence. If the special knowledge upon which the act of profession is based is wanting, then the whole relationship begins with a lie. The decision may even fortuitously turn out to be the "right and good" one for the patient, but if it does, it is based on chance, not knowledge. The patient has been deceived into believing the advice he received is the fruit of the physician's competence. The far greater likelihood is that the incompetent physician will not make the right or good decision. Then he becomes worse than a quack. The latter at least follows a system which makes no claim to being scientific, while the incompetent physician enshrouds his ignorance in a mantle of science.

The moral obligation to be competent is a lifelong one and an affair of daily concern. It begins with a sound medical education and house staff training, and goes on to a dedication to continuing education, a willingness to subject his decisions to peer review, an openness to criticism by one's colleagues, a willingness to confess ignorance or error to the patient, and a concentrated and sustained effort to deepen one's clinical craftsmanship. Competence, then, is a moral imperative, and a clear statement of that fact together with its fullest implications should be an essential element in any professional code. Competence is explicitly required by the first four principles of the latest revision of the AMA code. It is equated therein with "scientific" medicine. Such a formulation is correctly applicable to the technical steps involved in diagnosis, prognosis, and therapeutics. It includes also the art and skill needed to perform the recommended procedures safely and with a minimum of discomfort.

But in the complex anatomy of clinical judgment, competence is a necessary, but not sufficient, condition of a moral medical transaction and an authentic act of profession. Competence must itself be shaped by the end of the medical act—a right and good healing action for a particular patient. Competence must be employed in the best interest of the patient, and wherever possible that interest must conform with the patient's values and sense of what it is to be healthy.*

Technically correct conclusions may not necessarily be in the patient's best interest when that interest is defined in the patient's terms, for example, abortion for a Catholic, transfusion for a Jehovah's Witness, prolonging life in someone prepared to die, or "letting" another die who wants to live what may seem to the physician an unsatisfying life. A scientifically correct medical conclusion, its "oughtness," can range from "must," "should," "may," "need not," or "must not," depending upon the interacting moral agencies of patient and physician.

The physician has a special moral obligation to assure and facilitate the patient's moral agency, especially in the light of the patient's special vulnerability. To assure a fully participatory moral agency, the physician must repair to the extent possible the wounded humanity and state of inequality of the sick person. He does so only in part by curing, or containing, illness or relieving pain and anxiety. These must be complemented by disclosure of the information necessary for valid choice and genuine consent† and by guarding against manipulation of choice and consent to accommodate to the physician's personal or social philosophy of the good life.

A first requirement, therefore, is to remedy the patient's information deficit as completely as possible. Information must be clear and understandable and in the patient's language. He must know the nature of his illness, its prognosis, the alternative modes of treatment, their probable effectiveness, cost, discomfort, side effects, and the quality of life they may yield. Disclosure must include degrees of ignorance as well as knowledge and the physician's own limitations.

The physician who is conscious of the special nature of his act of profession will not easily excuse himself from the obligation of disclosure on the grounds that the patient cannot understand or will be harmed by the information. There are few, if any, evidences that such knowledge is deleterious, the Hippocratic warnings to the contrary. Indeed, in those rare instances where the matter has been studied, informed patients show a lower anxiety and complication rate than the uninformed.[32]

Reducing the inequality in information between patient and physician is essential in obtaining a morally valid consent which is the vehicle for expression of the patient's moral agency. More is required than the minimal conditions of a legally valid consent,

* We have established that ethics in medicine is not a relative piety adopted by its practitioners, but a necessary and productive basis for action. In this respect, see Eric Cassell.[30]

† "It is essential that the patient believe that he is an independent, worthy person entitled to the most clearly stated information possible".[31] In my view, the position is not only a claim derived from the principle of respect for persons, but a necessary moral principle of the physician-patient relationship.

which is after all, guarantee against the grosser violations of the patient's right to decide. A morally valid consent moves closer to the realization of both senses of the word "con-sent" (Latin: *consentire*), to feel and to know something together. Patient and physician, therefore, must each feel he knows and understands the available facts, and each must feel he is truly part of the decision making.

When the patient cannot participate in the decision, the physician must deal with the patient's surrogate—the family, guardian, or the court. The obligations to respect the patient's value system are the same. When dealing with surrogates, however, an additional obligation is imposed, and that is to be sure that they do in fact have the patient's interests at heart. In the case of the unconscious patient or the child, the physician must assure himself that the surrogate, parent, or family does not unconsciously with the patient's demise.

This state of feeling and knowing together places the actual locus of decision making somewhere between physician and patient, and not really with one or the other. As in any relationship between humans, medical or otherwise, obtaining consent requires persuasion, a mutual accommodation of wills. It is extremely difficult to set limits on the degree to which manipulation of consent is morally permissible. It is important for this essay only to indicate that the physician must be alert to those subtle choices of words, nuances of emphasis, or body language which tip the patient's consent in the direction of what the physician feels is "good." It is unrealistic to expect even the most ethically sensitive physician not to wish the patient would make certain choices. In some cases some degree of persuasion may even be ethically obligatory.

No set of rules could encompass all the subtle complexities of even the most ordinary relationship between two persons, much less the special dimensions peculiar to the medical transaction in which one person in special need seeks the assistance of another who professes to help. The morality of clinical judgment goes well beyond the merely technical and scientific probity of the craft.

There are times when the physician can and should exert moral agency for the patient and make the value choice in his behalf. One instance would be when the patient or family request him to do so even after the physician has attempted to provide the necessary information and has taken all pains to be clear and unequivocal about the choices. Some patients and families are either emotionally or educationally ill-equipped to deal with such difficult decisions. They may then ask the physician to "decide." The physician then has a mandate to assume moral agency, and it would be a failure of the authenticity of his act of profession not to say what should be done. The same applies when the situation is of such an urgent nature that to consult the patient or even his or her family would be impossible or would delay emergency treatment. In the operating and emergency rooms, the intensive-care and coronary-care units, the obligations we have stressed must be drastically modified because the patient's interest itself overrides even these fundamental requirements of medical morality. The retrospective examination of how, for what reasons, and according to what value sets the decisions were made is an essential antidote to overzealous assumption of moral authority even in emergency situations.

Here, too, a caveat is in order. For the physician to say simply that he would treat the patient as he would treat himself or a member of his family is morally unsound.

This misinterpretation of the golden rule would only reopen the possibility of overriding the patient's wishes. The golden rule in medical decisions is to be observed rather differently: We should so act that we accord the patient the same opportunity to express or actualize his own view of what he considers worthwhile as we would desire for ourselves.* This latter interpretation of the golden rule is fully consistent with the view of authenticity of the act of profession we have developed in this essay.

What obligations of this type require is a combination of conscious advertence to the meanings of the three elements—the fact of illness, the act of profession, and the act of medicine—with compassion. We do not think this has to involve the *iatrike philia,* the love of which Pedro Lain-Entralgo speaks as the fundamental link in his superb phenomenological study of the physician-patient relationship. It does require the capacity to "feel with" the patient something of the existential situation he is experiencing in the condition of illness, whether it is somatic or physical in origin. Not to be able to feel something of the patient's anguish and anxiety before the ontological assault of illness is to rely on only a rational adumbration of the obligations which inhere in the act of profession. But even this is superior to the more traditional conception of the physician as benevolent agent of both technical and moral decision making who decides what is "best" for the patient.

Many aspects of the physician's obligations which could be derived from the philosophy of the medical transaction proposed here have not been touched upon. Those chosen are meant to be illustrative, and not comprehensive. We have not discussed, for example, how to resolve conflicts in values between the physician's social and patient responsibilities, the obligations of the profession as a corporate whole, or the applicability of these principles when the physician functions in a collectivity as a member of a team, or an institution.

Also, on this view, there is a set of obligations which would bind the patient so that we can begin to develop an ethics of the "good" patient. If the physician construes his act of profession as a promise of a special kind given under special conditions, and if the patient understands it that way, then the patient incurs certain obligations as well. He must be truthful in the information he gives the physician; he must avoid manipulating the physician in consent; he must follow recommendations mutually agreed upon faithfully; he must educate himself sufficiently to comprehend the facts disclosed to him, and take the trouble to be sure he does understand; he must not consult another physician without informing his medical attendant unless he suspects dishonesty or malpractice. Further, he is partially obligated, by the fact that he is a member of the human race, to participate in reasonable experiments which are either aimed at healing his disease (therapeutic) or at discovering possible cures for this disease for others (nontherapeutic), provided the other rules for professional behavior are

* Although we have developed this "golden rule" from the philosophical reflections on the physician-patient relationship, it does carry similarities with general ethical points of view, particularly that principle of liberty developed by John Stuart Mill (On Liberty) which argues that one cannot interfere with the freedom of another unless they are a danger to others, and the ethical reflections of Gert.[33]

followed. We say "partially obligated" because the vulnerability of the patient excuses him from any absolute obligation.

The principle of autonomy and the principle of partial obligation enunciated above represent almost a classic example of the possible clash between two goods. On the one hand, the person who is ill is clearly given the opportunity and the freedom to attend to his needs for healing, a value which takes precedence over any altruism to be demanded of him. However, the ill person is also a member of the human race and has obligations to help foster the understanding of the disease so that either he or others might benefit.

The patient, in short, in the relationship we have described, owes the physician the same respect for his values and cannot demand that the physician violate them even when the patient might benefit. The patient cannot ask his physician to practice deception with insurance companies and governmental agencies. In sum, even though the vulnerability imposed by illness makes the patient more vulnerable, the tyranny of the patient is as wrong as the tyranny of the physician.

This construal of the patient-physician relationship calls, therefore, for mutual respect and compassion, even though it involves one person who is less free and more vulnerable. That is why the relationship cannot be regarded as a contract or even a covenant. It is not an agreement between two parties more or less equal, more or less free, who can negotiate terms for the delivery of some service or commodity. Medical care is not a commodity one may choose as freely as one chooses automobiles or television sets.

What we propose is a mutually binding set of obligations, predicated upon a special kind of human interaction and deriving its morality from the empirical realities in the relationship which specify it among human relationships. These specifications could be the basis for a philosophically justifiable statement of principles—a code—common to all physicians, indeed to all healers. If their implications are expanded, we can even hope for a more general code applicable to all the health professions at least in part since all health professionals make an act of profession in the sense we have defined it here.

The post-Hippocratic reconstruction of professional ethics is therefore possible. We need not return to the ethics of the good craftsman, as in our Greek beginnings. We can instead extend and build upon the idea of Scribonius Largus and Panaetius that there is an ethic specific to each profession, based in the nature of that profession, and philosophically justifiable.

CONCLUSION

Looked at historically, our line of reasoning has taken us away from the dominant sources of medical morality—that is, the Hippocratic *Corpus* and the oath especially, away from both the craft and privileged-status ethic. My inclination has been, rather, to the extension and elaboration of the idea of profession as it was advanced by Scribonius Largus and Panaetius and the middle Stoics. I have suggested a derivation of medical ethics from the specific relationship of three phenomena of the medical transaction rather than applying philosophical conceptions drawn outside of medicine to medicine. In contradistinction to Scribonius Largus, I have not made *humanitas* the specific end of medicine, nor as with Lain-Entralgo the *iatrike philia,* but rather a right and good healing action for a particular patient. This is what the physician professes, what the patient expects, and what must be offered in the presence of the state of wounded humanity we call illness. This is the foundation of professional ethics, the source of medical morality, and the leitmotiv of a more satisfactory professional code of how the physician should act *qua* physician. It is necessarily antecedent to whatever position may be taken in specific moral dilemmas. Indeed, sensitively attended to, it assures the morality of the personal transaction even when there is a difference between physician and patient or physician and physician about particular medical moral problems.

A summary of the obligations for a medical-professional code of ethics might be schematized as follows:*

1. Technical competence
2. Insuring moral agency of patient
    - Information
    - Consent
    - Proxy consent
3. Respect for the individualized nature of the transaction.

A corresponding set of patient obligations can be summarized as follows:

1. Trust in competence
2. Respect for the moral agency of the physician
3. Truthtelling about the illness
4. Caution in asking more of medicine than it can provide
5. Partial obligation to participate in medical research.

With these considerations in hand, we can examine and find fruitful solutions to some problems of contemporary medical practice that are rarely addressed.

* I am indebted to Dr. David Thomasma for his critique of this essay and his suggestion that these principles be extracted in this form as a résumé of essential elements in a reconstruction of medical morality.

CHAPTER THREE

PHILOSOPHY OF MEDICINE: Problematic and Potential

> *PHAEDRUS: Hippocrates the Asclepiad says that the nature even of the body can only be understood as a whole.*
>
> *SOCRATES: Yes friend, and he is right—still we ought not to be content with the name of Hippocrates, but to examine and see whether his argument agrees with his conception of nature.*[1]

Medicine and philosophy oscillate about each other like the strands of a complex double helix of the intellect. They are intermittently drawn together by their immersion in man's existence and driven apart by their often opposing preoccupation with that existence. Special tensions arise from their conflicting claims to universality—medicine divinizing the body and the particular, philosophy the intellect and the abstract.

The state of the relationship is, however, always of profound cultural significance. When medicine and philosophy converge, they can greatly advance man's search for a unified image of himself and the world; when they diverge, that image becomes fragmented, puzzling, and even absurd. Today the intersections of medicine and philosophy are fraught with uncommon possibility and urgency. The problematic state of that intersection is one of the most significant challenges our culture faces.

The ambiguities and the tensions inherent in the relationships of medicine and philosophy have been expressed in ancient and modern terms:

Plato, with his usual prescience, exposes these ambiguities. In the *Protagoras*, the *Gorgias*, and elsewhere, he stresses the close congruity of medicine and philosophy as practical disciplines, aimed at the promotion of the good life. For both Plato and Aristotle they share a concern with the normative—medicine prescribing the right conduct of the body, philosophy the right conduct of the soul as well as of the social and the political life.[2,3]

In the *Symposium*, however, the emphasis is on the antithetical claims of medicine and philosophy. Eryximachus, the physician, is a symbol of technicism in his promulgation of the cultivation of the body as the true end of human life: "And this is what the physician has to do, and in this the art of medicine consists: for medicine may be regarded as the knowledge of the loves and desires of the body, and how to satisfy them or not…".[4,5] But later on Diotima speaks for Socrates, of a higher form of Eros: "But what if man had eyes to see the true beauty—the divine beauty, I mean, pure and clear and unalloyed, not clogged with the pollutions of mortality and all the colors and vanities of human life?" (Plato 211, 1:335). Or, as Socrates says to Simmias, "…the body is always breaking in upon us, causing turmoil and confusion in our inquiries".[6]

These dichotomies are expressed in more modern terms as an opposition of method, the antithesis between contemplation and understanding and fact and observation. Claude Bernard stated what is still dominant medical view: "…philosophy does not teach anything, and is unable to teach anything itself, since philosophy makes neither experiment nor observation."[7] Scott Buchanan, calling for a philosophy of medicine, says "…it [medicine] stands at the head of the natural sciences, and does not know which way to go. It has a record maximum of knowledge and a minimum of understanding. It has art, and wonders if it has science. It is suffering from an intellectual imbalance of virtues."[8]

Medicine and philosophy have inherent tendencies to a special kind of hubris which has complicated their relationship for centuries. Medicine is pulled toward technicism, especially today when its technologic apparatus is so impressive. Philosophy leans toward detachment, as the emphasis in the recent past on speculative metaphysics or linguistic analysis has illustrated. Paradoxically, a deeper perception of the advantages of these tendencies has now revealed the need in both disciplines for a conscious balancing of these tendencies. Medicine is recognizing the need for understanding and critical reflection; philosophy has recently addressed itself to some of the more practical issues in legal, political, and social philosophy.

Contemporary medicine and philosophy are therefore at the moment in their intellectual histories when each needs the other to redress an internal imbalance. It is the context, the quality, and the perimeters of this new engagement of medicine and philosophy that I shall examine in this essay. In an expanded and more rigorous form, it is also the *raison d'etre* of the *Journal of Medicine and Philosophy.*

I will inquire into one problematic aspect of the ground between philosophy and medicine—the philosophy *of* medicine. Is a discipline under this rubric possible? Is there a formal discipline which has as its object the philosophical issues specific to medicine and medical phenomena? Can it be distinguished from other branches of philosophy? What particular problems does it subsume? What value does it have for philosophy itself, for medicine, and for society? In what ways specifically can philosophy engage medicine, and how can it avoid spurious and contrived relationships?

My aim will be simply to map out these questions as they appear to a nonphilosopher who believes that medicine must become increasingly an "examined" discipline—one which is critically justified as science and practice. My stance is that of the academic clinician, educator, and administrator, aware of the presuppositions upon which medicine is built and their exquisite significance for individuals and society. My hope is to engage bona fide philosophers in the examination of the conceptual bases of medicine, leaving to them the more rigorous and more distinctly philosophical treatment the issues demand—and this essay must necessarily lack.

MUTUAL BENEFITS AND ATTITUDINAL OBSTACLES

In every culture, medicine rests on a substructure of concepts which determine its character; that is to say, its method and practice as well as its ethos, ethics, and ideology. These are the ideas used to justify the expectations and the behavior of physicians, patients, and society. They are the source too, for an idea or image of man which inevitably flows from medicine to color the whole of culture. Never have the conceptual bases of medicine had a wider impact on mankind than today, and never has it been more urgent to examine them critically, dialectically, and speculatively (i.e., philosophically).

Philosophy, then, has a special cultural and social responsibility to help redress the "imbalance" of intellectual virtues in medicine to which Buchanan alluded. It possesses the intellectual tools—its own traditional and contemporary techne—to make the whole matter of medicine an examined activity. It can bring the understanding and clarification necessary to forestall the easy seductions of technicism. Few issues are more fundamental to human well-being than the humane use of medical knowledge. But the validity of the ends and means of medicine and of the models of man that emerge from them is a "transmedical" matter—one not susceptible to the methods of medicine itself.

Philosophy's engagement with questions raised by medicine is not without significant benefit to its own enterprise. Anglo-American philosophy, more so than European philosophy, has too assiduously eschewed a concern with the central issues of human existence. As it moves to reengage those issues, philosophy will need a fuller input from what medicine has learned about man's encounters with his body, his world, and his psyche. Medicine abounds in concrete, verifiable, and measurable data abut human life and offers these as grounds for cogitation and inquiry. Out of this ground, philosophers can find new stimuli to their traditional concerns for apprehending human being, thought, knowledge, and value. It is very much as Wartofsky has put it: "I believe philosophy has to get beyond philosophy to remain philosophical."[9]

For the dialogue to be mutually beneficial, each party will have to overcome its temptations to universality.

Philosophers must learn to see the immediate and grave issues in medicine as philosophically legitimate and no less respectable for their origin in such a practical domain as medicine to be of service to medicine, and to itself, philosophy must learn to turn to medicine even to understand some of the issues with which it is itself concerned. A refurbished and less precious—though no less rigorous—image of philosophy needs to be fashioned.

For its part, medicine must overcome its antiphilosophical bias and its own claims to preciosity and sacerdotal privilege. These barriers to a critical examination of the conceptual structures of medicine are already breached by the searching reevaluations of the social purposes of medicine now under way. The most effective way medicine can generate a new and more realistic image of itself is through the kind of scrutiny philosophy can bring. This scrutiny does not entail an abandonment of the scientific fundaments of medicine. In fact, a realistic appraisal of what medicine is, and must be, should reinforce the validity of the effort.

The dialogue between Eryximachus and Diotima is entering a new phase—one in which competing claims of medicine and philosophy to universality may have to be compromised in the interests of the mankind each presumably serves.

MEDICINE AND PHILOSOPHY: THE HISTORICAL ANTECEDENTS[10]

Medicine began as a discipline under the domination of religion and myth. In the Western world it freed itself from this influence by becoming a part of pre-Socratic Ionian natural philosophy, from which it imbibed an interest in the explanation of the natural world through reason as well as a fascination with the ideas of cause and effect and change. In this period physicians and philosophers—as well as medicine, science, and philosophy—were largely indistinguishable.

Medicine became an independent profession in the fifth century B.C. with the appearance of the Hippocratic School. As Edelstein[11] points out, medicine took on two distinct features—it emphasized the importance of basing its art in the observation of the individual patient and of doing so in an ethical frame.

Medicine and philosophy became independent and strong disciplines. Because of this fact Hippocratic medicine and Attic philosophy enjoyed their most fruitful relationship and one not equaled since. Each contributed conceptually to the other, and their congruence eventuated in *Paideia*, the ideal of Greek culture, as Werner Jaeger so well documents.[12] It was in the spirit of this felicitous conjunction that Hippocrates likened the physician who was a philosopher to a demigod,[13] Aristotle posited that philosophy properly ended in medicine,[14] and Galen insisted that the best physician was a philosopher.[15]

But even in that most salubrious of relationships, there were discordant notes. The treatise *On Ancient Medicine* in one sense fortifies the analogies between medicine and philosophy, as exemplified in the *Protagoras*. But in another sense that same treatise warns explicitly against speculations undisciplined by direct observation of patients.[16] Hippocratic medicine even developed some of the attributes of a philosophy of its own. Thus, even at the moment of their happiest conjunction the tensions which Plato symbolizes in the *Symposium* were clearly discernible.

The more usual pattern over most of its history was for medicine to come intermittently under the influence of whatever philosophical school had currency in a given era. It took the methodological potency of modern science to fortify medicine against overspeculation of philosophical domination.

In the Hellenic and Greek worlds, whole medical systems were fashioned out of bits and pieces of the philosophies of Aristotle, Plato, Pythagoras, or Zeno—as the multiple and successive schools of dogmatism, methodism, or eclecticism attest. In the

Middle Ages, scholasticism and Christian theology suffused medical thought and practice. Later, the power of Descartes's mechanistic biology became (and remains today) a powerful influence, from the iatromechanists, iatrochemists, and iatrophysicists of the seventeenth and eighteenth centuries to the biological reductionists of our time.

Of more recent memory is the influence of German idealist philosophy on the medical systematists of the eighteenth and nineteenth centuries like Hoffman, Stahl, John Brown, and William Cullen. Risse and Galdston have documented how such notions as nervous ether, animism, or vitalism could derive from readings—or misreadings—of Hegel, Kant, Schelling, or Fichte.[17,18,19] Systems of diagnosis and treatment unrestrained by empiric or scientific observations proliferated in the romantic era and for a time inhibited the growth of scientific medicine.

As a reaction to these transfers into medicine of poorly comprehended philosophical models, modern medicine has become distrustful of philosophical intrusions. Its historical susceptibility to the domination of philosophical systems derived from the lack, for so many centuries, of a scientifically verifiable base of knowledge. Thought unopposed by fact was too powerful to be gainsaid. But in the last century the triumph of Bernard's experimentalism and the infusion of the chemical and biological sciences into clinical medicine have reduced this susceptibility to a very large degree.

The philosophical temptation to medicine is no longer unrestrained system building, but excessive faith in positivistic modes of thought and explanation. Medicine is now strong enough and independent enough to engage philosophy without fear of domination.

Philosophy has successfully completed its century-long reaction to speculative overemphasis of idealist and romantic philosophical systems. Logical positivism and the analytic and linguistic emphasis of Anglo-American philosophy have served this purpose well. Many philosophers, among them the philosophers of science, have already recognized the need for grappling with some of the more traditional metaphysical concerns, as McMullin shows.[20]

There is a renewed interest in both medicine and philosophy in the recurrent and fundamental issues of purpose, value, and the meaning and mode of human existence. Medicine manifestly cannot grasp the full reality of its subject, man, or learn to use its knowledge morally without relaxing its positivist bias, even when philosophy has already taken the turn away from this positivist strain. Philosophy, in its turn, cannot deal adequately with the new questions about man without its own recent turn to the phenomena and the realities revealed in human biology and the medical encounter.

The serious normative issues in medical ethics, for example, demand more than can be extracted from "metaethics."

If these issues are not related philosophically, they will be resolved in the crisis of the clinical situation and by individual practitioners in the light of their own philosophical or pragmatic leanings. These issues are too important for society to be decided without serious critical reflection and the participation of thinkers outside, as well as inside, medicine. Philosophies are taking an interest in questions of the value and purpose of human life and on the uses of professions as instruments of personal and social purpose.

European philosophy, with its phenomenological and existential emphases, has turned to some of the nonscientific dimensions of human existence and has grappled with some of the issues medicine is examining. One thinks notably of the work of Marcel, Merleau-Ponty, Lain-Entralgo, Foucault, and E. Straus. These thinkers observe a conscious fastidiousness about ontological questions and eschew the ancient idea of a "first" philosophy which confronts the unanswerable, but perennially relevant questions. European philosophy, however, has on the whole been responsive to the fact that questions of another kind must now be addressed, and those questions must bear once again on this human condition, its meaning, and the central questions of what man "is." The grapplings of Marcel, Camus, and Sarte with the complexities and absurdities of the human existence at least face the questions, even if their solutions are not acceptable.

Even at this late date in the English-speaking world, there is no recognition of a formal discipline under the rubric of the philosophy of medicine. We do acknowledge the philosophies of law, education, science, religion, and history. But even Edwards's[21] comprehensive *Encyclopedia of Philosophy* has no article under this heading; indeed, its only reference to medicine is an article on Hippocrates.

In Continental Europe, the philosophy of medicine has had a more definable status. Beginning in the nineteenth century, a substantial number of studies under this category have appeared in Germany, France, Poland, Italy, and Russia, as Szumowski's valuable review attests.[22] A wide variety of topics is covered—such as the logic and epistemology of medicine, the concepts of health and disease, medical ethics, causality in medicine, the mind-body problem, mechanism and vitalism. Several chairs of philosophy were established in Polish universities in the twenties.

The significance of the European efforts is not to be denied. They represent, however, a rather all-encompassing notion which suffers from diffuseness and includes much that would not be strictly defined as the philosophy of medicine. They are notable exceptions to the predominantly antipathetic attitude of the majority of physicians toward philosophical exercises.

Doubtlessly, many thinkers in both fields will continue to see an impassable gulf. The stereotype of philosophy contemplating the world of untestable ideas and of medicine confined to practical and technical concerns are too comfortable to be speedily abandoned. The artificiality of these extreme positions is becoming plain in the light of the kinds of issues medicine now raises and in the kinds of questions philosophy must itself confront. As their interests reach beyond the peripheral intersections we now observe a true dialogue must emerge—one which will require each to break out of its immediately past traditions and biases.

The need for a genuine dialectic is increasingly obvious. The philosopher cannot really clarify the ontological status of man without reliance on the most accurate statement he can obtain on man's existence. Much of this can be found in the kind of data medicine alone can provide. The physician, on the other hand, needs an ontological conception of man which can give order and intelligibility to his objective search—and this is the business of philosophy. The ontological encounter between science and philosophy which de Waelhens feels is so important for our understanding of each, can have its paradigm in the encounter of medicine and philosophy.[23]

The possibilities inherent in such an encounter are exemplified by the increasing number of philosophers in recent years who have examined questions highly pertinent to medicine or the medical context. We can cite only a few to make the point: the deep interest in the philosophy of the body evidenced in the work of Marcel,[24] Merleau-Ponty,[25] and Spicker[26]; the philosophical foundations of psychiatry, psychology, and perception in works by Straus,[27] Straus, Natanson, and Ey,[28] and Grene[29]; Engelhardt's[30,31] concern with concepts of health and disease and philosophical bases of medical ethics; Buytendijck's[32] fusion of physiology and anthropology; Lain-Entralgo's[33,34,35] analyses of the patient-physician encounter; Warofsky's[36] inquiry into human ontology and medical practice, and Zaner's[37,38,39] series of papers underscoring the character of the human self, interpersonal bonds (as exemplified in medical contexts), and the concept of "enabling" in medical education.

These explorations speak eloquently to the genuinely philosophical nature of many medical issues. They underscore the need for an orderly and detailed inquiry into the matter of medicine, from its prelogical assumptions to its method and modes of thought and their applications to persons and society. Serious philosophers are now examining this totality with a variety of philosophical tools. The increasing frequency and depth of these engagements raise the possibility of the philosophy of medicine as a formal discipline, distinct from other branches of philosophy. The subject is still in an inchoate state. It is toward its maturation that Engelhardt and Spicker have established their series on philosophy and medicine,[40] this *Journal of Medicine and Philosophy* has been initiated, and the American Philosophical Association has formed a Committee on Philosophy and Medicine.

The historical wariness of the two disciplines is being overcome, and the ground between them is again being actively tilled. We are entering a new era of dialogue—perhaps one as promising as that between Greek medicine and philosophy. Given the historical antecedents, the relationship will be a delicate one nonetheless.

PHILOSOPHY OF MEDICINE: DISCIPLINE OR PHILOSOPHICAL MÉLANGE

Do the medical forays of philosophers in Europe and the current interest in the United States prefigure the emergence of a definable discipline—the philosophy of medicine? Opinions range from flat denial to all-encompassing acceptance. Jerome Shaffer categorically denies the possibility; Toulmin regards it as problematic, and Szumowski accepts the notion, going so far as to define it. We will first examine these opinions and then lay out the requirements the philosophy of medicine must satisfy if it is to be a distinguishable discipline.

Shaffer's denial of the possibility is unequivocal.[41] He doubts there are any problems common to medicine and philosophy. Those alleged to be at the interface are either misclassified or not philosophical problems at all. He would reduce all philosophical efforts in the medical context to philosophy of science, philosophy of mind, or moral philosophy. He freely acknowledges the significance of the issues for philosophy but sees nothing to distinguish medicine from a mere summation of biology and psychology.

Toulmin partially agrees with Shaffer by finding no real distinction between medicine and physiology.[42] Physiology is itself a derivative of physics and chemistry. Physiology, however, deals with "the special field of life" where the laws of physiology are not independent of chemistry and physics but still not fully equated with them. Thus the somatic elements in medical science are subsumed under the philosophy of science or of biology. Toulmin, however, allows for the possibility of philosophy of medicine based on the psychosocial dimensions of medical practice and the whole realm of values and choice which remain outside the concepts of medicine as science.

Szumowski, who traced the history of medical philosophy in Europe, is the least critical, and proposes a very broad definition as follows:

> The philosophy of medicine is a science which considers medicine as a whole; it studies its position in humanity, society, the state, and the medical school; it embraces at a glance the totality of the history of medicine; it sets forth the most general problems of philosophy and biology; it analyzes the methodological forms of medical thought, mentioning and explaining the logical errors committed in medicine; it borrows from psychology and metaphysics the knowledges and ideas of moment to the whole of medicine; it touches on medical praxiology; it discusses the principle values in medicine; it formulates the principles of ethics and medical deontology; finally, it discusses aesthetics in medicine.[43]

None of these views is really adequate. Shaffer ignores too much, Szumowski embraces too much, and Toulmin occupies a halfway house which on further analysis must go either with Shaffer or accept philosophy of medicine as a discipline, though not necessarily in the diffuseness of Szumowski's definition. Toulmin is right that the first stop is to distinguish medicine from science. Then we must show what specific philosophic issues are contained within medicine which are susceptible to comprehension by no discipline other than philosophy.

In recent times philosophy has examined many special disciplines for their meaning and essence, their modes of explanation, the metaphysical assumptions upon which they are based, and the possibility of some unifying theory of the realities they encompass. Thus the logical, epistemological, and metaphysical examinations of what historians, lawyers, or scientists do, and the meaning of what they study, comprise the philosophy of history, law, or science. One can ask the same questions about philosophy itself—the philosophy *of* philosophy. Indeed this has been a preoccupation of some of our major thinkers, like Ortega y Gasset,[44] Heidegger,[45] Merleau-Ponty,[46] and Husserl.[47]

Special difficulties do arise when we consider adding the philosophy of medicine to this list. Medicine does, in fact, derive much of its method, logic, and theory from the physical and biological sciences, and so it is to a certain extent a branch of those sciences. But medicine is also a praxis in the Aristotelian sense—knowledge applied for human ends and purposes. In this sense, medicine can be classed among the technologies. But medicine also sets out to modify the behavior of individuals and societies and thus has roots in the behavioral sciences. Finally, medicine operates through a personal, and therefore an ethical, relationship intended to "help" the person to "better" health. It is a value-laden activity, with roots in ethics and the humanities.

At first glance, it would seem that Shaffer's position is correct—medicine is totally derivative. It has no distinctive subject matter, and its "philosophy" is therefore nothing but the sum total of the philosophies of biology, mind, and moral science. But is this so? Let us see if we can distinguish medicine from science first and then from the social sciences and the humanities. Only then can we speak properly of a philosophy of medicine.

Medicine is in part a truly scientific endeavor. It shares with chemistry and physics the aim of understanding physical processes. Medicine as science studies man by observation, mensuration, hypothesis formulation, and experiment under controlled conditions. In studying *man* as *object* it follows the canons of good science—proper experimental design, validity of observation and method, correct logic, and verifiable conclusions. This surely is the content of the basic sciences of medicine, even though they pursue these ends in the most complicated of biological systems. Granting that the "special field of life," as Toulmin suggests, imparts special features to the laws of chemistry and physics, the basic sciences of medicine could indeed be subsumed under the philosophy of biology.[48]

But the basic sciences are not sufficient by themselves to constitute medicine either as clinical science or medical practice. As clinical science, medicine must study the human entity in which purpose, values, consciousness, reflection, and self-determination complicate the laws of chemistry and physics even more than do the special microenvironments of living things in general. Medicine, even as science, must encompass the special complexities of *man as subject* interacting with *man as object* of science. Physiology, unlike the clinical science of medicine, studies physical processes while ignoring the lived reality of the experimental subject—his or her self-perceived history, uniqueness, and individuality. Thus even when it functions as clinical science, medicine must correlate the explanatory modes of the physical sciences with those of the social and behavioral.

But neither the basic sciences nor the clinical sciences can be properly considered as medicine until they are used in a particular purpose to effect the attainment of health. The purpose of medicine *qua* medicine, then, transcends that of medical science per se, which is primarily to know. Medical science, basic or clinical, becomes medicine only when it is used to promote health and healing; that is to say, only when it is an intervention into an individual human life to alter the human condition. Medicine thus construed has a telos which distinguishes it from its component sciences, whose telos is to understand physical processes in as general a way as possible and certainly not to particularize that knowledge in an individual human life. For medicine *qua* medicine cannot deal with general scientific laws as such but must place them in a time, place, and person.

Medicine is, in short, a practical theory of human reality. It is a moral activity, since it operates through an interrelationship of persons in which physician and patient are coparticipants in defining the goal and achieving the goal—cure of illness or promotion of health. The patient is not a passive object to which a technique is applied, since the patient seeks help on what he "ought" to do and modifies his behavior in conformity with the physician's advice. This dimension of the "ought" impinges directly on the person and his values. It involves two persons interacting, each in his own sociohistorical moment. The intersection of their values together with those of medicine, science, and of society create a nexus of choices and priorities. It is the unraveling of that nexus for this patient, here and now, that constitutes medicine. The resultant synthesis is more than the sum total of the component sciences—physical, social, and moral—which contribute to that unraveling.

This synthesis, moreover, is constrained by the fiduciary responsibility which imposes itself on the physician by the very nature of the contract between him and the patient. He is *presumed* to help and not to harm and to advocate the "good" of the patient at all times. The patient presents himself in a state of wounded humanity. He has lost some of his freedom since he must come to the physician; he must give consent when he is in pain and discomfort, and he does so in the presence of an information gap which can never be closed fully. Medical science, therefore, becomes medicine only when it is modulated and constrained in unique ways by the humanity of the physician and patient. Its telos takes it out of the realm of *téoria* and puts it into the realm of *praxis.*

It is the totality of this unique combination which constitutes the clinical moment and the clinical encounter, without which authentic medicine does not exist. No simplistic neo-Cartesian reduction of medicine to sciences of mind, arithmetically added to sciences of the body and tied together with a ribbon of moral science, is adequate to explain this synthesis. Nor is this merely biology. Neither plants nor animals—granting that they become ill as well as humans—can enter into a relationship with the healer in which the patient participates as subject and object simultaneously. Plants and animals can be simply the objects of applied scientific knowledge, and in that sense botanical and veterinary medicine are simply applied biology.

Medicine might be considered in one sense a technology, since its purpose is the application of knowledge to meet specific human needs. But technology cannot be the same as medicine, since the way technology is used is determined by the clinical encounter as we have outlined it above and not by technology itself. Technology, like the sciences, becomes part of a larger synthesis when it is used within medicine. The further question of "usefulness for what" is beyond both medicine and technology and resides in philosophy, as Jonas points out.[49]

We have thus far said nothing of medicine as art. Here, too, medicine has an autonomy very much like that of music, for example. Music depends upon physics, acoustics, and mathematics. But it operates with an autonomy which results in an entity called "music," which is not completely definable in terms of its derivatives.

The same kinds of distinctions can be made between medicine and the social sciences and humanities, upon which it also depends. Medicine differs from psychology because it works on and through the body to affect health, while psychology works through the senses only to affect the psyche—as does religion to affect the spirit.

Medicine differs from the humanities, which also deal with values and human existence. But they do not do so with the direct purpose of affecting health or curing illness through manipulation of the body. The philosophy of medicine, therefore, is not congruent with the philosophy of the humanities any more than it is with the philosophy of sciences.

Finally, we must add the social dimensions of medicine as medicine—the applications of medical knowledge on an aggregate of humans rather than an individual. This "social encounter" is a parallel of the clinical encounter with an individual patient. Without taking the time to carry out a parallel analysis, it is clear that scientific knowledge can also be used to improve the health of the community. Here medicine is concerned with values, choices, and priorities which relate to the "good" of society. Such issues as the distribution of health services, the purposes for which medicine is used and for whom, who decides the aims and upon what principles services are based would constitute the elements of a social philosophy of medicine.

Medicine, then, is an activity whose essence appears to lie in the clinical event which demands that scientific and other knowledge be particularized in the lived reality of a particular human, for the purpose of attaining health or curing illness, through the direct manipulation of the body, and in a value-laden decision matrix. It is in this sense that medical theory is a theory of practical reality and not just the theory of the sciences which contribute to it.

Up to this point, I have tried to distinguish between three levels of meaning of the term "medicine": (a) the basic sciences component, which seeks to understand physical processes in a living being, healthy or ill; (b) the clinical sciences component, which seeks to understand physical processes in a perceiving subject in whom mind and body are united; and (c) medicine per se, or medical praxis, in which the clinical and basic sciences are particularized in the clinical moment or encounter, with all the complexities outlined above. In medicine *qua* medicine the sciences are not only means of understanding but means to intervention in the lives of persons or societies.

Thus I would agree, with Shaffer, that the basic science portions of medicine are derivative and that their philosophy is the philosophy of biology or the sciences. Clinical sciences, however, attempt to understand a larger totality which includes the entities of mind and psyche. The contemporary Cartesian would consider even clinical science to be completely derived from physical sciences and psychology and its philosophy to be some combination of the philosophies of biology and psychology. My preference is to see clinical science as a level of synthesis which cannot be encompassed by biology and psychology, so its philosophy would be philosophy of clinical science. Finally, medicine as medicine (i.e., medical practice as we have outlined it in the clinical encounter) could not be totally congruent with either basic or clinical sciences, and hence the philosophy of medicine could not be congruent with the philosophy of biology, plus the philosophy of mind, plus moral science.

I might summarize my line of reasoning in Aristotelian terms in this way: the *final* cause of all disciplines, scientific and otherwise, is understanding. The *final* cause of the physical and biological sciences is understanding of man in the human context, and of the social sciences man in the social context. The distinguishing *final* cause of medicine is the understanding of physiological processes in a human being who is a part of the human context and who exists in a social milieu—particularly as his being is modified in health and disease. The *efficient* cause of all the disciplines is "to know," and in this medicine is not unique. The *material* cause of medicine is the body of the individual or the "body" politic. The *formal* cause of medicine—its unique feature which is not shared with other disciplines—is the clinical encounter, operationally delineated above.

Medicine clearly is a domain of activity which is distinctive and distinguishable as science, art, and praxis. It comprises a set of legitimate philosophical issues and questions which derive from the unique nature of the clinical encounter. This is the singular ordering concept which distinguishes medicine from the sciences and which is the ground for the logic, the epistemology, and the metaphysics of medical practice. It cannot be reduced to the philosophy of science, mind, and morals, as Shaffer proposes; nor is it so all embracing, as Szumowki's definition would have it. By failing to place emphasis on the clinical moment, Szumowki's definition would include everything about medicine—not only its philosophy, but its sociology, economics, politics, education, and aesthetics. In his definition, both philosophy and medicine are too loosely used.

PHILOSOPHY AND THE MODES OF ENGAGEMENT WITH MEDICINE

The philosophy of medicine must emphasize genuinely philosophical questions, and these must be defined with care. These are the questions not answerable by medicine itself or by any of the other scientific or humanistic disciplines which enter into it. It is important, therefore, to elaborate somewhat the sense in which the term "philosophy" is used here. The term has been particularly misused by medical writers, as Temkin's observations about even so revered a figure as William Osler make clear.[50] Osler's *Way of Life* is an example of a large number of works of opinion and belief written by eminent physicians about medicine which are commendable but which have been too gratuitously termed "philosophy."[51]

The nonphilosopher cannot presume to enter into the question "what is philosophy," which has engaged almost every major modern philosopher. Nor would I exalt one mode of philosophizing above the others as most suitable to the specific issues raised in medicine. The number and variety of problems are sufficient to challenge the whole range of philosophical methods. Some problems are best approached phenomenologically, others analytically, and others speculatively. This is not to sanction an undiscriminating collage of philosophical notions or some mysterious process of intellectual *épluchage.* However, in the nascent state of the inquiry a pluralistic methodology has certain advantages. The precise nature of the questions may be more clearly revealed by divergent modes of inquiry—particularly if they eventuate in similar formulations.

There is little room for an autocratic notion of philosophy sitting in judgment above the special disciplines. This tendency is too easily manifest in dealing with medicine, whose immersion in the practical may range from the sublime to the sordid.

There is already something of a backlash among medical people as a consequence of misunderstanding the intent of some philosophers who have ventured into the troublous arena of bioethics.[52]

What is needed is a systematic set of ways of articulating, clarifying, defining, and addressing the philosophical issues in medicine. The philosopher can contribute by his capacity for critical discussion of the physician's thought and action and by dialectical dissection of the presumptions behind them. The aim is the same as in philosophizing about any human activity: to grasp something of its reality, of the value of the things which comprise it, and of the nature of man as it is revealed in the medical act, the clinical encounter. It is the act of philosophizing on the whole domain of the clinical moment that is essential, not the particular mode of that philosophizing.

There are three distinct ways by which philosophy can engage medicine. I have devoted most attention to one of them—the philosophy *of* medicine—because it is the most problematic and also the most in need of delineation. There are two others—philosophy *in* medicine, and philosophy *and* medicine. They can be distinguished by the ways in which medicine and philosophy address each other and the types of issues with which they deal.

These distinctions are a modification of the distinction my colleague Robert Straus has made between sociology *in*, and *of*, medicine.[53] He did not make a third distinction, sociology *and* medicine, which I shall add in the case of philosophy.

Philosophy *and* medicine comprises the mutual considerations by medicine and philosophy of problems common to both, or problems which exist in medicine but are not limited to the special rubric of the philosophy of medicine as we have outlined it above. Here, the effort is collaborative. Medicine and philosophy retain their identities. Each draws on the resources of the other, is enriched, and elaborates some new medical or philosophical concept of its own. Some of the recurrent problems of philosophy—the mind-body debate; the meanings of perception, consciousness, language; the special or nonspecial character of chemical and physical laws in living things—are susceptible to this type of collaborative attack. The findings of neuropathology, neurosurgery, the physiology and pharmacology of the nervous system are essential, for example, to any serious deliberation on the philosophy of mind or psyche. Out of the interaction of medicine *and* philosophy may come part of a synthesis of the constellation of interpretations which now constitute the idea or image of man. A true philosophical anthropology must start in the full range of observations medicine makes of individual men in health, in illness, and facing death. It cannot end there, of course.

Philosophy *in* medicine refers to the application of the traditional tools of philosophy—critical reflection, dialectical reasoning, uncovering of value and purpose, or asking first-order questions—to some medically defined problem. The problems can range from the logic of medical thought to the epistemology of medical science as science, the problem of causality, the limitations of observation and experiment, and of course, the whole range of vexing issues in the active field of biomedical ethics. These are problems which medicine shares with other sciences, professions, and technologies. The philosopher serves an invaluable function *in* medicine; that is to say, in the medical setting as educator and trained thinker exhibiting the way philosophy can illuminate and examine critically what physicians do in their everyday activity.

This is a common form of interaction in the United States, especially on those medical campuses and hospitals which have formal programs in medical ethics. Philosophers in these medical settings are making significant contributions without necessarily addressing the question of the theory of medicine as medicine. Most of the problems of the basic clinical sciences as sciences can fall under this rubric.

When philosophy turns to the meaning of medicine as clinical practice and examines its conceptual foundations, its ideologies, its ethos, and the philosophical bases for medical ethics, then it becomes the philosophy *of* medicine. The questions examined by philosophy *in* medicine are then carried to the unique realm of the clinical encounter with a human being experiencing health, illness, neurosis, or psychosis, in a setting which involves intervention into his existence. The questions then transcend the philosophy of science per se and grapple with the meaning of medicine, its nature, concepts, purposes, and value to society—what can be called the philosophical problem of medicine. The philosophy of medicine seeks explanations for what medicine *is* and *ought* to be, in terms of the axiomatic assumptions upon which it is based. This is the realm of the transmedical meaning of medicine, the realm which neither medicine nor any other science can explore itself. "And yet, there is another side in every science which that science as such can never reach: the essential nature and origin of its sphere, the essence and essential origin of the manner of knowing which it cultivates… ."[54]

These three types of engagement are rarely separable in actual fact, and philosophers can, and do, engage in all three. We have dissected them free to underscore the central importance of the philosophy of medicine: the philosophical issues imbedded in the theory of medicine as a practical human activity. Ultimately, the more proximate issues dealt with by philosophy *and* medicine, and philosophy *in* medicine, must rest on the philosophy *of* medicine.

SOME URGENT PHILOSOPHICAL ISSUES ARISING IN MEDICINE

Whatever mode or level of philosophizing one chooses, there is a series of interesting and genuine philosophical problems arising in contemporary medicine. I will choose only a few to illustrate some of the points I have been making thus far.

First, there is a set of questions which medicine shares with the philosophy of science—such as the analysis and meaning of medical language and explanation, the verifiability criteria of medical theories, the notion of causality, the logic of discovery and experimental design, and the limitations of statistical and stoichastic analyses. These questions are modulated in medicine, since they must be examined in reflecting, conscious subjects in the clinical context. Some mode of explanation must be found which overcomes the pretensions of reductionism and vitalism. How, if at all, is the scientific enterprise to be modified in medicine?

There is another set of questions, not usually part of the philosophy of science, which demands philosophic inspection. These relate to the unique existence of humans as a unity of mind and body. The meanings of the phenomena of embodiment and corporeality and their perception by the subject have a deep impact on medical theory and practice. Both Cartesian dualism and monistic materialism are glaringly deficient in satisfactory explanations of these phenomena. Still, no alternative to these polarities is at hand. Resolution of the deficiency is fundamental to any theoretical development of medicine.

To what extent are the methods and modes of explanation of sociology, psychology, and philosophy valid in grappling with the realities of man's existence as a thinking being? Is intelligence, for example, reducible to engineering concepts and totally simulable as artificial intelligence by the computer? Or, as Dreyfus suggests, are the metaphysical assumptions upon which such an assertion rests, in error?[55] Medicine and philosophy should be able to reinforce each other in dealing with such issues. Philosophy is still far from drawing fully on the large base of neurophysiologic, neuropsychiatric, and neuroendocrinologic data medicine has collected; medicine has yet to appreciate the insights metaphysical or phenomenological analysis can contribute to the interpretation and intelligibility of these data. This conjunction should help to reconcile the scientific with the commonsense images of man.

This reconciliation is a most important step in the persistent search for a philosophical grasp of the idea of man. Philosophical anthropology is still a diffuse exercise of quite recent origins. The "image of man" is fractured and in need of restoration, as Scheler,[56] Cassirer,[57] and Buber[58] have told us. There is a growing need to weave together the numerous separate strands of information about human existence (Stent, an unusually philosophical biologist, has sketched the limitations of both the positivist and structuralist formulations of man).[59] Difficult as the effort may be, such a scientific-philosophic synthesis is fundamental, and prior, to the choices we must make about human life, death, health, and disease. There must be some idea of man to order our definition of what is "good" for the person and society and for the optimal relationships between them. Individual and social bioethics both derive from this context of our idea of man.

Intimately related to the philosophical conception of man are the definitions of health and disease, of cure and of disability. The presuppositions physicians hold about these conceptions shape medical theory and practice. Since health is the end and purpose of medical knowledge, the clearer definition we can give to that term, the more order and priority we can give to our uses of medical knowledge. The intersection of human, societal, and historical values which characterizes the medical encounter can only be dealt with rationally if both physician and patient understand each other's presuppositions about the purposes and perfection of human existence.

The idea of man underlies a whole set of humanistic issues which arise out of the technological potencies of modern medicine. Matters formerly the concern of the speculative and imaginative intelligence are now technological realities. For example, medicine can prolong or terminate life, control conception and fertility, elevate our moods, or blunt our pain and anxieties. To apply these measures is to challenge traditional meanings of the value and dignity of individual life, of the family, of suffering and dying, or of individual versus social good. The ancient metaphysical question of what is "the good" has resurfaced with an unprecedented urgency. We cannot use medicine for the attainment of health or "the good life" unless we clarify these conceptions in the light of our technological possibilities.[60]

The philosophical foundations of contemporary biomedical and professional ethics also derive from the ideas of man, the person, and the balance which should obtain between the life of man as an individual and as a member of society. Samuel Gorovitz has sketched out a very complete topography of the philosophical issues at the heart of medical ethics. He underscores the urgent need for a closer examination of the assumptions about the primarily philosophical questions which underlie medical decisions and calls for their examination by philosophers. In fact, Gorovitz puts the matter squarely in terms of social responsibility: "That science exists in the final analysis, for the pleasure and for the benefit of society, is a point to which philosophers generally accede reality. What is perhaps less often noted by them is that philosophy, too, is a social enterprise supported in the final analysis by the public, to whose interest it accrues."[61]

But what value system should we use in addressing these humanistic questions? Do we follow the ideology of modern science, which has influenced so many medical men today? Bronowski and Holton have ennobled the community of science, and the pursuit of science is an ethic of unique proportions in itself. Bronowski praises the value system of science—the capacity to tolerate dissent, to foster freedom and independence of thought.[62] Holton holds that the scientist has no choice but to pursue creativity and new knowledge, even if we have not the means at hand to cope with the challenges to human values created by the scientist's activity.[63]

Hans Jonas, on the other hand, calls for an ethic of limit, prudence, and restraint to balance the ethics of endless progress.[64] The more a technique has the possibility for modifying human life, the less free is the scientist to pursue it without some restraint. This is the direct contradiction to the freedom which the ethics of science holds as a fundamental requisite: "The demand of each discipline to choose its own problems and fit them to its own concepts and techniques and instruments, suggests that science is not eager to undertake to solve the problems of society, as society would define them."[65]

The ethos, as well as the ethics, of science and medicine demands critical examination. How do we reconcile the image medicine has developed of itself and the concept society holds of its functions? The ideology of science has taken firm hold in medicine. But can medicine provide answers to the questions it creates using only the method of science? Medicine must be reintegrated with all the humanities, as I have argued elsewhere.[66] Isolation of technique from purpose poses an antinomy whose perpetuation can only confuse, and possibly subvert, the humane use of medicine.

The process of modernization is associated with bureaucratization and technology, which have become values in themselves. They are prime shapers of the cognitive style of our culture and of modern medicine. They are part of what Foucault calls our *epistemé*—the aggregate of history of a human endeavor which enables it to occupy a specific space in a given culture.[67] Has the *epistemé* of medicine arising from its own bureaucratization already determined what society seeks from medicine and created a self-reinforcing cycle carrying man ever further from what is distinctly human? Will this distorted "view" contribute further to man's philosophical infirmity?[68]

These are some of the questions which might constitute the content of the philosophy of medicine as a formal intellectual endeavor. This topography is necessarily incomplete. What it illustrates is that there are several sets of truly philosophical questions which medicine can neither pose clearly nor discuss critically if it relies only on its own modes of inquiry. These questions are susceptible to deeper exploration by the methods of ancient and modern philosophy. The choice of any particular set of questions and the emphasis placed on them will depend upon the philosopher's own conception of his subject and of the act of philosophizing.

WHAT THE PHILOSOPHY OF MEDICINE OUGHT NOT TO BE

Several dangers lie at the surface in any effort to use the critical and speculative intellect on the matter of medicine. Risse and Galdston, as noted above, both have shown how medical theory, when not securely based in the data of experimental science, can become a vast speculative enterprise which inhibits the growth of medical science. These authors use the example of the German physicians of the eighteenth century who hoped for "ultimate" causes of life, health, and disease. The resulting conflict between those physicians who sought truth in speculative constructs and those who sought it at the bedside was a vigorous one, felt even today. The deleterious effects of thus making medicine into philosophy have been only too evident in the history of medicine. The greatest disservice to modern medicine would be done by a resurgence of that error today. Medicine should not become bad philosophy, or philosophy bad medicine.

MacIntyre recently warned against the unrealistic expectation the public and physicians might have of philosophy.[69] The philosopher, and the particularly the ethicist in medicine, cannot hope to provide ready answers or formulae for all the moral problems of modern medicine; nor can ethicists be society's only monitors over the actions of health professionals. Some medical people are too eager to delegate moral guidelines to philosophers or ethicists, while others would resist even the asking of ethical questions by those outside medicine.

Philosophers cannot, on the other hand, avoid their responsibility as "delegated intellects." They must not, however, compromise the integrity of their discipline or be lured by sudden prominence and attention to indulge in pontifications beyond the limits of the method they master. Philosophers are as susceptible as others to the temptation of all intellectuals to see their special mode of inquiry as the universal way to truth. One way to balance this tendency is to place philosophers in medicine in the company of other humanists. Historians, theologians, and specialists in literature are also entering the medical setting. Their interaction with philosophers may be salubrious for all.

Nor should the philosophy of medicine become *medical* philosophy; that is to say, the musings, ruminations, and meditations of physicians on the state of medicine, the professions, health, or other related matters. These intuitions serve a hortatory, interpretive, and inspirational purpose, important in education and practice. They might become a matter for the pondering of the philosophy of medicine, but they must not be confused with the philosophy of medicine.

The philosophy of medicine should also not become a quest or crusade for *the* philosophy—some unified theory for all medicine which would explain all human, biological phenomena. We seek rather to emphasize the continual examination of the crucial philosophic questions which arise in the substance of medicine, not a final system of medicine which will put an end to all questioning. We can conceive of a philosophy of medicine—some theoretical construct put forth tentatively to be tested against experience on the one hand and dialectical reasoning on the other. A philosophy of medicine as a set of propositions *about* medicine is valid only as hypothesis is valid in experimental science.

The philosopher contemplating medicine must be careful to avoid the twin seductions of overly serene detachment on the one side and total submersion in medicine on the other. He should remember the unfortunate plight of some social scientists who have lost their identity in the medical setting, losing credibility as social scientists and contributing little to the medical milieu. The philosopher will be helpful to medicine and advance his own discipline only if he remains a bona fide philosopher

SOME EDUCATIONAL IMPLICATIONS

If there is any cogency in this explication of the necessity and nature of the philosophy of medicine, then its nurture becomes of concern to educators and practitioners as well as scholars. Wartofsky's recent analysis of the impact of human ontology in shaping the concept of disease, and thus of medical practice, illustrates clearly how important the seemingly academic considerations of the philosophy of medicine can be in the practical world.[70]

The questions subsumed under the three forms of engagement of medicine with philosophy outlined here will have varying degrees of immediacy for physicians and other health workers. Practitioners need, most of all, to develop some capacity for critical examination of their own value systems and their concepts of man. Teachers of medicine will require a deeper understanding of theological and epistemological questions in medical science and clinical practice. Those who make public policy decisions will require a better grasp of the social ethics of medicine. The medical scholar will want to probe the more ontological and metaphysical issues.

It would be palpably unwise to attempt to make every physician a philosopher, in Galen's or Plato's sense. But every physician, since he is involved with values, concepts, and ideas of medicine, must have some philosophical *sense.* It does seem reasonable to expose every student to critical discussion of the issues outlined here, particularly those relating to medical and professional ethics. Medical schools are becoming more cognizant of the centrality of issues of human values in medical practice. Approximately twenty schools have developed programs to integrate ethics, philosophy, and the humanities into professional education.[71] Similar efforts have been initiated to involve the practicing physician as well.

A minimal aim for all students in the health professions should be to sensitize them to the reality and meaning of their personal value presuppositions so they can understand more clearly the basis of their own daily decisions and recommendations. Some exposure to the rigor of philosophical inquiry may possibly balance some of the antiphilosophic bias of medical education. For those students who wish to probe more deeply, opportunities for extended study, research, or a career in the problems at the interface of medicine and philosophy may help to expand the number of physicians able to take responsibility as educated men in the consideration of how medicine shall be used to advance human purposes.

What is needed is the cultivation of the humanities and philosophy in the medical and health-care setting with something like the vigor we dedicate to the basic sciences. Indeed, for the greater number of practitioners the utility and importance of humane studies equals that of the clinical and basic sciences. Charles Fried has shown how philosophical, legal, and economic values and principles overlap in practical decision making—not only in human experimentation, but in person health care and in the social ethics of medicine.[72] Few physicians who wish to be more than technicians can ignore the philosophic bases of these practical, daily choices so integral to their authenticity as professionals.

SUMMARY

The congruence between medicine and philosophy which we find in the *Protagoras* and the *Treatise on Ancient Medicine* as well as the tensions symbolized in the dialectic between Eryximachus and Diotima will always be with us. The congruence and the divergence of these ancient disciplines are both important to human well-being. By opposing one another, medicine and philosophy can each balance the other's pretension to universality. By converging, they illumine some of the most important questions of human existence.

This essay has examined ways in which medicine and philosophy can converge in our times as philosophy *and* medicine, philosophy *in* medicine, and philosophy *of* medicine. The present moment in our intellectual history is particularly propitious for the nurture of the engagement of medicine and philosophy. The most fruitful form of that interaction may be in the philosophy *of* medicine, which is a definable discipline with a set of issues specific to it. If the obvious intellectual dangers can be avoided, those who practice medicine, those who think about it, and those who are served by it can gain deeper insight into the nature and the purpose of medicine as well as the nature of the profession and of man himself.

Perhaps—positioned as it is, at the intersection of the sciences, the humanities, and technology—medicine can become "…a medium and the focus in which the problems of wisdom and science meet."[73]

CHAPTER FOUR

THE GOALS AND ENDS OF MEDICINE: How Are They to be Defined?

Medicine today is in an unprecedented state of confusion about its identity, about its role and the role of physicians in contemporary society. Philosophers and judicial opinions are disassembling the Hippocratic Oath and ethic; medical care has become a commodity translated as a business and organized as an industry; insurance companies see in medicine an investment opportunity; scientists and engineers see it as the subject of technical prestidigitation.

All of this puts patients and physicians in a quandary. Is the physician still a helper, healer, and caregiver? Or are physicians something else—gatekeepers, guardians of society's resources and employees, "managed" by gag rules and restrictive clauses, or entrepreneurs and co-investors in the commerce of health care? There may be legitimacy in some of these roles but not in all of them. If there is legitimacy, how are conflicts among them to be resolved? What priority should be given to each?

There are the questions society and the profession must face. To answer them requires the reformulation, or at least the reassessment of medicine's ends, purposes, and goals. This reassessment is the challenge Daniel Callahan has so clearly and precisely set before us in his project on the goals and priorities of medicine. It is a timely, inescapable challenge. How we respond will determine not only what physicians will be, but what will happen to the care of sick people.

In this essay I want to reexamine one issue with which the project had to grapple at the outset, namely, how are ends, goals, and purposes to be derived, justified, and placed in some order of priority? What is determinative in selecting or rejecting goals and purposes? Is it something *internal* to medicine itself, something inherent in its nature as a particular kind of human activity? Or are the goals of medicine set *externally* by some form of social construction, relative to the values of culture, place, or time in history? Should medicine be continuously redefined and reformulated, or are there elements that do not, and should not change?

After careful deliberation, the report concludes that both approaches have merit, and that a certain tension between them is healthy, provided only that neither perspective is absorbed by the other. I believe this conclusion merits some reexamination for three reasons: First, it may not do full justice to the depth of logical opposition between the two modes of goals derivation; second, it does not distinguish between goals, purposes, and ends; and, third, it leaves unanswered the questions of priorities: (a) between and among conflicting goals; and (b) between the two modes of goal derivation when they are in conflict. Some further clarity on these points seems requisite in preparation for the fuller discussions that the Hastings Center project is sure to stimulate in the years immediately ahead.

My aim is to compare and contrast what I prefer to call an "essentialist" with a socially constructed method of setting goals. My emphasis is on how goals are defined, not on the goal or ends themselves. This comparison is more than simply an exercise of methodology for its own sake. It is central to the enterprise the Hastings Center wants us to undertake. Before we can balance one goal or purpose against another, we need a way to justify one choice over another, and to place our choices in a priority order. Given the urgency and complexity of the problem, it is of practical importance to examine the presuppositions on which any solution is to be based. A middle-ground approach that places too much faith in Hegelian dialectic seems likely to end up in a synthesis which conflates internal and external ends and purposes in just the way the Hastings Center project wants to avoid.

I will develop this thesis in three stages: First, by comparing and contrasting the essentialist and socially constructed modes of determining goals and purposes; second, by defining the ends of medicine and their priority order *internally*, that is, in terms of the essential nature of medicine as a special kind of human activity; and third, by relating the ends of medicine internally construed to the societal purposes and goals to which medicine and physicians may be put.

ENDS AND GOALS: ESSENTIALIST VS. CONSTRUCTIONIST DEFINITIONS

The Essentialist Definition: Ends before Goals

The essentialist approach is grounded in the nature of medicine, in what sets it apart from other activities as an enterprise of a special kind, and defines it as something in the real world independent of the construction society might put upon that reality. This approach is based in a real definition, a grasp of some extramental reality from which we abstract that which makes a thing what it is and separates it from all those other characteristics it possesses: its so-called accidents, or that which is not crucial to what a thing is.

Before defining the content of this essentialist approach, it is important to take note of the strong objections leveled against any essentialist position today.

First, many contemporary thinkers accept Wittgenstein's rejection of real definitions as imaginary or impossible. For Wittgenstein any congruence between the real world and the language we use to describe it is merely a matter of grammatical articulation. As he puts it, "Essence is expressed as grammar."[1] "Grammar tells what kind of object anything is."[2] On this view, Aristotle's definition of a thing by its essence, and all of Socrates' "What is…" questions, are illusory. They cannot get at real world essences.[3]

Second, if real definitions are not possible, we cannot define ends or goals intrinsic to medicine. We can only define goals by deciding the uses to which we want to put medicine. By defining the goals we choose we can define what medicine is. On this instrumentalist view the ends of medicine can only be a project for social construction, generated by what we want to achieve socially, politically, economically, and legally. Theoretically we could "construct" medicine in such a way as to divert it totally, or in part, from its dedication to the care of the sick, or we could add to it, any function we might wish like gatekeeping or assisting in state-ordered executions, or involuntary or nonvoluntary euthanasia.

A third objection is that an essentialist definition puts arbitrary limits on the goals of medicine. Goals, it is argued, could be independent of traditional goals of healing, curing, caring, and helping individual patients. On a socially constructed model, the limits of medicine can be expanded or contracted by societal fiat. Thus, the majority opinions of both the Second and the Ninth Circuit Court include physician assistance in suicide as part of the practice of medicine.[4,5] This inclusion is a sociolegal construction of practice. If the opinions are upheld by the Supreme Court, assisted suicide may be offered to patients as the "standard" of practice. Or a patient or a society could stretch the limits of medicine to include provision of whatever treatment a society might want even if it is scientifically futile or even harmful to individual patients.

A final objection, which any attempt to derive essences must confront, is the problem of separating what to include in the "essence" from what to leave out. On the view I shall present, this determination is not arbitrary; that is, what is essential is derivable from the phenomena of medicine itself, from the concrete realities of the physician-patient relationship, or from what healing, helping, caring, and curing entail a point—I will develop in more detail later in this essay.

Here is not the place to engage in an epistemological and metaphysical rebuttal of the objections against essentialism. It suffices for my present purposes simply to compare and contrast the logical consequences of essentialism and social construction since the question is which one should have primacy in determining the ends and goals of medicine.

Social Construction: Goals before Ends

An influential approach today in the definition of reality and morals is through social construction. The foundation of this approach so far as goal setting goes is that there is little likelihood of agreement on such things as essences, definitions, or ethical norms. In consequences, there can be no universalizable ends of purposes.[6] Rather, these must be defined by each community in terms of its own values and perceptions of reality.[7] On this view, reality itself, knowledge, and nature are social constructs. Medicine becomes primarily a social endeavor since its concepts of disease, illness, healing, and health are all socially defined. Social construction comes in many forms as varied as the social reality of Schutz's everyday world, and Marxian praxis.[8,9] Social constructions have in common an emphasis on subjectivity, intersubjectivity, process, dialogue, and consensus as the sources of social realities like morality, medicine, and social good.

In any case, the term "social construction" as used in the Goals of Medicine project report is not taken in this strictly formal philosophical sense. One therefore need not engage its full epistemic or ontological implications. Rather, social constructionist is used in the project report to apply to a process definition of the goals of medicine, arrived at by social dialogue, consensus formation, political process, or negotiation. It is in this latter, more general sense, that I will take the term when comparing it with the essentialist viewpoint.

This is not the place to discuss the various forms of social construction. But there are certain conceptual difficulties common to social construction in general. I will confine myself to the difficulty they present to defining the goals of medicine.

First of all, to accept social constructionism is to accept that there is ultimately nothing permanent or universalizable about medicine. If so, its goals can be defined only in an ephemeral manner. They will change with each new construction and have no permanence. The whole project of goal setting is perilous as a result. If we are continually redefining medicine and its goals, how far beyond the present social moment can we look in confronting the issues the project report so well identifies?

The second difficulty with constructed models is that they conflate the meanings of ends, goals, and purposes and use these terms interchangeably. In the social construction models, goals can stand for whatever political, economic, physician, citizen, or other groups determine them to be. On this view, the ends are simply the uses to which medical knowledge or physicians can be put. It is in this sense that many use the term "goals" when they speak of reshaping the goals of medicine.

Ends are not the same as goals. Ends in the classical sense of the *telos* are tied to the nature of medicine, to its essence. Ends serve to define medicine. Without certain ends, the activity in question does not qualify as medicine. The ends of medicine distinguish it from other arts and sciences that have different ends. To convert the ends of medicine to the purposes of economics, politics, or professional prerogative, transforms medicine into economics, politics, or professional preference.

Medical science for example can be used to advance the ends of medicine, but medical science is not per se medicine. It becomes medicine only when it is used to advance the ends of medicine, that is, only in the clinical encounter, with the needs of a particular patient. Medical knowledge per se has uses other than cure, care, help, or healing of the sick. It can be used to cure animals, or manipulate their genes, synthesize new organic molecules, attain economic goals or political advantage, and so on. Only when medical knowledge is focused on the healing of *this* patient, here and now, or on promoting the health of society as a whole is it medicine per se.

Goals and purposes, unlike ends, are not formally tied to the essence of medicine. They may conform to the ends of medicine, but they may not. The goals and purposes to which we put medical knowledge or activity may even destroy medicine or frustrate its proper ends. The list of possible distortions of the healing purposes of medicine is a long one: torturing political prisoners, genocide, "cleansing" society of the unfit or handicapped, participating in state ordered executions, making political converts, punishing political dissidents, or managing medical care for nonmedical purposes such as profit or political power. Goals and purposes are therefore unrestrained by the specific ends intrinsic to what medicine is. They are subject to many social interpretations, some quite inimical to the ends of medicine.

Socially constructed goals—as long as they have social sanction—open medicine to possible subversion by economics, politics, social ideology, or government and this openness is an ever present threat to the integrity of medicine as a practice. The ends internal to medicine are the compass points by which goals and purposes can be measured. Ends provide the mooring for medical ethics. The enormous extent of medicine's technical power is vulnerable to the pathological use a disordered society may wish to make of it unless it is restrained by the ends proper to medicine.

Finally, which community of values shall determine the goals of medicine? We all belong to many communities—family, neighbor, school, church, profession, political party, and social group—and the values of these overlapping communities may conflict with each other. Which shall have primacy when this occurs? How do we decide to choose one community's values over another? Is there such a thing as a good society and good medicine? If so, then we are back at a dilemma: either we strive for an essentialist definition of the good society and good medicine, or we submit to constant revision of the ends of both medicine and society.

An Essentialist Construction: Ends over Goals

On the essentialist view, the ends of medicine are defined internally out of the nature of medicine itself. They grow out of the phenomenology of medicine, that is, out of that which is more fundamental than medicine itself—the universal human experience of illness. It is the universality of this experience, its existence beyond time, place, history, or culture—and the need of sick persons for care, cure, help, and healing—that gives medicine its essential character. These ends make medicine what it is. On this view, the ends of medicine are the same for Hippocrates among the Ancient Greeks, the Maimonides in the Middle Ages, Sydenham in the eighteenth century, Osler in the nineteenth century, and for the nameless physicians who will take care of those who are ill on the first spaceship to penetrate intergalactic space.

Several things are notable about this way of defining the ends of medicine. First, it depends on a real not a nominal definition of medicine, one which describes something in the real world, not just a language game or simply the way we use the word "medicine." Second, the ends of medicine are built into the reality of medicine as a special kind of human activity. Third, the limits of medicine are also built into its ends. When those ends are not longer achievable—when treatment is not effective or beneficial, or when cure cannot be achieved—care and helping become primary ends.

These are the ends of medicine, and they are as old as medicine itself. They define medicine. They are its essence. From the beginning they had to be defined to answer those who denied that medicine existed as a separate endeavor, or that it qualified as an art. For example, the Hippocratic authors had to make clear that medicine was distinct from both religion and philosophy, that it was "invented" to care for the sick and had its own practitioners to achieve this end.

> Let us consider also whether the acknowledged art of medicine, that was discovered for the treatment of the sick, and has both a name and artists has the same object as the other art and what its origin was. In my opinion, as I said at the beginning, nobody would have even sought for medicine if the same ways of life had suited both the sick and those in health.[10]

Elsewhere the Hippocratic author(s) provide a more specific definition of the ends of medicine, noting its limitations as well.

> First I will define what I conceive medicine to be. In general terms, it is to do away with the suffering of the sick, to lessen the violence of their diseases, and to refuse to treat those who are overmastered by their diseases realizing that in such cases medicine is powerless.[11]

Later on, in the same treatise, the Hippocratic author places limits on what the patient may expect from medicine, and insists that it ought not be used when it is futile, that is, when its ends cannot be attained.

> Whenever, therefore, a man suffers from an ill which is too strong for the means at the disposal of medicine, he surely must not even expect that it can be overcome by medicine.[12]

But even if a case is not medically curable, the patient is not abandoned. Other ends than cure are recognized as ends for medicine.

> Why forsooth trouble one's mind about cases which have become incurable? This is far from the right attitude. The investigation of these matters too belongs to the same science; it is impossible to separate them from one another. In incurable cases we must contrive ways to prevent their becoming incurable...while one must study incurable cases so as to avoid doing harm by useless efforts.[13]

In later centuries the ends of medicine were spelled out a little differently but in fidelity to the Hippocratic definition with emphasis on the phenomena of healing and helping. Here is one example.

> It is the duty of the doctor in the first place to cure us; in the second to be kind to us; in the third to be true to us; in the fourth to keep our secrets; in the fifth to warn us and best of all to forewarn us; in the sixth to be grateful to us; and in the last to keep his time and his temper.[14]

Objection may be made at this point that the ancient texts do not speak of prevention specifically as one of the ends of medicine. This is true, but it does not mean that prevention was not recognized or respected as an end of medicine. Indeed, in the Hippocratic era, the culture of health was closely tied to the whole idea of education.[15] Gymnastics, diet, hygiene were critical for the Hippocratic physicians and intrinsic to the education of citizens of the Greek state. Prevention was thus the concern not only of medicine but of a good life of body and mind.

Clearly we have in these ancient sources intrinsic definitions of the ends that set medicine apart as a certain kind of human activity. At the same time, we are introduced to the limits of medicine—to the now much discussed notion of futility—to those times when medicine ought not be used since its ends are no longer attainable. But even then, care and help were recognized as ends intrinsic to the art of medicine.

I would expand the derivation of the ends of medicine by an extension of these concise definitions of the Hippocratic writers. Like them, we must assert the obvious: medicine exists because humans become sick. It is an activity conceived to attain the overall end of coping with the individual and social experience of disordered health. Its end is to heal, help, care and cure, to prevent illness, and cultivate health. Medicine itself is a true art because it pursues its ends with knowledge and understanding for the good of its object—the sick person or social group—and in a practical way.[16]

In its everyday clinical practice, the ends of medicine are technically right and morally good decisions and actions made by, and with, the person who is ill. Both the technical and moral good are essential to the craft of medicine if it is to achieve its ends of healing, helping, caring, and curing.[17] It may achieve those ends by a variety of means, but those means are always constrained by the ends.

On this view physicians do not determine the ends of medicine; it is their task to realize these ends in a specific clinical encounter with a particular patient. Physicians are charged with ascertaining, together with the patient, the content of the end of healing. Note, the content of healing is not a social construction of the end but it accepts healing as an end. It is healing which is specific to this patient, not healing as an end. For this healing, technical knowledge is essential, but not sufficient. That knowledge must also be applied within the context of the patient's notion of health and well-being. Thus, medicine could not be defined solely as knowledge-based, but as knowledge, based and directed to a specific end—knowledge directed by an architectonic principle—healing or helping a sick person become whole again.

This forum is not the place to expand on the details of the nature of the healing relationship. Thomasma and I have done so in extenso elsewhere.[18] Here I wish only to note that the ends of medicine are related to the reasons humans established medicine—that is, as a response to a universal and common experience of illness.

It is this healing end of medicine in the context of patient vulnerability that determines not only the technical practice of clinical medicine but also the ethic of medicine. The physician offers to help, professes to have the needed craft and to use that craft in the interests of the person confronting the experience of illness. The ends of medicine thus define the moral obligations, the virtues, duties, and principles that constitute medical ethics. This role is their justification, not the fact that doctors have constructed ethical codes or that society has mandated legal regulation of the profession. Clinical medicine, preventive medicine, nursing, public health, and social and community medicine each have ends arising out of specific health needs. These too are derivable from the phenomena with which they deal. By analogy with our analysis of the ends of clinical medicine, each health profession is shaped by a specific set of ends that set it apart and give it a needed role in the larger spectrum of "health care."

This line of reasoning does not assume that defining the ends of medicine as intrinsic to medicine necessitates that physicians are the arbiters of those ends. In the essentialist view, physicians themselves are bound by the ends internal to medicine as a specific kind of human activity. They can make, have made, are making, and will make errors in defining those ends. If the ends of medicine are derived from a critical examination of the nature of medicine, I argue, these errors can only be identified and corrected by reference to the inherent ends of medical action which are in turn derived from the phenomenon of healing.

But if physicians have no epistemological sovereignty in defining the ends of medicine, neither do economists, politicians, policymakers, or ordinary citizens. What all of us must do is determine how to use medical knowledge and skill to bring the goals and purposes we assign to medicine into conformity with its intrinsic ends. It is the telos or goal of the medical craft that provides the ethical restraint in the way medicine is used. No social mechanism, regal fiat, legislative, or professional decree should be immune to the test of congruence with the ends internal to medicine as a special kind of human activity.

Whenever medicine is used for any purpose or goal—however defined—that distorts, frustrates, or impairs its capacity to achieve its proper ends, it loses its integrity as a craft and its moral status as a human activity. This consequence is true whether the distortion is generated by physicians, economics, politics, or exigency of any kind.

We have socially crucial reasons for maintaining the internally defined ends of medicine. Without ends, there is no source of criticism, no counter to the most malevolent uses of the power of medical knowledge and skill by individuals, societies, or governments. To the extent that they are genuinely faithful to the ends of medicine. Physicians must set limits on what they will do in the name of medicine no matter what the social construction of medicine may demand of them. They must know when to say "no." This refusal is what the Nazi and Soviet physicians failed to muster. It is their infamy—not to have resisted a malevolent social construction of medicine.

Economics, politics, cultural and social values, and mores are important. But they are not sovereign. They are subject to restraint, criticism, and even refusal when they seriously impair the ends of medicine. Once we accept a socially constructed external definition of those ends, we eradicate these restraints at the peril of the sick and of society itself.

Relating Inherent Ends and External Goals

Medicine does not exist in isolation from societal policy and constructs. Nor is it self-justifying. It must, as the Hastings Center report suggests, be in dialogue and dialectic with the society it serves. As the report properly concludes, the socially constructed and essentialist models will always be in tension with each other. But that tension can be productive without necessarily agreeing that the two models are equal when it comes to setting the goals of medicine. The ends of medicine are ontologically related to what medicine is. To open them to social constructionist interpretation is to compromise the integrity of medicine as the kind of human activity it is.

Purposes and goals of medicine, however, are more malleable. They are open to societal construction and may be altered in different times, places, and cultures. What is essential is that as medicine, they are subject to judgment by the *ends* of medicine. This distinction is not trivia. It means that proposed public policies regarding medicine must ultimately return to the ends of medicine. Societal policy must not frustrate the ends of medicine—healing, helping, curing, caring, and cultivating health—but rather enhance those ends.

If these distinctions are kept clear, a valid relationship can be established between the ends of medicine essentially defined, and the purposes and goals that society may wish to attain through medicine. These relationships can be illustrated by examining the levels at which physicians can function:

When serving the ends of medicine as medicine, the physician's focus must be his covenant with the patient. The physician is then bound by a covenant of trust which must not be compromised by other roles of, for example, the physician as gatekeeper, entrepreneur, guardian of social resources, or by the economic pressure to undertreat. Unnecessary treatment is by definition morally prohibited. The welfare of the patient, jointly determined between physician and patient or patient's morally valid surrogate must continue to be the end of medicine in the clinical encounter and first in the order of priorities for the physician's role.

At a second level, physicians are members of a moral community. They have a collective role of advocacy, to stand for the welfare of all sick persons when social policy threatens that welfare. To do so successfully, physicians must protect the ends of medicine by giving collective support to those ends when they are threatened. The sources of threat are many and varied: unfettered fee-for-service, for-profit medicine, gag rules, financial incentives that pit the physician's self-interest against the patients, making the physician a participant in state ordered executions, interrogation of prisoners, torture even in time of war, or placing the physician in positions of conflict of interest in forensic psychiatry, or renal institutional medicine. Less obvious but equally demanding are the collective obligations of the profession to advocate just distribution of physicians, health care resources, and facilities. A role of advocacy in distributive justice is a collective moral obligation of physicians.

These are all areas in which a social construction of the physician's role can distort and frustrate the intrinsic ends of medicine, destroying the integrity of medicine and the protection it affords those whom physicians attend. The profession as a whole has been insufficiently responsive to these distortions of the ends of medicine. All too often it has responded in terms of self-interest rather than the interests of those for whom medicine was "invented," as the Hippocratic authors put it. The community of physicians has often failed to use its moral power to bring aberrant social policies into conformity with what the ends of medicine should be.

A third way physicians can play a role of societal responsibility is as technical experts and as scientists. If social policy is to be rational, if choices are to be made on evidence, then policymakers require reliable data about diseases, treatments, and procedures. Here a social construction of the physician role is legitimate. It serves the ends of medicine as well so long as manipulation of data for some political, economic, or commercial purpose is precluded. This caveat, of course, applies as well to medical research which is an obligation of the profession but which must not be subverted to political purposes.

Finally, physicians participate as individual citizens in the social construction of goals and purposes. Some of these goals may be consistent with the ends of medicine and others may not. As a citizen, not as a physician bound to the welfare of a particular patient, physicians may sponsor or vote for a variety of forms of practice, financing, and distributing care in accordance with their personal, political, and social philosophies. But, even here, as citizens with a special knowledge of medicine, there is some restriction on the kind of social philosophy they might espouse. Some social ideologies like the totalitarian, or the laissez faire free market approach are inconsistent with the ends of medicine. A physician could not be authentically a physician if he tolerated a dichotomy in his life which espoused the ethical ends of medicine when caring for patients, and tolerated political incursions into the integrity of medicine in his public life.

In the end, as Daniel Callahan has so well pointed out, the choices we make in the way we distribute our societal resources are reflective of our values as a society.[19,20] These values will shape whatever social construction of the goals of medicine we may elaborate. Societies do reveal their deepest values—that is, the kinds of people they are and want to be—by the way they treat the sick, the aged, and the poor. Preserving the ends of medicine, and not just the goals society may construct for medicine, is an essential safeguard not simply for the integrity of medical ethics and practice, but for the safety and well-being of all the vulnerable members of society.

In preparing his challenging report, Callahan has served us well. He has taken seriously "the philosopher's privilege… to render the taken for granted the object of critical reflection."[21] He has laid out an agenda to which we must address ourselves as health professionals, policymakers, and as the patients or potential patients we all are or will be.

CHAPTER FIVE

THE RELATIONSHIP OF THEORY AND PRAXIS IN THE PHILOSOPHY AND ETHICS OF MEDICINE*

INTRODUCTION

In the last decade or so, at least in America, clinical bioethics has developed as a sub-branch of the larger field of biomedical ethics. Clinical bioethics is presumed to focus on the concrete, particular decisions which must be made daily "at the bedside" in the practice of medicine, nursing, and the other health professions. It is distinguished by its practical orientation and its urgency because clinicians must *make decisions.* There is no possibility of abstaining from moral choice in the clinical arena. These choices are ubiquitous: they affect the welfare of patients. They are complicated by the multiplicity of moral agents who may participate—physicians, nurses, other health workers, patients, their families, institutions, and organizations.

Clinical bioethics and the resolution of ethical conflicts and dilemmas are intrinsic to the clinician's role. For this reason, clinicians have an obligation to develop knowledge and skills in ethical analysis, both for the benefit of their patients and for the preservation of their own moral integrity. The skills of moral analysis, therefore, are as

* A revised version of E.D. Pellegrino, *Praxis as a Keystone for the Philosophy and Ethics of Medicine: The Need for an Arch-Support: Some Comments on Toulmin and Wartofsky*, in R.A. Carson - C.R. Burns (eds.) *A Twenty-Year Retrospective and Critical Appraisal*, Kluwer Academic Publishers, Dordrecht 1997 (Philosophy and Medicine Series, 50), pp. 69-84.

essential to the clinician as the skills of the arts of medicine—i.e., history-taking, physical examination, evaluation of laboratory data, prognostication, and therapeutics.

The theoretical substructures of clinical biomedical ethics are in the earliest stages of development. Three views are currently expressed. (1) Some see clinical bioethics as simply the application of ethical theory of particular cases using standard, pre-existing ethical theory as the source for principles, duties, rules, etc. (2) Others see clinical bioethics as a field with special qualities in which concrete details, cases, and practices interact with, and influence, ethical theory in a mutually supportive and reciprocal way. (3) A third view, advanced most recently, is that clinical ethics gives life to ethics, provides an antidote to abstract theories and principles, and, indeed, provides the normative foundation, in itself, for the ethics of medicine, eliminating the need for foundational theories.

As clinical bioethics emerges, the key philosophical is the proper relationship between theoria and praxis, and it is to this question that I wish to direct my remarks in this essay.

Praxis and Ethics in Medicine

Medical ethics embraces at least two broad categories of moral questions. One has to do with the conduct of the healing relationship, with the obligations of physicians-*qua*-physicians in their relationships with those who seek their help. This is the realm of the ethics of medicine as a practice or *techne* with specific goals and purposes which define it as a certain kind of human activity.

There is, however, another entire realm of much more profound questions which must be decided in the course of medical praxis, problems of greater profundity than praxis per se can ever encompass. This is the realm of ethics *in* medicine. I refer, here, to the whole vexing range of "bioethical" and "biomedical" ethical issues from abortion, euthanasia, embryo research and eugenically motivated genetics, to care of the environment, allocation of scarce resources, and the corporate responsibilities of managed care organizations. Those questions are beyond medical praxis as such, even though physicians play a role in their implementation. Here, we must wrestle with ultimately metaphysical questions—the nature and moral status of persons, fetuses, brain-damaged humans, or higher primates. We cannot expect to find answers to these questions by a contemplation of practices.

As Burleigh shows, the "practice" of physicians before and during the Holocaust was inspired by the belief that everything was relative, including codes of medical ethics, and that there were lives unworthy of life which were owed a merciful death.[1] A pragmatist with a utilitarian end-point might project the consequences of acts of genocide and infanticide using the ethical methodology of James or Dewey and be convinced these were the right things to do. Dewey and James, and most pragmatists, would certainly shrink from such an atrocious distortion of their methodology. But without metaphysical foundations, it is difficult to avoid such distortion. The same holds for such utility-driven possibilities as the use of humans in permanent vegetative states, rather than healthy primates, for experimental purposes.[2]

One need not succumb to the temptations of Descartes' kind of Foundationalism to argue for the necessity of certain universal, metaphysically-based concepts like the dignity of each human person, or the inalienable right to freedom and to life. To be sure, the critical examination of these issues must also be based in concrete reality, but the examination must also transcend the particular and the concrete to get at the more general moral truths without which everything eventually becomes relative.

Proponents of pragmatism, of course, object that metaphysics has no place in medical ethics, that metaphysical differences do not necessarily result in different ways of acting in practical moral situations.[3] Parkin refutes this view by showing that ethical theories and metaphysical presuppositions are relevant and inescapable.[4] Indeed, for the second category of medical-ethical issues mentioned above, if ethics is to be at all philosophical, it cannot avoid confrontation with concepts, arguments, justifications, principles, and values as well as the notions of person, life, death, etc.

This type of foundationalism is compatible with a respect for, and engagement with, practices and particularities. None of this implies acceptance of Cartesian foundationalism. There is a place for the "philosophic turn" in all practices. Amelie Oksenberg Rorty suggests, for example, that philosophers should enter all aspects of institutions and public affairs (government, corporations, and schools of education, medicine, and law).[5] Rorty hopes philosophers engaged in such institutions and practices can help to determine how the epistemological and metaphysical alternatives would affect those institutions and practices. Rorty wants philosophy to engage practices because understanding the "foundational" problems of practices might help to resolve them.

Praxis and the Ethics and Philosophy of Medicine

The only way out of the circularity of an ethic with its origin and terminus in praxis is to resort to some criterion other than the criterion of praxis itself. For medical ethics at least, the way out of this circularity is to ground medical ethics in a philosophy *of* medicine, one which begins with medical praxis but looks for understanding of what medicine *is*, that is to say, what sets it apart as the specific kind of human activity it manifestly is. This would be a philosophy *of* medicine in the classical sense of that term.[6-9]

The great post-Cartesian, Hippocratic physicians of the seventeenth and eighteenth centuries, Thomas Sydenham (1624-1689), Giorgio Baglivi (1668-1706), and Herman Beorhaave (1668-1738), all recognized the failure of Descartes' attempt to deduce the whole of medicine from universal truths. They called for an end to speculation about disease just as the Hippocratic authors had done. In its place, they insisted on reliance on observation and experience subjected to reason.[10]

They did not repudiate theory entirely. In fact, they adhered to a theory of medical praxis, one based in the inductive science of Bacon and the experimental method of Galileo. They took Aristotle's *Posterior Analytics* for granted as the method of reason to be applied to careful observation so as to make medicine a verifiable, and not a speculative, activity. Their theory of medicine was the direct antithesis of the prevalent Galenic philosophy. Like Descartes, Galen proposed to ground medicine firmly in philosophical premises.[11,12] In a sense, the Galenists and Hippocratics were re-debating the same issues the Hippocratic treatise *Ancient Medicine* was presumed to have settled centuries before.[13]

Both the Galenists and Hippocratics, however, were in agreement in the ethics of medicine. They saw no need to link a philosophy *of* medicine with the central moral reality of medical praxis, i.e., the physician-patient relationship. They were agreed on the viability and validity of the Hippocratic, patient-centered ethos. This is decidedly not the case for our time. The Hippocratic Oath had been reinterpreted, altered, even repudiated, and each of its precepts, dismantled.[14]

In many ways, the Hippocratic ethic, like philosophy, has sustained the same kind of deconstruction and anti-foundationalist attack as philosophy. The task of medical ethics, today, is to rebuild something from the shards of a shattered ancient tradition. I do not think that praxis itself can provide the requisite building material or the grouting that can hold it all together.

Ethics based solely in practices suffers certain disabilities, i.e., over-emphasis on methodology, conflation of scientific method and philosophic reflection, and circular reasoning since both the origin and terminus of ethics are located in the practices themselves. It is impossible to avoid self-justification which is just as dangerous in praxis-based ethics as it is in principle or rule-based ethics. Any recourse to theory beyond praxis as a way out of the dilemmas is precluded by the current fascination with the anti-foundationalist credo.

A limited set of choices seems available: (1) abandonment of any universally binding precepts of professional ethics in favor of whatever precepts are institutionalized at any historical moment or place; (2) replacement of professional ethics by positive law removing any claim to the integrity of professional ethics; or (3) a reconstruction of medical ethics out of some 'foundation' (small 'f') other than praxis per se.

The last option is the most viable. To be successful, it will have to begin in the realities of praxis. But it cannot end there. It must also be grounded in a philosophy of medicine, one which also starts with the realities of praxis but seeks to discern from those realities what makes medicine the kind of activity it is, and what obligations follow from those realities for physicians, patients, and society.

Thomasma and I have pursued the linkages between a philosophy of medicine and its ethics in a series of works.[15,16,17] In that effort, we believe we are following the Aristotelian mode of thought, something which Toulmin also seeks to restore. Our philosophy of medicine, and hence the ethics we derive from it, is teleologically structured. It is derived *a posteriori* from the universal realities of the clinical encounter, i.e., healing, helping, caring, health. Toulmin seems to start where we start with the universality of the phenomenon of illness when he speaks of the fact that broken bones, bleeding, pneumonia, etc., and their treatments are "for clinical medicine and its moral practice the same in California, Central Africa, and Spain."[18] The "right" procedures are generalizable, Toulmin says, not because they are so *a priori*, but because clinical demands and equity transcend cultural and societal differences.

Toulmin raises the possibility of as *a posteriori* as against its *a priori* derivation in a rationalist schema. This is consistent with the "Aristotelian hunger for concreteness."[19] Aristotle's search also went beyond the concrete, beyond these aspects of the concrete that so fortuitous accidental. "....[T]hat there is no science of the accidental is obvious; for all science is either of that which is always, or of that which is for the most part. For how else is one to learn or teach another?"[20] We can only learn what "is for the most part" by examining the concrete realities of whatever world we are interested in. In the case of medicine, this is the world of the clinical encounter.

Medicine is not theory-free. As Plato, and Aristotle after him, repeatedly asserted, medicine is a *techne.* It is knowledge realized only when put into practice. It is a practice based not just on experience (the realm of the empiricist), but on understanding of the real nature of its object, (a capacity of explain its procedures and serve the good of its object.) A *téchne* needs general rules and fixed knowledge. It differs from theory in always being linked to concrete practices. To the extent that there are generalizable rules for a *téchne,* it has a theory, but not a theory in the sense of *epistéme* or first philosophy.[21]

Those generalizable rules of a *téchne* provide the basis for an ethic of medicine because they define the conditions without which the ends of medicine cannot be achieved. In this way, the ethics of medicine connects with the concreteness of the ends of the clinical encounter. These ends in turn spell out the ethical obligations internal to the practice of medicine. Thus, a theory of medicine links the *téchne* of medicine with the practice and ethics of medicine in a continuous mutual and reciprocal relationship. This is a foundation (small "f") without the disabilities of *a priori* Cartesian Foundationalism. I share Toulmin's skepticism about "grand" theories in medicine but I would not exclude theory as a foundation (small "f") for medical practice and ethics.

Given that there are rules to a praxis or *téchne,* these do not constitute a complete moral *epistéme.*[22] No rule can encompass all the particularities and concrete details under which moral actions are taken. Nor, on the other hand, is a knowledge of the particulars sufficient. It is the task of practical reason, of *phrónesis* to link the proper rule to the particular action.

But *phrónesi*s not the same as praxis. *Phrónesis* is a virtue possessed by the *phrónimos,* the person of practical wisdom who through character and experience can judge "with an eye *to* the occasion"—to what is the precise fit between rule and particular action. The practitioner is not automatically the *phrónimos.* He or she may lack the virtue of *phrónimos* or fail to develop the moral experience and character necessary to make right and good judgements. After all, there are "good" and "bad" practitioners, technically and morally.

But the *phrónimos* cannot exercise the virtue of *phrónesis* without rules and principles which he or she fits to the occasion of moral action. Without rules or norms, the practitioner becomes the norm, and herein lies the danger of the hegemony of praxis without general rules. Incomplete though such rules may be, as moral *epistéme,* they are essential to moral praxis.

Thus, medical ethics, like ethics more generally, will need a proper balance of norms and principles, of *phrónesis* with praxis, of moral theory with application to particular moral acts and agents. Toulmin is right to assert the importance of praxis which is surely Aristotelian in spirit but he seems to slight theory which also had its significant place in Aristotle's ethics and metaphysics. A medical ethic faithful to the Aristotelian mode of reasoning would aim at proper ordering of the relationship between theoria and praxis and general and particular moral *epistéme.* Here, theory would not have merely the instrumental function it has been allocated in modern science.[23] In its purest form, theory is knowledge for its own sake, abstracted from things. As Aristotelian "first philosophy," it is "… the active possession of thought as thought."[24] Again, to grant this is not to succumb to Cartesian rationalism but to return to the Aristotelian mode of philosophy, which ranges from experience to art to wisdom—each level with its own kind of knowledge and degree of abstraction.[25]

In the long run, we cannot escape the "desire to know," as Aristotle put it, and that desire will not be satisfied without a reach for ultimacy, a reach to attain "...knowledge about certain principles and causes of thing,"[26] to know "the first principles and causes of things." This was the aim of philosophy for Aristotle as it was for Plato. Whereas Plato grounded his thinking in eternal forms, Aristotle sought to extract the knowledge of the ultimate from the immediate, the real and the practical in ethics, metaphysics, rhetoric, biology, and especially, medicine. Praxis and theory come together in a human effort to know in the fullest sense of that term.

Medicine is Aristotle's "paradigm" case. Aristotle emphasizes that the physician treats individuals not "man." If a person has a theory without a grounding experience and recognizes the universal but does not know the individual included in it, that person will often fail to cure, for it is the *individual* that is to be cured.[27]

Aristotle and Plato agree that the highest life would be the life of pure *theoria.* Both recognized- Aristotle more convincingly than Plato- that human beings are not gods and that the best life for humans is one which combine *theoría* and praxis.[28] A life (and medicine) based in Cartesian *theoría* is unrealistic and unbalanced. The current turn to praxis—to action and doing in medicine—is welcome and needs to be heeded in medicine, ethics, and philosophy.

In the emerging field of clinical bioethics, we need a proper balance between theory and practice. For this, medicine occupies the special place of a *téchne* between empiricism, on the one hand, and speculation, on the other. Medicine is a *téchne*—a practice, grounded in experience, guided by rules and by a knowledge of what *is*, what ought to be done, the way it ought to be done, and the reasons for which it should be done in that way. In these realities lie the substance of a genuine philosophy and ethics of medicine. For Aristotle, medicine, like ethics, is a science of the practical, and that is its special point of view.[29] It is a point of view most pertinent for clinical bioethics as it emerges in bedside decisions.

CHAPTER SIX

BEING ILL AND BEING HEALED:
Some Reflections on the Grounding of Medical Morality

Medicine is a special moral enterprise because it is grounded in a special personal relationship—between one who is ill and another who professes to heal. Illness is an altered state of existence arising out of an ontological assault on the humanity of the person who is ill. Healing is a mutual act that aims to repair the defects created by the experience of illness. The moral authenticity of the healing act is thus measured by the fullness with which it remediates the afflicted state that illness represents. Medical morality therefore is grounded in a philosophical conception of the healing transaction.

THE EXPERIENCE OF ILLNESS

For technological man illness is a more insistently painful experience than it was for his ancestors. It penetrates the freneticism of his work and pleasures to remind him that immortality is still an illusion. For each disease that science extirpates, a new one takes its place—like some perverse hydra—to remind us of the ultimate fragility of our existence. Because we have conquered so many diseases, it is more difficult than ever to accept the disease that attacks us now. The experience of illness is far more terrifying, far more disabling—more of an absurdity—to modern man than it ever was for his less technologically capable ancestors.

For the man of faith, illness can have transcendental meaning and justification. But even the believer today imbibes the dominant ethos and is offended and shocked when he becomes ill. Why me? Why now? What did I do to deserve this? They may

Copyright 1982. "Being Ill and Being Healed: Some Reflections on the Grounding of Medical Morality". In: Victor Kestenbaum. *The Humanity of the Ill: Phenomenological Perspectives.* Knoxville, Tennessee: The University of Tennessee Press; 1982: pp. 157-166.

construe the experience of illness differently, but both believer and nonbeliever perceive illness as an assault on the person—a wounding of their very humanity.

Illness forces a change in existential states. It thrusts man into contact with the reality of the via dolorosa that all eventually must traverse. It is only in part defined medically as a concrete organic or psychosocial aberration. It is the perception of the change in existential states that forms the central experience of illness—the perception of impairment and the need to be made whole again—to be cured, healed, or cared for. That perception is personal and unique, since each person has a different meaning for health and illness.

We feel healthy when we are in a state of equilibrium between our already experienced shortcomings and our aspirations and thus have adjusted our goals to the gap between them. Health is a state of accommodation, defined in different terms by each person. Illness rudely upsets that equilibrium. It is an undesired, unsought, capricious irruption demanding a new equilibrium—one that may be drastically different. It may mean the loss of personal image, identity, or existence itself. The ill person becomes *homo patiens*—a patient—a person *bearing* a burden of distress, pain, or anxiety; a person set apart; a person wounded in specific ways.

The uniqueness of illness among human experiences is rooted in its ontological assault on the unity of the being of the one who is ill. One aspect of that assault is the rupture of the unity we ordinarily experience between self and body—facing the world and others and interacting with them as one being. Illness interposes the body—or the mind—between the self and reality or our perception of reality. The body is in pain, suffers a disability, or malfunction, that no longer makes it the willing instrument of the self. It impedes choices and actions: it is no longer the willing servant of transbodily purposes—work, amusement, pleasure. The body stands opposite to the self; it demands to be served—to take center stage. It stands in opposition to the self while still partially inseparable from self.

For the emotionally ill person the rupture of ontological unity may be subtler and deeper. The psyche or spirit is interposed as an impediment between the self and its intents and purposes as well as being interposed between self and body. The resultant fractures of the unity of the person are deeper and more complex. Of course, even in what is presumably "only" bodily illness, these oppositions of body, self, mind, and external world also occur to varying degrees. What is essential to our current concern is the fact that illness—whether bodily, emotional, or both, as is usually the case—attacks the fundamental unity of being associated with the state we perceive as health.

Further, illness erodes the images we have constructed over the years, often painfully, of ourselves and our world. That image is our personal effort to harmonize our deficiencies and our strong points. It is our personal definition of our situation in respect to others and the world, our unique relationship to work, play, or salvation. That image is laboriously fabricated and delicately balanced against the changing exigencies of life. It must be modulated subtly in almost every human encounter. Illness threatens this carefully wrought self-image. It forces a radical reappraisal; it opens up new, and relights old, anxieties.

No one has captured so well as Ortega y Gassett the fact that each of us is engaged in a personal project—to fashion a life of our own out of the circumstances in which we find ourselves.[1] Each person confronts the realities of his unique situation and humanizes it, attains his equilibrium with it. "In short the reabsorption of circumstances is the concrete destiny of man."[2] Illness moves us the other way—toward the absorption of man by circumstance. Healing is the attempt to find a new balance, to move back in the direction of our personal project.

These ontological crises must be confronted in a peculiarly vulnerable existential state. In illness we lose most of the freedoms we ordinarily associate with being able to act as a fully human person. Homo patiens is impeded in making rational and personal choices, since he does not understand what is wrong; how it can be cured, if at all; what the future holds; or whether the one who professes to heal can in fact do so. The ill person has not the knowledge or skills requisite for curing his own bodily or mental illness or to gain relief from his pain or anxiety. His freedom to act as a person is severely compromised. He may not even be free to reject medicine when he is the victim of overwhelming trauma, pain, shock, or coma.

Unless the person wishes to ignore his illness, or to rely wholly on his own healing powers, he must seek the help of another. The ill person is condemned to a relationship of inequality with the professed healer, for the healer professes to possess precisely what the patient lacks—the knowledge and power to heal. The healing relationship is thus inherently one of inequality which the patient enters in a special state of vulnerability and wounded humanity not shared by other states of human deprivation and vulnerability.

To be sure, the poor, the imprisoned, the lonely, and the rejected are also deprived of the full expression of their humanity, so much so, that men in these conditions may long for death to liberate them. But none save saints seeks illness as the road to liberation. In no other deprivation is the dissolution of the person so intimate that it impairs the capacity to deal with all other deprivations. The poor man can still hope for a change of fortune, the prisoner for a reprieve, the lonely for a friend. But the ill person remains impaired even when freed of these other constraints on the free exercise of his humanity.

Even when one is "cured" the experience of illness leaves its imprint. Body and self are never again quite so comfortably united, for the person who has been ill recognizes that at any time his body or mind may again come into opposition with the self. The proof of man's mortality is felt in the experience of illness in a way it can never be felt vicariously even in the illness and death of one we love.

Homo patiens is, therefore, man in an altered state: wounded, vulnerable, needing help, and afflicted with a special anguish that must be adequately ameliorated in a bona fide healing relationship with other human beings. It is this fact that defines the healing relationship—between homo patiens and those who profess to make him whole again. Genuine healing must be based on an authentic perception of the experience of illness in *this* person. It must aim at a repair of the particular assaults which illness makes on the humanity of the one who is ill.

OBLIGATIONS OF THE HEALER

It is the needs arising from the experience of illness in *this* person that provided the source of the professional morality of those who profess to heal. Their moral obligations are rooted in the phenomenology of illness, since the experience of illness gives rise to expectations in the one who is ill. These expectations become promises each time the professional presents himself or herself to the person who is ill and offers to help. The promise of help shapes the nature of every healing act and defines the requirements for successful healing—even when cure is not possible. To heal is "to make whole again" and that entails confronting and ameliorating the ways illness wounds the humanity of the one who is ill.

This is precisely what is promised, when the professed healer presents himself before the ailing person. He promises that he has authentic knowledge and skill—competence; that he will put them at the service of the patient, will act in the patient's best interest. This is the true meaning of the act of pro-fession—a promise made to man as homo patiens. This voluntary act on the part of the healer signifies willingness to make that promise authentic.

Patients and physicians seem to be at odds increasingly today about what constitutes authenticity in the healing relationship. Physicians often fail to comprehend what the patient understands by the promise of healing; patients often fail to understand what the physician thinks he is promising. Physicians seem to be moving toward a restricted sense of the promise, emphasizing technical competence, whereas patients seek technical competence plus compassionate help with the experience of illness as an assault on the person. This gap promises to widen as specialism increases and the demands of competence become more urgent. The wider it becomes the more remote is a genuine healing relationship grounded in the experience of illness. The stronger, too, will be the urge for patients to seek alternatives to the "medical model." The opposite danger—that of losing the benefits of scientific competence—then presents itself.

A balance between competence and compassion—interpreted here as the capacity to *feel* something of the experience of illness *with* the patient—must be struck. The promise implicit in the act of pro-fession, the promise of the healer, and the expectations the patient derives from the promise, can be aligned properly only if the assault of illness on the person of the patient is fully comprehended and ameliorated. I have suggested elsewhere that in contemporary medicine this alignment is possible only by the partition of the task between generalist and specialist.[3] But both the specialist and the generalist must comprehend—one within a narrow sphere, the other in a broader sphere—the requirements of a fully authentic healing relationship.

What are those requirements as they emerge from the experience of illness and the implied promise of the professed healer? Obviously, competence must be present or the relationship begins in a lie that damages it irreparably. Competence is a necessary but not sufficient condition, however. It must be shaped at every step by the purposes of the healing acts—by the good of the person who is ill—his bodily good, of course, but also his concept of health, his value system, and his sense of the kind and quality of life he thinks worthwhile.

The physician, therefore, has the obligation to protect the moral agency of the patient, to enhance it even in the face of the special vulnerabilities of being ill. The physician is obliged within the possibilities of the clinical situation, to assist the patient to recover as much as possible of the freedom he has lost by the fact of illness. The defect in knowledge about the illness—what is wrong; how serious it is; what can be done;

what should be done; what it costs in time, discomfort, money; what alternatives are available; the physician's own capability to treat this illness—these must be disclosed. The patient must be assisted, to the extent he wishes, to make conscious choices and thus to at as a human person rather than become the object of technical manipulation.

Closing the information gap is the essential first step in enhancing the patient's capacity to act as a human person in the healing relationship. It must aim at a morally valid consent—a mutual decision between patient and physician that one course or another should be followed. On this view consent is a feeling and knowing together what is to be done—it, too, is a moral obligation arising out of the special experience of illness. Only with morally valid consent can the patient's right to determine what shall happen to his body and what kind of life he wishes to live be safeguarded.

It is often objected that the patient may be harmed by knowing the nature of his illness when it is grave or life-threatening. There is little clinical evidence for such an assertion. But even if there were, it would not vitiate the greater obligation to respect the moral agency of the patient which, because it is in the moral order, transcends other considerations.

Only the patient, or his surrogate, may modify or release the physician from these obligations. If the patient prefers not to know or if he is too ill, too confused, or too ill-educated, he or his surrogate may ask that the physician decide the course of treatment. The physician then has a clear mandate to assume moral agency for the patient. But this obligation must not be assumed hurriedly to save time or trouble for the physician. The patient is owed a fair chance to decide the degree to which he cares to participate in his own healing.

None of this excuses the physician from saying what he feels is the right and good decision as long as he first fulfills the requirement to close the information gap. When the patient is very seriously ill or incompetent and cannot participate, or when no one is there to act as surrogate, the physician must do what he thinks best. Even then, his every effort must be to do what he thinks might be best for *this particular patient*, not what he would like for himself or his family were he in like condition.

When dealing with families and other surrogates, physicians have the extremely difficult task of ensuring that the surrogate is really acting in the best interest of the patient. The physician's promise is to the patient, not to the surrogate, the family, or the court. When the patient is fully competent, the physician cannot avoid his obligation to deal with the patient by "speaking to the family" about diagnosis or prognosis. The experience of illness is personal; it cannot be "felt" by someone else—even if that someone is a dearly loved member of one's own family. Only if the patient consciously delegates him to do so can the physician enter decision-making relationships with others.

General rules for the moral conduct of persuasion are virtually impossible to elaborate. Just where the line is crossed between justifiable persuasion and subtle coercion is a variable matter with each patient. The physician must strike the right balance for *this* patient between freedom that might be self-injurious and coercion that would impair a human decision. The physician must reflect on the existential and ontological nature of illness and his own healing acts if he is to sense when and to what degree persuasion is morally defensible. What counts most is his willingness to accept the moral obligation to allow the patient to make a choice. He need not be so neutral that he does not indicate what he considers the proper choice. To stand idly by when the patient makes a patently bad choice without some effort at persuasion is a form of abandonment. What must be guarded against is persuasion that becomes coercion because of the subtle slanting of evidence or incomplete disclosure or the substitution of the physician's values for the patient's.

A morally valid consent is the vehicle for the patient's expression of moral agency. Legal consent is a protection only against the grosser violations of consent. It cannot substitute for the degree of sensitivity to the patient's moral agency that a proper grounding of medical ethics ensures. It is precisely this preservation of moral agency in the face of the vulnerability of the agency in the experience of illness that constitutes the necessary grounding for professional ethics.

It is also to the proper grounding for the social ethics of medicine—the obligations of physicians to society, the obligations owed by institutions to those who are ill, and the obligations that bind collective decisions in health care.

THE SOCIAL ETHICS OF MEDICINE

There is growing pressure today for physicians to become instruments of social or even economic policy. In the larger sense this may mean a call to greater concern for equity in the distribution of services, for avoiding the horrors of nuclear war, or for halting the ravages of environments and occupational health hazards. In such matters the physician as citizen and expert in health has legitimate and essential roles to play which do not conflict with his healing obligations to individual patients.

Very significant conflicts occur, however, when physicians are asked to take social and economic consideration into account in their clinical decisions. They cannot appoint themselves as arbiters of whether the life of an incurable adult, a malformed infant, or a mentally defective child is socially useful or worthwhile. When he agrees to care for *this* patient the physician must have this patient's "good" in mind. As nearly as possible that good is to be equated with the patient's definition and not society's or the physician's. Only in being sensitive to the grounding of medical morality in the experience of illness and the promise he makes in the face of that experience can the physician respond morally to the conflicts between the good of his patient and the good of society.

Physicians who feel morally compelled to be instruments of social or economic policy and who thus wish to impose their personal evaluations of the quality of life on their patients must announce the fact in advance. In this way, the patient's consent will enable the physician to act as an agent of society as well as the patient's agent. To presume that this is so is to violate the moral agency of the ill person.

This is not to deny that considerations of cost, burdens on the family, and suffering of the patient are not important. In carefully defined circumstances—where it is clear that the patient is incurably ill, the death is imminent, and that the only thing keeping the patient alive is the physician's intervention—if the patient and/or the family or other surrogate participate fully, decisions can be made weighing factors of cost or expense and impact on family. But even here the decision is made in the interest of *this* patient and/or *this* family—those to whom the physician has made his promise—not society.

A hospital (or other health agency, such as an individual health professional) also makes a promise to those who are ill simply by presenting itself to the community. In doing so it declares it will place its resources at the service of those in need of them and that it will act for their "good." It becomes in some sense a moral agent interacting with another moral agent—the patient

The hospital, therefore, incurs the same obligations as the individual physician to take into account the ontological and experiential affliction that illness brings, to attend to the obligations arising from the inherent inequality of the healing relationship and to preserve the integrity of the moral agency of the person who is ill. This obligation binds the staff, administration, and board of trustees in different ways and to varying degrees, difficult as yet to delineate precisely.

The same can be said for the members of the many formal and informal patient care teams who collectively make clinical decisions about individual patients. Team members participate in a collective promise and each shares an obligation to make that promise authentic. The obligation binds different team members in differing degrees depending upon their closeness to the clinical decision and the authority they bear in the team. Elaboration of a theory of collective morality and its distribution among team members is one of the more urgent tasks in bioethics today.[4]

Governments and societies, too, if they claim to be humane, have obligations that arise from the nature of illness in human persons. Health may be placed lower than other human needs by social decisions when resources are limited. But the nature of the experience of illness, its universality, its unique assaults on the humanity of persons afflicted, and its essentiality for the enjoyment of all other human goods—all these impose special obligations on any government that presumes to call itself concerned or civilized or purports to "serve" its constituents

With the collective decisions of government the questions are far more complex and even less well examined than in the case of health care teams. Usually only the grossest aberrations of morality are noticed. Yet governments are moral agents in the collective sense, making promises and eliciting expectations as a result. Those who exercise the powers of government may advert to their legal obligations but rarely if at all to their moral obligations as part of a decision-making collectivity.

Being ill and being healed are so fundamentally grounded in the human condition that governments, too, must examine the moral obligations they incur when they promise to meet medical and health needs. They make an act of pro-fession just like the health worker, the health care team, or institution and must be held to stricter moral account than law or public opinion alone can guarantee.

RECAPITULATION

There are many more implications of the grounding of medical morality in the ontological and experiential phenomena of human illness and healing. I have attempted here only to establish that ground by emphasizing how profound phenomenologically is that transition from a state of healthy existence to one of illness. The fact of illness afflicts our humanity and diminishes it and renders us less able to function as moral agents and as human persons. Illness wounds, diminishes, and compromises our very humanity and places us in a uniquely vulnerable situation in relation to the professed healer. The relationship of healing is inherently one of inequality, vulnerability. The obligations of those who profess to heal directly—the health professionals—and those who profess to provide the conditions requisite for healing transactions—hospitals, teams, or governments—are grounded in the phenomenon of illness as it is experienced by human persons—and this is the philosophical source of professional morality.

CHAPTER SEVEN

THE HEALING RELATIONSHIP:
The Architectonics of Clinical Medicine

> *Thus the Art of Medicine rules and orders the Art of the chemist because health with which medicine is concerned is the end of all the medications prepared by the chemist. The arts that rule the others are called Architectonic, as being the ruling arts.*
>
> *Thomas Aquinas,* Summa Contra Gentiles, *Bk. 1, Ch. 1.*

INTRODUCTION

In his devastating novel of the destructive force of human passion, the Spanish philosopher-novelist, Miguel de Unamuno y Jugo, records this conversation between the painter, Abel Sanchez, and the doctor, Joaquin Monegro:

- The habit of giving titles to paintings is peculiar to the literati; something like the doctor's habit of giving names to diseases they can't cure.
- And whatever told you that the real purpose of medicine was to cure illnesses?
- What is it, then?
- Knowledge, a knowledge of disease. The end of all science is knowledge.
- I had thought it was knowledge to cure. What use otherwise of having tasted the fruits of good and evil, if not to free ourselves of the evil?
- And the end of art, what is that?
- That is its own end; it contains its purpose. It is an object of beauty and that's enough.[1]

In this brief exchange de Unamuno captures the central dilemma of modern medicine—What is it? What is it for? What knowledge does it need?

It is paradoxical, and frustrating, that after so many centuries we are still uncertain about what we mean by medicine, illness, and health.[2] Yet, all our debates about medical practice, education, and ethics still must center on the unsettled question of nature of medicine.

This is more than a trivial or contrived dilemma. What we think medicine is, determines what we think physicians ought to do, what they need to know, and what they should be taught. Each philosophy of medicine creates its own model of disease and health, of resource allocation and public policy. Most critically it also shapes the relationships of physicians to patients and society. It makes a real difference therefore what philosophy we espouse. Unless we are clear about what medicine *is*, we risk deceiving ourselves, our patients, and our society.

The resolution of the dilemma has never been more difficult or important. The capabilities of modern medicine, its frightening costs, its ethical challenges, and its influence on society and culture force us to grapple with the philosophical issues. That is why the philosophy of medicine has become an expanding and legitimate field of inquiry.[3*] A wide range of competing philosophies is being advanced and must somehow be sorted out. At one extreme is Donald Seldin's restrictionist view that medicine is applied biology[4]; at the other, the global pretensions of the WHO definition.[5] In between, we find a spectrum of definitions—the bio-psychosocial model, the holistic concept, and theories grounded in medicine's social and cultural context or in some *a priori* definition of health.[†] Each depends upon some partial truth about modern medicine. Medicine has indeed advanced prodigiously because of its marriage with science; it has learned to benefit patients by a knowledge of psychobiology and psychosociology; it has improved human existence immeasurably by its preventive and public health contributions; it is learning how familial, social, and cultural contexts are implicated in the genesis of illness and its treatment.

The problem is not the denial of these obvious truths but rather, how much should be included under the rubric of medicine? How much is the physician's responsibility? How much belongs to other professions, to individuals, and society? How do we delimit what properly should be counted as medicine? We know we must practice some economy in our pretensions. Yet, we must also afford the patient what he or she needs, to be cured, healed, or helped.

What competing philosophies of medicine are seeking is an architectonics—some ordering or organizing principle whereby the boundaries of medicine can be determined. They seek it in a variety of places and ways. Some regard medicine primarily as a body of knowledge and confine it within the perimeters of a predetermined set of disciplines. Others define medicine in terms of its end or purpose or some predetermined concept of health for which medicine is the means. Still others would define medicine as the negotiated outcome of the physician-patient relationship.

My purpose, in this essay, is to sort out some of these theories, examine their logical and epistemological difficulties, and place them in some orderly relationship with

* Two journals now deal solely with this subject, *The Journal of Medicine and Philosophy* and *Theoretical Medicine*, both published by D. Reidel, Dordrecht.

† This recent anthology collects a series of essays defining medicine, illness, health, and disease. The range of definitions past and present indicates how problematic these key concepts remain.[6]

each other. I will also propose an organizing principle derived from an empirical and phenomenological examination of medicine as a human activity of a special and unique kind. My thesis is that it is in the nature of the healing relationship that we will find what is unique about clinical medicine, what is its immediate end, and what will serve as its architectonic principle.

SOME THEORIES AND MODELS OF MEDICINE

Medicine as a Body of Knowledge

The commonest approach to a definition of medicine is to identify it with some body of knowledge useful in the treatment of illness. The dominant example of this genre is the so-called biomedical model, well articulated by Donald Seldin. Seldin defines medicine as biology applied to the cure and prevention of disease and the postponement of death. He specifically excludes social concerns, psychosocial elements, and bioethics as beyond the boundaries of the physician's knowledge base, though he does not deny their importance in society.[7] Seldin summarizes his view this way:

> Medicine is a discipline which subserves a narrow but vital arena. It cannot bring happiness, prescribe the good life, or legislate morality. But it can bring to bear an increasingly powerful conceptual and technical framework for the mitigation of that type of human suffering rooted in biomedical derangements.[8]

Seldin articulates clearly the dominant view of today's practitioners, teachers, and students. It has the virtue of limiting medicine to what it can do well, excluding what it does inadequately, and defining disease in terms of etiologies that are measurable and quantifiable. So attractive is the biomedical model that some investigations urge that it be the paradigm for psychopathology as well as somatic disease.[9]

The limitations of this model are several. For one thing, it is flagrantly reductionistic, limiting medicine to biology, chemistry, and physics. It suffers, therefore, from the logical and epistemological deficiencies of all reductionism.[10] It commits the error of circuitous reasoning—what we need for the proof is itself in need of proof by the settlement of the question we are asking. We cannot prove medicine is only biology unless we know first what medicine is—and that is the question.

The result is that the aims of medicine are determined by a preselected body of knowledge instead of medicine determining what knowledge it needs to achieve its ends. The error of reductionism is that it cannot logically exclude alternative reductions of medicine to applied sociology, psychology, or anthropology. Since these are admittedly elements of illness, why not assign them to the physicians and relegate the biological aspects to the biologists?

Even if we were to accept Seldin's reduction he does not tell us who is to provide the other kinds of knowledge needed to treat patients. How can those other dimensions be related to medicine? Who adjudicates the conflicts? Who decides what *should* be done for the patient? Since man is more than a biological being and his illness is more than biology, who manages the relationships between those different bodies of knowledge needed to heal? Seldin does not deny that human illness may rise in personal, familial, or social contexts or that they cannot be treated by biological means alone. What makes the patient "whole" again—since this is what healing means?

The most serious empirical limitation of the biomedical model is its one-dimensionality, its abnegation of the complexity of the experience of illness and therefore of the complexity of healing those who are ill. François Jacob, the molecular biologist, shows how limited this one dimensionality can become:

> The one-dimensional sequence of bases in the genes determines in some way the production of the two dimensional cell layers that fold in a precise way to produce the three dimensional tissues and organs that give the organism its shape, its properties, and, as Seymour Benzer puts it, its four dimensional behavior.[11]

Since disease and illness involve all four dimensions, it is hard to see how biology *qua* biology can be satisfactory as an explanatory principle to say nothing of a therapeutic one.

George Engel responds to the defects in the biomedical model by proposing one that includes biology as well as sociology and psychology and, he says, "will include the patient and his attributes as a person."[12] He (the doctor) must weigh the relative contributions of social and psychological as well as biological factors implicated in the patient's dysphoria and dysfunction as well as his decision to accept patienthood and with it the responsibility to cooperate in his own care. "It is the doctor's, not the patient's, responsibility to establish the nature of the problem and decide whether it is best handled in a medical framework." "Hence the physician's basic professional knowledge must span the social, psychological and biological for his decisions on behalf of the patient involve all three."[13]

Engel goes further and offers general systems theory as an explanatory model rather than biology. In this way, he proposes to resolve the controversies between reductionists and holists. Systems theory, he says rather expansively, should be the "...blueprint for research, a framework for teaching and a design for action in the real world of health care."[14] Having expanded the model of medicine he then confines it in a new mold - not of biology but of applied systems theory. The logical difficulties differ in degree but not in kind from Seldin's.

Engel's model has the virtue of including more of the realities of human illness, and vesting in the physician the task of fusing them in treating patients. It remedies some of the grosser deficiencies of the biomedical model but it still defines medicine in terms of a knowledge base, albeit a broader one. Indeed, so broad is this definition that it errs in the other direction, it leaves out very little. It would not take much analysis to stretch the biopsychosocial model to embrace almost as much as the much criticized WHO definition of health as complete physical, social, and emotional well-being.

Significantly, Engel does leave out one dimension—that is the spiritual, unless he includes it under the social and psychological. This is a dimension that the proponents of "holistic" medicine feel is also a part of medicine and healing.[15*] Since religion, or at least some stance with reference to the transcendental, is part of the fabric of human existence, what justifies its exclusion?

Engel's theory along with Seldin's and the others that define medicine in terms of a knowledge base always ends up begging the question: What is medicine? Is it only the disconnected sum total of the kinds of knowledge it uses? If so, why is one combination of disciplines more pertinent than any other? The question can only be answered by recourse to something more fundamental, in the nature of medicine itself, something which shapes what knowledge is needed and for what purpose. Engel, for a brief moment, touches this question when he refer to what patients are seeking in their encounter with the physician.[16] He quickly leaves it to expatiate on the value of general systems theory as an organizing principle.

Systems theory may well provide a useful explanatory model for the interacting hierarchies of form and function that characterize human health and illness. But to make it, as Engel does, the "blueprint", "design", "framework" of the whole of medicine is to trade on one kind of reductionism—the biological—for another. Granting the utility of such a step, it can become a shackle on medicine. The explanatory utility of a paradigm does not qualify it as a theory of medicine. It has always been perilous to transpose the method and language of one discipline beyond its operational boundaries. We need only mention the misleading and even deleterious effects of the appropriation of such concepts as Darwinian evolution, entropy, relativity, Freudian or Jungian metapsychology, or Wilsonian sociobiology by social, political, and administrative theorists to illustrate this point.[17]

Neither Seldin's restrictionist nor Engel's expansionist theories are adequate as organizing principles. We are still left with the question: What is the nature of medicine, what knowledge does it need, what does it do?

Medicine Defined in Terms of Its End

An alternative approach to viewing medicine as a body of knowledge is to define it in terms of its end, its purpose, the terminus toward which medicine is directed as a human activity. The end then becomes the determining principle that defines what kind of knowledge medicine needs. Leon Kass is one of the few theorists of medicine who analyzes the nature of medicine this way—a genuinely philosophical way. He declares the healthy human being the only "reasonable" goal of medicine. He rejects such goals as happiness, social adjustment, behavior modification, or the simple prolongation of life. "Health" is the end of medicine and not "...pleasure, happiness, civil peace and order, virtue, wisdom, and truth."[18]

Kass admits that he cannot define health precisely but he offers "wholeness" and "well-functioning" as approximations. Health is, he says, a "finite and natural norm," the "...well working of the organism as a whole, an activity of the human body in accordance with its specific excellence."[19] It is not only a somatic norm but a psychic one as well. Indeed, "our whole way of life" influences our health.[20]

On Kass's view, attainment of the end of health is the doctor's only business. His role should be limited to the use of only the technology and knowledge that advance

* See also [32].

therapeutic purposes. It is the physician, not the consumer or the government, that must define health care and the standards of practice. He questions expenditures for costly procedures like dialysis, and doubts the validity of such concepts as the right to health and the benefit of national health insurance. Health, while it is a good end in itself, is not the only ingredient of a good life. Those other ingredients are not the domain of medicine.

Having tried to contract the domain of medicine, Kass then opens it up again. He says health is everybody's business—not only the physician's. Medicine itself must become "whole" again by attending to health maintenance as well as cure of illness. He urges more research in "healthiness", disease prevention, and health maintenance and that these become the determinants of health policy.

Kass's analysis has the virtue of defining medicine philosophically in terms of the purpose for which it is ordained or acts. Physicians and patients do in fact seek health through the acts of medicine. That is why health has been recognized as the end of medicine since Hippocrates. The weakness of this theory lies in the indefiniteness of the definition of health. While Kass limits the physician to the attainment of health for his patient, his notion of health has such wavering boundaries that it could include even those things Kass specifically excludes. How, for example, can we place social adjustment or behavior modification outside medicine? Can emotional or psychological illness be ameliorated without some attention to social adjustment? Can prevention which requires a change in lifestyle be achieved without some modification of established behavior patterns? The doctor is enjoined to seek "wholeness" and well function of psyche and soma. These ends require the same breadth of concern and knowledge that Engel includes in his theory.

Defining medicine by its end is more sound philosophically than defining it as a knowledge base. But unless the end itself can be delineated the boundaries balloon again when we try to realize that end in actual practice. Selfin's view at least has the virtue of specificity in its end—those illnesses susceptible to biological cure or amelioration. Furthermore, health is an abstract notion, an ideal toward which the doctor is supposed to work. As an ideal it is never fully attained. What is the doctor's function when health is not even relatively restorable, when the illness can only be ameliorated symptomatically, or contained? What is the end of medicine when even these limited goals are not attainable? Surely one of the "ends" of medicine is to help the patient to cope with chronic illness or disability, or even to live the last days of life as comfortably and humanely as circumstances will allow.

Kass recognizes that responsibility for health is not solely medicine's. Everyone has some part in promoting his own health and society's. If this is so, we face the recurrent question: When is the pursuit of health the physician's duty and when not? Kass's theory never answers this question satisfactorily. It warns against using technology for "non-medical ends" but this depends on defining "medical" - something Kass does not do. As with Seldin and Engel, the central question remains.

Defining Medicine in the Patient-Physician Encounter

To obviate some of the difficulties of the knowledge and end-determined theories of medicine, one can approach the question more phenomenologically. Mark Siegler, for example, focuses his theory on the nature of the physician-patient relationship—on "...how clinical medicine works in the realities of daily practice."[21] He criticizes most theories because they are "context-free" and deductive, to which he opposes his own concept which is "context dependent" and inductive.

Siegler's major thesis is that "...a problem becomes one for clinical medicine only when the patient and doctor agree that it is one."[22] Siegler sees the definition of medicine as the result of a negotiated agreement between individual patients and physicians. He sees the negotiation in four stages: (1) The decision by the patient that he is ill; (2) the physician's application of the clinical method to answer the patient's question of whether he is sick or has a serious disease; (3) the doctor-patient "accommodation" in which each decides whether or not to enter the relationship with the other; and (4) the doctor-patient "relationship" in which an exchange of trust occurs and a stable and prolonged relationship is established.[23]

Except for the second stage, Siegler feels that theories of health and disease have relatively little influence on the definition of clinical medicine. Its nature is defined principally by the resolution of individual doctor-patient accommodations. In that accommodation Siegler clearly leaves the final determination to the physician. He says that "every patient presentation generates a claim to be heard by physicians."[24] But it is the physician who determines whether he will manage *this* problem in *this* patient.

Siegler's formulation has the signal advantage of seeking a definition of medicine in the phenomena of clinical medicine itself—indeed, in what is most characteristic of medicine, the encounter between physician and patient. His description of the four clinical "moments" is sound so far as it goes. I too have use the term "clinical moment" in defining what is unique about medicine—but in a rather different sense from Siegler's.[25]

Unfortunately, Siegler does not really define clinical medicine. What he does is to describe the *process* whereby physician and patient agree to enter the clinical relationship, but not the essence of the relationship itself. The process of negotiation decides whether or not physician and patient will accept each other for what each claims to be—one claims to be sick, one claims to be able to heal. This would make medicine anything the physician and patient want it to be. Even if this were defensible in individual clinical encounters, it could not serve as a basis for public policy.

Siegler's four stages are propaedeutic to some end or purpose. It is what occurs after the decision is made that constitutes the clinical moment that sets medicine off from other activities. Doctor and patient may reject each other but presumably at some point each engages in some other therapeutic relationship—and what happens once the engagement occurs is what defines clinical medicine. The process of negotiation cannot exhaust what we mean by clinical medicine, hence it cannot *define* clinical medicine. This is not to deny the utility of Siegler's description of the preludes to clinical medicine but the prelude is not that which is essential to medicine as a human activity. Let us assume that the physician denies the patient's "claim" to be ill. If the patient accepts this decision he has been relieved, reassured, and educated. He has been healed, cured, or helped. Something more than a mere negotiation has occurred. If the patient does not accept the denial of his claim to be ill, the reason he consulted the doctor remains unattended. He will seek another physician who does agree to go beyond the negotiation. In either case some end beyond negotiation of a claim about illness must be served.

The potential latitude of a definition by negotiation makes it difficult to translate into public policy, education, or ethics. The narrowest and the broadest interpretations would be equally tenable. On which of these bases do we establish the physician's ethical obligations, the education he should receive or the extent of what society should support as medical care?

Siegler's insistence on a definition based in the reality of clinical medicine itself is superior to the knowledge, or end-oriented definitions. It does not go far enough, however, into the central phenomenon of the physician-patient encounter. Since it leaves the ultimate definition to the physician who evaluates a patient's claim to be ill, the physician's philosophical conception of medicine is far more influential than Siegler allows.

Siegler shares with Seldin, Kass, and Engel the conviction that it is the physician's specific duty to define what is health, a view Whitbeck and others would contest. Whitbeck defines health as "...the psycho-physiological capacity to act or respond appropriately in a variety of situations."[26] She argues that medical expertise is not relevant to many health decisions and concludes that some of these decisions are best made by the person whose health is at stake. One might raise the same question about the definition of illness which is, after all, a subjective experience which the physician penetrates only partially and incompletely.

Fabrega takes the external definition even further, showing how social, personal, and cultural norms determine health, disease, and illness.[27] Since medicine is part of the socio-cultural and ethnic fabric of societies it is related to the dominant characteristics of society. This view has merits for homogeneous cultures with univalent value systems. For multivalent systems like ours, the question remans: What is medicine? If it is defined externally, which of the many possible value systems should predominate?

Every society and era does indeed provide some system of succor for its members who, because of illness or trauma, cannot function in their accustomed social roles. The social and cultural definitions of health and illness may vary but the need for healing is a constant. It is in that constant fact that we should seek our organizing principle—the universal fact that humans become ill, and in that state seek and need help, healing, and cure. However the cultural milieu may differ, this fact is common to all medical systems. Thus the immediate and practical end of medicine is an action taken in behalf of one who is ill, who has decided that his unease is significant enough to warrant a decision to seek medical help. Health is a more remote end. It is attainable only if the special human relationship of healing is a successful one. It is that relationship which provides the architectonics of medicine as medicine, and not health which may not even be attainable for many who seek help and healing.

THE HEALING RELATIONSHIP AS ARCHITECTONIC PRINCIPLE

No single theory can reconcile the conflicting definitions of medicine currently locked in debate. Granted their conceptual deficiencies, each derives from some truth about medical reality and thus has some heuristic value. But it is a long way from heuristics to a universal description of clinical realities. No single theory, including my own, can close this gap completely. I do believe, however, that the closer a theory comes to the phenomena of medicine as a relationship of persons the closer will it discern medicine's true nature.

I have offered elsewhere a model of medicine based in the clinical reality of the healing relationship.[28] I believe this is what distinguishes medicine from other human activities like baking bread, taking one's car to the mechanic, or buying clothes.[29*] The healing relationship is a genuine architectonic principle for it shapes, directs, and bounds the physician's work, education, and ethics. In propounding this view, I can agree with selected aspects of the several theories I have discussed: with Seldin on the need for an economy of medical pretensions, with Engel on including the patient as well as the illness, with Siegler on the importance of clinical realities, with Kass on the need to define ends, and with Whitbeck on including the patient's assessment of what constitutes health. I am not proposing a "please everybody" eclecticism; rather I acknowledge the validity of my colleagues' insights but differ substantially from most of them.

It may be objected that healing is not limited to medicine—and this is true. Psychologists, ministers, friends, and families can provide healing relationships. But they do so over a limited range of human need. Ordinarily the person who seeks extra medical healing does not consider himself sick—only troubled or anxious. Sickness implies embodiment, the distinctly human phenomenon of a conscious self in a lived body.[31*] When a person experiences some disturbance in his accustomed state of balance between body, psyche, and self he counts himself as sick. It is the fact of embodiment that creates the need for the physician. Only he can unravel the connections between the subjective experience of illness and its linkages to bodily function. Without denying the part others play, the physician comes closest to what healing means—to restore wholeness or, if this is not possible, to assist in striking some new balance between what the body imposes and the self aspires to.

What the sick person seeks is restoration to his or her definition of wholeness, that state in which Galen said we are unimpaired in doing the things we wish to do. This is as realistic a definition of health as we are likely ever to get. It depends as much on the patient's assessment as the physician's. If full restoration is not possible, then amelioration of suffering, adaptation, or coping with chronic or fatal illness become the ends of the healing relationship.

These are the ends specific to clinical medicine that distinguish it not only from other human activities, but also from other activities in which physicians may be engaged. Thus, medical science seeks the causes and pathogenetic mechanisms of disease and its end is knowledge. The end of preventive medicine seeks to promote the health of individuals and groups. Social medicine seeks the health of the entire population and its end is the public good. Physicians play important roles in all these activities but they can be accomplished without clinical skills. Only healing requires the physician as physician because its end cannot be achieved by others in society.

* The author likens the proprietary ownership of medical knowledge to the knowledge of baking bread. Michael Bayles[30] says there is no distinction between the physician-patient relationship and that between the car owner and his mechanic.

* See also [31].

The end of clinical medicine, therefore, is a technically right and good healing action—one taken in the interest of a particular patient who is in need of, and seeks, help.* To help that person the physician must answer four questions—What is wrong? What will it do to me? What can be done for me? What should be done for me? These are the clinical questions and they converge on the choice of an action. The moment of decision is the true clinical moment of truth, and in that moment what is most characteristic of medicine comes into existence.

Let us examine more closely what is involved in making a decision to act in a way that will be both technically right and good for *this* patient. This is far more than can be encompassed in the notion of medicine as applied biology or even as bio-psycho-sociology. Having a body of knowledge that may be pertinent to a clinical dilemma does not mean that the end of the healing relationship will be served. That knowledge must be directed to a specific practical end in a personal relationship in which one person is ill, vulnerable, and anxious and seeks the help of another who has knowledge that must be made to serve the interests of one who is ill.

Clinical medicine therefore only comes into existence at the moment of clinical truth, when a decision is taken and an action initiated to heal or help a particular patient. The true physician is the one who takes upon himself this responsibility, not as a negotiated task, but as an imperative built into the very nature of clinical medicine.

Medicine is therefore praxis and not theory. It contains its end within itself. Medical knowledge is incomplete as knowledge until it translates into action. It is also ethical knowledge because it is used for a good end. Although it uses science and art, medicine is closer in its moment of decision to the ancient definition of a virtue—an exercise in prudent action.

A technically right healing action must conform to several criteria. First, it must conform to the best available scientific information. Then it must draw on whatever sources are pertinent to the clinical state of this patient. This information must then be adjusted to the particularities of illness in this patient, taking into account all those things that make this patient an individual—sex, age, occupation, race, social, economic, cultural, and family context. Finally, the information must be shaped at every step by the end, choosing what is good for this patient.

The inherent logical difficulty here is that this patient is something more than an

* Given the multiple interpretations in meaning of the terms "right" and "good" it is necessary to define my use of them in this essay. Both words are used idiosyncratically, and specifically in relationship to the moment of clinical decision. "Right" refers to a decision that is technically correct, that squares with empirical and scientific fact, adjusted to the particularities of *this patient.* It is derived objectively by the physician. "Good" refers to what this patient perceives as worthwhile and valued in his life. It is personally derived. Physicians ordinarily see a "good" decision as covering both aspects, but patients, in fact, may not. It is to account for both domains—the physician's and the patient's—that the distinction is made. This is not to accept normative relativism but to focus on the moral management of value differences between physician and patient. No argument is made for a particular ontology of "right" and "good".[32,33]

instance of the operation of some scientific principle, although scientific principles are at work in him. Most of the statements we make in clinical medicine are statements of probability applicable to a population of patients sharing certain characteristics with this patient. We can never know in advance where on the frequency distribution curve this patient will be. Yet, to be right, our actions must predict as closely as possible where he is located in the universe from which our probability statements were derived.[34,35]

Optimization of decision and action in the face of uncertainty is the central characteristic of clinical decisions. That is why centuries ago Celsus called medicine an "art of conjecture." The degree of uncertainty can be reduced by access to the best available information, by meticulous attention to the clinical arts—history taking, physical examination, by critical use of probabilistic and modal logic, and mastery of the art of clinical dialectics. As I have shown elsewhere, the anatomy of a clinical decision is a complicated interplay of several different modes of reasoning and inquiry, not just a scientific one as the biomedical model supposes. Moreover, each step in clinical judgment must be modulated by value desiderata—those that advance the best interests of the one who is ill.[36,37]

These value desiderata are what convert a technically right decision into a good one. A good decision not only cures the illness but does so in harmony with the patient's conception of the conditions of an acceptable life. The choices must be responsive to the way the patient wishes to spend *his* life. This is a moral imperative particularly when the illness is untreatable or fatal. A good decision in this sense is impossible without restoring to the extent possible those human capacities eroded by illness—the capacity to make autonomous choices based on knowledge and free of coercion. An unequivocal criterion of a good decision is the enhancement of the patient's moral agency even when this flies in the face of what science or even a rational bystander might dictate. The patient is the one who must balance his vision of the good life with the realities illness forces upon him.

A good decision must be grounded in some sense on the meaning of illness to this patient. Illness challenges the meaning of life, suffering, and our relationships with others and with God. A patient's whole biography is at stake in any serious illness. Healing is impaired without some attention to that biography. There is a pattern to even the most seemingly chaotic life. The physician must grasp that pattern if his decision is to fit the patient before him. Yet he can do so only partially because the experience of illness is always unique and not penetrable to others.

To be technically right a decision must be objective; to be good it must be compassionate. It is in the fusion of these opposing attitudes that the end of clinical medicine is fulfilled. On the one hand the physician must be able to stand back, analyze, classify, measure, and reason. On the other, he must be able to feel something of the experience of illness felt by this patient. He must literally suffer something of the patient's pain along with him for that is what compassion literally means. Often the physician heals himself while healing the patient; oftentimes he cannot heal until he has healed himself. Thus the most ancient of admonitions—physician heal thyself![38]

The medical actions to which right and good clinical decisions lead must be carried out safely, efficiently, and competently. Herein lies the "art" of medicine strictly speaking. An art consists in the perfection of the execution of a product or art.[39,40] Medicine cannot be defined solely as an art because we can and do delegate specific medical acts to others. It is the decision to undertake a treatment or operation under the conditions of the healing relationship that makes medicine, in Aquinas's sense, a "ruling art." Great surgeons are not only good artists but also prudent decision makers about the use of surgery.

IMPLICATIONS OF HEALING AS AN ARCHITECTONIC PRINCIPLE

The significance of any theory of medicine lies in its influence on medical practice, education, and ethics. Perhaps some of the differences in substance between theories can be underscored by an examination of a few of the implications of the healing relationship as an ordering principle in these three areas. I have discussed in part the implications for education elsewhere.[41]

Medical Practice

If the distinguishing mark of clinical medicine is the healing relationship then it becomes the central function of all physicians as physicians. Specialists and generalists exercise this function in different ways which must, however, be complementary to each other. Each must answer the four questions that concern any human who is ill: What is wrong? What will happen to me? What can be done? What should be done? The answers to these questions lead to the right and good decision the patient seeks.

The specialist can undertake the healing relationship over only a narrow spectrum defined by the organ, organ system, or technique which bounds his specialty. He is freer than the generalist to define and negotiate the boundaries of his decision making: to help the patient find help in those dimensions of illness outside his specialty.

To the extent that the specialist narrows the boundaries of his field, to that extent he becomes less a physician and more a technician. Also the further his technique takes him from personal encounters the less he is a physician. This is invidious unless the specialist presumes to be a physician in the fuller sense I have defined it here or if he disdains the larger concerns of the generalist his patient may need.

The generalist cannot take refuge in the limitations of his specialty. For hm the healing relationship must be entered in the fullest sense. His claim is that he is the "personal" physician and he must indeed care for the special dimensions of his patient's experience of illness. He must help, care for, comfort, and ease when the specialist has nothing to offer. He often starts with a patient whose needs are not yet categorized. He must outline their configuration and devise some plan that places them in some order of priority. The patient often has made the rounds of the specialties; he is still ill, still needing answers to the key clinical questions. Even if the patient's illness has been "negotiated" out of medicine by other physicians, someone must remain who can help.

The generalist, on this view, is the physician par excellence since he has the most intimate relationship with the healing and helping functions of medicine. A specialist, especially if his domain is a technique, might get away with only scientifically right decisions; but a generalist, never. His most crucial task is to manage the experience of illness, coordinating the recommendations of specialists, interpreting them and, perhaps most important of all, serving as a critic of those recommendations. This critical function flows directly from the need to assist the patient in deciding whether a recommended treatment is worthwhile. It is not often enough performed and obviously a difficult assignment. Yet it is morally unavoidable. The generalist must confine himself to a critical analysis of the value questions in the decision. The technical aspects may be questionable too but they cannot be resolved by the generalist. The opinion of another specialist is needed.

On the view I am proposing, it is clear that contemporary medicine demands a complementary relationship between specialists and generalists. Each has a healing function. As medicine becomes further specialized in the future, the responsibility for the act most specific to medicine—deciding what is right and good for this patient—becomes increasingly the responsibility of the generalist. In this respect Engel's model is more realistic for the generalist, Seldin's for the specialist. Neither suffices unless ordered by the patient's needs for a healing relationship.

Medical Ethics

Once we have decided what medicine *is* and from that what kind of functions physicians perform, we can derive what they ought to do—that is the content of medical ethics. I have suggested a reconstruction of medical morality of the interaction between three facets of the healing relationship—the fact of illness, the act of profession, and the act of medicine.[42] My discussion in this paper has focused only on the third of this triad of relationships—the act of medicine, the right and good healing action for a particular patient.

Obviously the first moral requirement for any ethics of medicine must be competence because without it the physician's promise to help is a lie. Competence is the indispensable requirement for technically right decisions and the first requirement for a good decision as well.

The moral center of medicine, however, occurs at the moment when, having weighed all the things that can be done the physician recommends what *ought* to be done—what is in the best interests of the patient. It is here that value decisions must be made, where the values of physician and patient must intersect and conflict, where their respective moral agencies must be given equal respect. The physician has a moral obligation to conduct the decision reaching process so that the patient's capacities to make his own decision are enhanced to the degree the illness permits. Disclosure of the information needed to make this decision, telling the truth about the patient's condition, doing no harm, keeping promises, helping the patient to make a decision that is free, unmanipulated, and authentically his own. Much of this is submerged in the obligation to maintain a morally valid consent and doing no harm. These are all indispensable to the good clinical decision as I have defined it in this essay.

There is an obligation to take the pains necessary to assure that the patient understands the alternatives, the dangers and benefits, the costs, chances of success, limitations of the procedure or treatment. The patient must be helped, too, to make a decision that is authentic, that reflects his values, and he must be helped to discern and identify those values before he decides.

Finally, there is an obligation to help the patient cope with or adjust to a disease that is incurable, progressive, or imminently fatal. The physician need not do all of this himself but he has a major responsibility to see that these dimensions are exposed, and attended to by family, friends, or spiritual advisers. To do this requires some measure of compassion—the capacity to feel something of this patient's experience of illness. Compassion therefore is not just a romantic residuum of ancient medicine, it is a moral imperative of all medicine.

If the healing relationship is the organizing principle of medicine, it imposes moral obligations that go beyond the application of biology to clinical problems. The physician is therefore not entirely free to define medicine as he wishes. Medicine arises in a universal human need that transcends the physician's idiosyncratic definition of its boundaries. It is one thing to determine that a patient does or does not have a medically definable disease—that is the physician's responsibility. It is a different matter to say the patient is not ill. Society supports medicine because it promises to heal and help those who are ill. Society has more than a casual interest in how medicine is defined.

A 'CONCLUDING POSTSCRIPT'

It may be objected, properly, that this essay ignores the responsibilities of medicine beyond those of the clinical encounter. There are, indeed, legitimate functions for medicine such as its social responsibilities, its capacity for biological research, for promoting health and preventing illness, and serving as a source of criticisms of the way we live—individually and collectively. These are socially and culturally important responsibilities for medicine but not necessarily for *clinical* medicine. I have limited myself to what clinicians do, not only for want of space, but also because I wanted to concentrate on what is uniquely the physician's function, one that is unchanging because it is grounded in the universal human need for help and healing of those who are ill. I have addressed some of the other dimensions of medicine elsewhere.[43,44] I recognize that they must be taken into account in any full theory of medicine.

SUMMARY

That theories have practical consequences is no revelation except to the most absolute pragmatists. Equally true is the fact that theoretical confusion lies behind confusion in public and social policy. Nowhere are these truisms more clearly illustrated than in medicine.

Our theories tell us what medicine is, and on this basis we build our models of medical practice and morals. Today we face a vigorous reexamination of all our models of medicine. The consequences for the care of patients and for social and public policy are most significant. Some of the most crucial dilemmas about medicine cannot be resolved without some consensus on what we think medicine is, what it is for, what physicians ought to do, and how they ought to do it.

This essay offers a critique of the major contending theories of medicine—agreeing in part with some and disagreeing substantively with others. An architectonics of clinical medicine is offered which is based in the nature of the healing relationship. This is the most permanent, universal, and compelling phenomenon of clinical medicine; it gives shape to how medicine should be practiced, what its morals should be, and how its practitioners should be educated.

It is true, as John Burnham has recently emphasized, that the "Golden Age" of medicine seems to be in decline. The socio-cultural reasons he adduces for this fact are cogent. I would add to them the confusion about theories of medicine which have undergone significant alteration in the same period.[45,46]

II

Other Philosophical and Ethical Issues Confronting the Medical Profession

These articles and essays will give the reader a sense of why so many physicians have been influenced by Dr. Pellegrino's thoughts and insights through the years.

CHAPTER EIGHT

THE VIRTUOUS PHYSICIAN, AND THE ETHICS OF MEDICINE

Consider from what noble seed you spring: You were created not to live like beasts, but for pursuit of virtue and of knowledge.
Dante, Inferno *26, 118-120*

INTRODUCTION

In the opening pages of his *Dominations and Powers*, Santayana asserts that "Human society owes all its warmth and vitality to the intrinsic virtue of its members" and that the virtues therefore are always "hovering silently" over his pages.[1] And, indeed, the virtues have always hovered over any theory of morals. They give credibility to the moral life; they assure that it will be something more than a catalogue of rights, duties, and rules. Virtue adds that extra "cubit" that lifts ethics out of its legalisms to the higher reaches of moral sensitivity.

Yet, as MacIntyre's brilliant treatise so ably attests, virtue-ethics since the Enlightenment has become a dubious enterprise.[2] We have lost consensus on a definition of virtue, and without moral consensus there is no vantage point from which to judge what is right and good. Virtue becomes confused with conformity to the conventions of social and institutional life. The accolades go to those who get along and get ahead. Without agreeing on the nature of the good, moreover, we can hardly know what a "disposition" to do the right and good may mean.

These uncertainties force us to rely on ethical systems built upon specific rights, duties, and the application of rules and principles. Their concreteness seems to promise protection against capricious and antithetical interpretations of vice and virtue. But the concreteness turns to illusion once we try to agree on what is the right and good thing to do, in a given circumstance.

Despite the erosion of the concept of virtue, it remains an inescapable reality in moral transactions. We know there are people we can trust to temper self-interest, to be honest, truthful, faithful, or just, even in the face of the omnipresence of evil. Sadly, we also know that there are others who cannot be trusted habitually to act well. We may not be virtuous ourselves, we may even sneer at the folly of the virtuous man in our age, yet we can recognize him nonetheless. It is as Marcus Aurelius said, "...no thing delights as much as the examples of the virtues when they are exhibited in the morals of those who live with us and present themselves in abundance as far as possible. Wherefore we must keep these before us."[3]

And, in fact, the virtues are again being brought before us in the resurgence, among moral philosophers, of an interest in virtue-based ethics.[4-14] For the most part the resurgence is based in a re-examination, clarification, and refurbishment of the classical-medieval concept of virtue. On the whole, the contemporary reappraisal is not an abnegation of rights or duty-based ethics, but a recognition that rights and duties notwithstanding, their moral effectiveness still turns on the disposition and character traits of our fellow men and women.

MacIntyre has expressed his pessimism about the possibilities of an ethic of virtue in our times. He ends his tightly reasoned treatise with a surprisingly romantic hope for "...a local form of community within which civility and the intellectual and moral life can be sustained in the rough new dark ages which are already upon us."[15] One can accept MacIntyre's astute historical diagnoses without waiting too quietistically for the appearance of his new and "doubtless very different" St. Benedict to lead us into some new moral consensus. Even in the "dark age," it may be possible to incorporate the remnant of the classical-medieval idea of virtue into a more satisfactory moral structure that also includes rights and duties.

This essay examines the possibility in the limited domain of professional medical ethics. Using the classical-medieval concept of virtue; it attempts to define the virtuous physician, to relate his virtue to the ends of medicine and to the usual principles applied in medical ethics, as well as to the prevailing rights and duty-based systems of professional ethics.

This essay is part of a larger effort to link a theory of the patient-physician relationship, a theory of patient good, and theory of virtue in a unified conceptual substructure for the professional ethics of medicine.[16,17]

THE CLASSICAL-MEDIEVAL CONCEPT OF VIRTUE

What is virtue? What are the virtues? Are they one or many? Can they be taught? These are still the fundamental first order questions for any virtue-based ethical theory. And, as with so many of the perennial philosophical questions, they were first examined in an orderly way in the Platonic dialogues. In the first dialogues, Socrates raises them with his characteristic to, and fro, probing. Given his circumambulation of definitions, and the difficulties of translating from ancient languages, Socrates' precise meaning remains somewhat problematic.

Most commentators, however, focus on his equilibration in the *Meno*, *Protagoras*, and *Gorgias* of virtue (*areté*) with knowledge (epistemé).[18-21] Virtue is here synonymous with excellence in living the good life. This excellence depends upon knowledge of good, evil, and self. It is not specialized knowledge directed to any one activity but rather to living one's whole life well. It must, like an art, be perfected through practice. The individual virtues—courage, justice, temperance, wisdom, and piety—order life toward excellence. But they too depend on knowledge so that, on this view, vice is the result primarily of ignorance.

How much of this intellectualist definition of virtue is Socrates' and how much Plato's is debatable. In the later dialogues, the *Laws* and the *Republic*, more attention is given to justice as a central virtue and to proper ordering of state.[22] Wisdom is still a virtue but for the statesman it is knowledge of what is good not just for the individual good life but the good of the whole state. The aim of laws should be virtue but the chief of these is wisdom, so that wisdom is the knowledge that "presides" over justice (*Republic*, Bk. IV).

In the *Republic*, still exploring definitions, Plato draws the analogy of virtue with bodily health—"Virtue then as it sees would be a certain health, beauty and good condition of a soul and vice a sickness, ugliness and weakness" (*Republic*, Bk. IV). He likens virtue to the order and balance between the parts of the body that characterize health. For Socrates that ordering results from intellectual perfection of the art of living a good life. Plato, as Aristotle pointed out, paid more attention than Socrates to the non-rational elements in human life. Virtue, for him is as much a matter of disposition to act in the right way, as it is a desire for the good, arising from knowledge of the good.

Aristotle reacted to Socrates' over-intellectualization of virtue. He devoted large portions of the *Nicomachean Ethics* to his concept of virtue. His own work, Aristotle said, "...does not aim at theoretical knowledge like the others (for we are inquiring not in order to know what virtue is, but in order to become good, since otherwise our inquiry would have been of no use), we must examine the nature of actions, namely, how we ought to do them" (*Nicomachean Ethics*, 1099a, 10-11). He does not reject the role of intellect; he judges it a proper part of virtue, but not its whole. Thus he emphasizes that virtue is also concerned with feelings and actions—"...just acts are pleasant to the lover of justice and in general virtuous acts to the lover of virtue" (*Nicomachean Ethics*, 1099a, 10-11).

But virtue is not just feeling. It is of two kinds: intellectual and moral—"Intellectual virtue in the main owes both its birth and growth to teaching (for which reasons it requires experience and time) while moral virtue comes about as a result of habit, whence also its name *ethiké* that is formed by a slight variation of the word *ethos* (habit)" (*Nicomachean Ethics,* 1103a, 14-18). Virtue is not simply a passion, or a function, but a "...state of character" (*Nicomachean Ethics,* 1106a. 11), Virtue is that state of character "which makes a man good and which makes him do his own work well" (*Nicomachean Ethics*, 1106a, 22-24).

But states of character must be in accord with the "right rule." Hence the intellectual virtues play a part in making a man virtuous. Practical wisdom is that aspect of intellect that enables a man to direct his life to its chief good. The "right rule" is reached, as Ross says, "by the deliberative analysis of the practically wise man and telling him that the end of human life is to be best attained by certain actions which are intermediate between extremes. Obedience to such a rule is moral virtue."[23]

Aristotle's doctrine of the mean and his divisions and subdivisions of the intellectual and moral virtues are too complex to engage us here.[24] What is significant for the present discussion is the balance Aristotle strikes between moral virtue and reason, feelings, dispositions, and right action. These are Aristotle's modifications and extensions of the Socratic notion of virtue.

Aristotle made more explicit the Socratic orientation of virtue to ends. Thus "...every virtue or excellence both brings into good condition the thing of which it is the excellence and makes the work of that thing to be done well..." (*Nicomachean Ethics*, 2, 5, 1106a, 15-17). The end of virtue for both Socrates and Aristotle is the good life. What constitutes the good life is for both of them the fulfillment of the potentiality of human nature.

Aristotle summarizes the essential elements which distinguish the virtuous man: "...in the first place he must have knowledge, secondly, he must choose the acts and choose them for their own sakes, and thirdly his actions must proceed from a firm and unchangeable character" (*Nicomachean Ethics*, 11, 4, 1104, 6, 31-34). This combination of character, knowledge, and deliberate choice makes for a virtuous person. Actions themselves are virtuous when they emanate from just such a person (*Nicomachean Ethics*, 1105a, 5-6). For Aristotle, then, virtue resides not only in the act or in the knowledge of virtue, but the act itself must also be done virtuously, as a virtuous man would do it. "...But as a condition of the possession of the virtues knowledge has little or no weight, while the other conditions count not for a little, but for everything. Nor does virtue reside in the act itself" (*Nicomachean Ethics*, 1105b, 1-4).

Aquinas' treatment of the virtues is best understood in the context of his total enterprise, to reconcile, emend, and amend the ancient philosophers though the revealed truths of the Christian experience. Precisely to what extent his emphasis on the cardinal virtues coincides with, or departs from, Aristotle is difficult to say. Aquinas too had to surmount the problem of trying to apprehend the nuances of words in an ancient language no longer in daily use. MacIntyre calls him a "marginal figure" not representing the general opinion of the virtues extant in his time. He does, however, recognize that Aquinas' interpretation of the *Nicomachean Ethics* "has never been better."[25]

For Aristotle, the intellectual and moral virtues were requisite for the full development of man's natural capacities. But for Aquinas, man's natural end was itself insufficient because he had a spiritual destiny that transcends the merely natural.[26] Man is destined to union with God. To this end not only the natural virtues but the supernatural are needed, and these can be known only through the Christian revelation. For the Christian the perfection of the natural virtues is not sufficient.[27]

Like Aristotle, Aquinas held virtue to be grounded in good habits, in dispositions to do the right and good thing, but always in association with the right reason. Thus he says, "It belongs to human virtue to make a man good and his work according to reason."[28] "Through virtue man is ordered to the utmost limit of his capacity."[29] It is a condition of the perfection of human life. Or said another way, "Virtue is called the limit of potentiality...because it causes an inclination to the highest act which a faculty can perform."[30]

Virtues for Aquinas are habits and dispositions that enable a man to reason well (the intellectual virtues) and to act in accordance with a right reason (moral virtues)—*recta ratio agibilium.*[31] These two kinds of virtue can be independent of each other, but in the virtuous man, who strives for the perfection of his human potentiality, they are joined. And they are joined most firmly in the one virtue from which the others derive—prudence, the standard of right willing and acting, the form and mold for the other virtues.[32]

Josef Pieper among modern commentators has most clearly expounded Aquinas' teaching on prudence and the other cardinal virtues.[33] Without attempting to restate that teaching here, suffice it to say that for Aquinas all virtue is necessarily prudent, acting in accord with right reason in conformity with the reality of things. This is not prudence in the pejorative modern sense of caution, timidity, rationalized cowardice, cunning, or casuistic deviousness. Rather, it is the analogue of Aristotle's wisdom, the capacity and disposition to will and act rightly in particular, practical, and uncertain circumstances. As such, prudence informs, measures, guides, shapes, and generates the other virtues, by inclining us to choose good means to good ends for man.

The post-medieval transformation of the classical concepts were many: Rousseau opposed virtue to society; for Shaftesbury virtue lay in the pursuit of public interest; Hutcheson and Hume identified it with a "moral sense"; to Montaigne virtue was "an innocence, accidental and fortuitous"; for Descartes, strength of soul; for Malebranche, love of order; and for Spinoza, the soul directing itself by a universal and clear idea; Mandeville paradoxically defended the utility of the vices. MacIntyre shows with a wealth of detail the continuing emotivist and intuitionist trends of philosophies of virtue since the Enlightenment.

In the last several years the classical concept has been reexamined by a growing number of moral philosophers. They have underscored such things as the differences in meanings of the word *arete* in Greek, *virtus* in Latin, and "virtue" in English, the distinctions between virtues and skills, the difficulties in defining such words as "disposition" and "habit" as used in the traditional definitions, the relationships between the natural and the supernatural virtues, the relations of virtue, values and concepts of the good, the unity or non-unity of the virtues, whether they are teachable or not, their relevance to health and medical care, and their relationship with duties, rights, and obligations.[34-39]

MacIntyre, for example, extends the Aristotelian concept from qualities internal to practices, to role reference and to community good.[40] Hauerwas relates them to the narrative of a particular people.[41] Some commentators are more critical, some more accepting of the classical concepts. In the end, the great majority say almost the same thing as the ancients but in more modern language. One is tempted to say of virtue, as it has been said of pornography, "I can't define it but I know it when I see it."

THE VIRTUOUS PERSON, THE VIRTUOUS PHYSICIAN

Through these multitudinous definitions a set of common themes seems discernible. Virtue implies a character trait, an internal disposition, habitually to seek moral perfection to live one's life in accord with the moral law, and to attain a balance between noble intention and just action. Perhaps C. S. Lewis has captured the idea best by likening the virtuous man to the good tennis player: "What you mean by a good player is the man whose eye and muscles and nerves have been so trained by making innumerable good shots that they can now be relied upon.... They have a certain tone or quality which is there even when he is not playing.... In the same way a man who perseveres in doing just actions gets in the end a certain quality of character. Now it is that quality rather than the particular actions that we mean when we talk of virtue."[42]

On almost any view, the virtuous person is someone we can trust to act habitually in a "good" way—courageously, honestly, justly, wisely, and temperately. He is committed to *being* a good person and to the pursuit of perfection in his private, professional, and communal life. He is someone who will act well even when there is no one to applaud, simply because to act otherwise is a violation of what it is to be a good person. No civilized society could endure without a significant number of citizens committed to this concept of virtue. Without such persons no system of general ethics could succeed, and no system of professional ethics could transcend the dangers of self-interest. That is why, even while rights, duties, obligations may be emphasized, the concept of virtue has "hovered" so persistently over every system of ethics.

Is the virtuous physician simply the virtuous person practicing medicine? Are there virtues peculiar to medicine as a practice? Are certain of the individual virtues more applicable to medicine than elsewhere in human activities? Is virtue more important in some branches of medicine than others? How do professional skills differ from virtue? These are pertinent questions propadeutic to the later questions of the place of virtue in professional medical ethics.

I believe these questions are best answered by drawing on the Aristotelian-Thomist notion of virtues and its relationship to the ends and purposes of human life. The virtuous physician on this view is defined in terms of the ends of medicine. To be sure, the physician, before he is anything else, must be a virtuous person. To be a virtuous physician he must also be the kind of person we can confidently expect will be disposed to the right and good intrinsic to the practice he professes. What are those dispositions?

To answer this question requires some exposition of what we mean by the good in medicine, or more specifically the good of the patient—for that is the end the patient and the physician ostensibly seek. Any theory of virtue must be linked with a theory of the good because virtue is a disposition habitually to do the good. Must we therefore know the nature of the good the virtuous man is disposed to do? As with the definition of virtue we are caught here in another perennial philosophical question—what is the nature of the Good? Is the good whatever we make it to be or does it have validity independent of our desires or interest? Is the good one, or many? Is it reducible to riches, honors, pleasures, glory, happiness, or something else?

I make no pretense to a discussion of a general theory of the good. But any attempt to define the virtuous physician or a virtue-based ethic for medicine must offer some definition of the good of the patient. The patient's good is the end of medicine, that which shapes the particular virtues required for its attainment. That end is central to any notion of the virtues peculiar to medicine as a practice.

I have argued elsewhere that the architectonic principle of medicine is the good of the patient as expressed in a particular right and good healing action.[43] This is the immediate good end of the clinical encounter. Health, healing, caring, coping are all good ends dependent upon the more immediate end of a right and good decision. On this view, the virtuous physician is one so habitually disposed to act in the patient's good, to place the good in ordinary instances above his own, that he can reliably be expected to do so.

But we must fact the fact that the "patient's good" is itself a compound notion. Elsewhere I have examined four components of the patient's good: (1) clinical or biomedical good; (2) the good as perceived by the patient; (3) the good of the patient as a human person; and (4) the Good, or ultimate good. Each of these components of patient good must be served. They must also be placed in some hierarchical order when they conflict within the same person, or between persons involved in clinical decisions.[44]

Some would consider patient good, so far as the physician is concerned, as limited to what applied medical knowledge can achieve in *this* patient. On this view the virtues specific to medicine would be objectivity, scientific probity, and conscientiousness with regard to professional skill. One could perform the technical tasks of medicine well, be faithful to the skills of good technical medicine per se, but without being a virtuous person. Would one then be a virtuous physician? One would have to answer affirmatively if technical skill were all there is to medicine.

Some of the more expansionist models of medicine—like Engel's biopsychosocial model, or that of the World Health Organization (total well-being)—would require compassion, empathy, advocacy, benevolence, and beneficence, i.e., an expanded sense of the affective responses to patient need.[45] Some might argue that what is required, therefore, is not virtue, but simply greater skill in the social and behavioral sciences applied to particular patients. On this view the physician's habitual dispositions might be incidental to his skills in communication or his empathy. He could achieve the ends of medicine without necessarily being a virtuous person in the generic sense.

It is important at this juncture to distinguish the virtues from technical or professional skills , as MacIntyre and, more clearly, Von Wright do. The latter defines a skill as "technical goodness"—excellence in some particular activity—while virtues are not tied to any one activity but are necessary for "the good of man."[46] The virtues are not "characterized in terms of their results."[47] On this view, the technical skills of medicine are not virtues and could be practiced by a non-virtuous person. Aristotle held *techné* (technical skills) to be one of the five intellectual virtues but not one of the moral virtues.

The virtues enable the physician to act with regard to things that are good for man, when man is in the specific existential state of illness. They are dispositions always to seek the good intent inherent in healing. Within medicine, the virtues do become in MacIntyre's sense acquired human qualities "...the possession and exercise of which tends to enable us to achieve those goods which are internal to practices and the lack of which effectively prevents us from achieving any such goods."[48]

We can come closer to the relationships of virtue to clinical actions if we look to the more immediate ends of medical encounters, to those moments of clinical truth when specific decisions and actions are chosen and carried out. The good the patient seeks is to be healed—to be restored to his prior, or to the better, state of function, to be made "whole" again. If this is not possible, the patient expects to be helped, to be assisted in coping with the pain, disability or dying that illness may entail. The immediate end of medicine is not simply a technically proficient performance but the use of that performance to attain a good end—the good of the patient—his medical or biomedical good to the extent possible but also his good as he the patient perceives it, his good as a human person who can make his own life plan, and his good as a person with a spiritual destiny if this is his belief.[49,50] It is the sensitive balancing of these senses of the patient's good which the virtuous physician pursues to perfection.

To achieve the end of medicine thus conceived, to practice medicine virtuously, requires certain dispositions: conscientious attention to technical knowledge and skill to be sure, but also compassion—a capacity to feel something of the patient's experience of illness and his perceptions of what is worthwhile; beneficence and benevolence—doing and wishing to do good for the patient; honesty, fidelity to promises, perhaps at times courage as well—the whole list of virtues spelled out by Aristotle: "...justice, courage, temperance, magnificence, magnanimity, liberality, placability, prudence, wisdom" (*Rhetoric*, 1, c, 13666, 1-3). Not every one of these virtues is required in every decision. What we expect of the virtuous physician is that he will exhibit them when they are required and that we will be so habitually disposed to do so that we can depend upon it. He will place the good of the patient above his own and to seek that good unless its pursuit imposes an injustice upon him, or his family, or requires a violation of his own conscience.

While the virtues are necessary to attain the good internal to medicine as a practice, they exist independently of medicine. They are necessary for the practice of a good life, no matter in what activities that life may express itself. Certain of the virtues may become duties in the Stoic sense, duties because of the nature of medicine as a practice. Medicine calls forth benevolence, beneficence, truth telling, honesty, fidelity, and justice more than physical courage, for example. Yet even physical courage is necessary in treating contagious diseases, violent patients, or battlefield casualties. Doing the right and good thing in medicine calls for a more regular, intensive, and selective practice of the virtues than many other callings.

A person who is a virtuous person can cultivate the technical skills of medicine for reasons other than the good of the patient—his own pride, profit, prestige, power. Such a physician can make technically right decisions and perform skillfully. He could not be depended upon, however, to act against his own self-interest for the good of his patient.

In the virtuous physician, explicit fulfillment of rights and duties is an outward expression of an inner disposition to do the right and the good. He is virtuous not because he has conformed to the letter of the law, or his moral duties, but because that is what a good person does. He starts always with his commitment to be a certain kind of person, and he approaches clinical quandaries, conflicts of values, and his patient's interests as a good person should.

Some branches of medicine would seem to demand a stricter and broader adherence to virtue than others. Generalists, for example, who deal with the more sensitive facets and nuances of a patient's life and humanity must exercise the virtues more diligently than technique-oriented specialists. The narrower the specialty the more easily the patient's good can be safeguarded by rules, regulations, rights, and duties; the broader the specialty the more significant are the physician's character traits. No branch of medicine, however, can be practiced without some dedication to some of the virtues.[51]

Unfortunately, physicians can compartmentalize their lives. Some practice medicine virtuously, yet are guilty of vice in their private lives. Examples are common of physicians who appear sincerely to seek the good of their patients and neglect obligations to family or friends. Some boast of being "married" to medicine and uses this excuse to justify all sorts of failures in their own human relationships. We could not call such a person virtuous. Nor could we be secure in, or trust, his disposition to act in a right and good way even in medicine. After all, one of the essential virtues is balancing conflicting obligations judiciously.

As Socrates pointed out to Meno, one cannot really be virtuous in part:

> Why did not I ask you to tell me the nature of virtue as a whole? And you are very far from telling me this; but declare every action to be virtue which is done with a part of virtue; as though you had told me and I must already know the whole of virtue, and this too when frittered away into little pieces. And therefore my dear Meno, I fear that I must begin again, and repeat the same question: what is virtue? For otherwise, I can only say that every action done with a part of virtue is virtue; what else is the meaning of saying that every action done with justice is virtue? Ought I not to ask the question over again; for can any one who does not know virtue know a part of virtue? (*Meno*, 79)

VIRTUES, RIGHTS, AND DUTIES IN MEDICAL ETHICS

Frankena has neatly summarized the distinctions between virtue-based and rights- and duty-based ethics as follows:

> In an ED (ethics of duty) then, the basic concept is that a certain kind of external act (of doing) ought to be done in certain circumstances; and that of a certain disposition being a virtue is a dependent one. In an EV (ethics of virtue) the basic concept is that of a disposition or way of being—something one has, or is not does—as a virtue, as morally good; and that of an action's being virtuous or good or even right, is a dependent one.[52]

There are some logical difficulties with a virtue-based ethic. For one thing, there must be some consensus on a definition of virtue. For another there is a circularity in the assertion that virtue is what the good man habitually does, and that at the same time one become virtuous by doing good. Virtue and good are defined in terms of each other and the definitions of both may vary among sincere people in actual practice when there is no consensus. A virtue-based ethic is difficult to defend as the sole basis for normative judgments.

But there is a deficiency in rights- and duty-ethics as well. They too must be linked to a theory of the good. In contemporary ethics, theories of good are rarely explicitly linked to theories of the right and good. Von Wright, commendably, is one of the few contemporary authorities who explicitly connects his theory of good with his theory of virtue. This essay, together with three previous ones, is part of the author's effort in theat direction.[53-55]

In most professional ethical codes, virtue and duty-based ethics are intermingled. The Hippocratic Oath, for example, imposes certain duties like protection of confidentiality, avoiding abortion, not harming the patient. But the Hippocratic physician also pledges: "...in purity and holiness I will guard my life and my art." This is an exhortation to be a good person and a virtuous physician, in order to serve patients in an ethically responsible way.

Likewise, in one of the most humanistic statements in medical literature, the first century A.D. writer, Scribonius Largus, made *humanitas* (compassion) an essential virtue. It is thus really a role-specific duty. In doing so he was applying the Stoic doctrine of virtue to medicine.[56,57]

The latest version (1980) of the AMA "Principles of Medical Ethics" similarly intermingles duties, rights, and exhortations to virtue. It speaks of "standards of behavior," "essentials of honorable behavior," dealing "honestly" with patients and colleagues, and exposing colleagues "deficient in character." The *Declaration of Geneva*, which must meet the challenge of the widest array of value systems, nonetheless calls for practice "with conscience and dignity" in keeping with "the honor and noble traditions of the profession." Though their first allegiance must be to the Communist ethos, even the Soviet physician is urged to preserve "the high title of physician," "to keep and develop the beneficial traditions of medicine" and to "dedicate" all his "knowledge and strength to the care of the sick."

Those who are cynical of any protestation of virtue on the part of physicians will interpret these excerpts as the last remnants of a dying tradition of altruistic benevolence. But at the very least, they attest to the recognition that the good of the patient cannot be fully protected by rights and duties alone. Some degree of supererogation is built into the nature of the relationship of those who are ill and those who profess to help them.

This too may be why many graduating classes, still idealistic about their calling, choose the Prayer of Maimonides (not by Maimonides at all) over the more deontological Oath of Hippocrates. In that "prayer" the physician asks: "...may neither avarice nor miserliness, no thirst for glory or for a great reputation engage my mind; for the enemies of truth and philanthropy may easily deceive me and make me forgetful of my lofty aim of doing good to thy children." This is an unequivocal call to virtue and it is hard to imagine even the most cynical graduate failing to comprehend its message.

All professional medical codes, then, are built of a three-tiered system of obligations related to the special roles of physicians in society. In the ascending order of ethical sensitivity they are: observance of the laws of the land, then observance of rights and fulfillment of duties, and finally the practice of virtue.

A legally based ethic concentrates on the minimum requirements—the duties imposed by human laws which protect against the grosser aberrations of personal rights. Licensure, the laws of torts and contracts, prohibitions against discrimination, good Samaritan laws, definitions of death, and the protection of human subjects of experimentation are elements of a legalistic ethic.

At the next level is the ethics of rights and duties which spells out obligations beyond what law defines. Here, benevolence and beneficence take on more than their legal meaning. The ideal of service, of responsiveness to the special needs of those who are ill, some degree of compassion, kindliness, promise-keeping, truth-telling, and non-maleficence, and specific obligations like confidentiality and autonomy, are included. How these principles are applied, and conflicts among them resolved in the patient's best interests, are subjects of widely varying interpretation. How sensitively these issues are confronted depends more on the physician's character than his capability at ethical discourse or moral casuistry.

Virtue-based ethics goes beyond these first two levels. We expect the virtuous person to do the right and the good even at the expense of personal sacrifice and legitimate self-interest. Virtue ethics expands the notions of benevolence, beneficence, conscientiousness, compassion, and fidelity well beyond what strict duty might require. It makes some degree of supererogation mandatory because it calls for standards of ethical performance that exceed those prevalent in the rest of society.[58]

At each of these three levels there are certain dangers from overzealous or misguided observance. Legalistic ethical systems tend toward a justification for minimalistic ethics, a narrow definition of benevolence or beneficence, and a contract-minded physician-patient relationship. Duty- and rights-based ethics may be distorted by too strict adherence to the letter of ethical principles without the modulations and nuances the spirit of those principles implies. Virtue-based ethics, being the least specific, can more easily lapse into self-righteous paternalism or an unwelcome over-involvement in the personal life of the patient. Misapplication of any moral system even with good intent converts benevolence into maleficence. The virtuous person might be expected to be more sensitive to these aberrations than someone whose ethics is more deontologically or legally flavored.

The more we yearn for ethical sensitivity the less we lean on rights, duties, rules, and principles, and the more we lean on the character traits of the moral agent. Paradoxically, without rules, rights, and duties specifically spelled out, we cannot predict what form a particular person's expression of virtue will take. In a pluralistic society, we need laws, rules, and principles to assure a dependable minimum level of moral conduct. But that minimal level is insufficient in the complex and often unpredictable circumstances of decision-making, where technical and value desiderata intersect so inextricably.

The virtuous physician does not act from unreasoned, uncritical intuitions about what feels good. His dispositions are ordered in accord with that "right reason" which both Aristotle and Aquinas considered essential to virtue. Medicine is itself ultimately an exercise of practical wisdom—a right way of acting in difficult and uncertain circumstances for a specific end, i.e., the good of a particular person who is ill. It is when the choice of a right and good action becomes more difficult, when the temptations to self-interest are more insistent, when unexpected nuances of good and evil arise and no one is looking, that the difference between an ethics based in virtue and an ethics based in law and/or duty can most clearly be distinguished.

Virtue-based professional ethics distinguishes itself, therefore, less in the avoidance of overtly immoral practices than in avoidance of those at the margin of moral responsibility. Physicians are confronted, in today's morally relaxed climate, with an increasing number of new practices that pit altruism against self-interest. Most are not illegal, or, strictly speaking, immoral in a rights- or duty-based ethic. But they are not consistent with the higher level of moral sensitivity that a virtue-ethics demands. These practices usually involve opportunities for profit from the illness of others, narrowing the concept of service for personal convenience, taking a proprietary attitude with respect to medical knowledge, and placing loyalty to the profession above loyalty to patients.

Under the first heading, we might include such things as investment in and ownership of for-profit hospitals, hospital chains, nursing homes, dialysis units, tie-in arrangements with radiological or laboratory services, escalation of fees for repetitive, high-volume procedures, and lax indications for their use, especially when third party payers "allow" such charges.

The second heading might include the ever decreasing availability and accessibility of physicians, the diffusion of individual patient responsibility in group practice so that the patient never knows whom he will see or who is on call, the itinerant emergency room physician who works two days and skips three with little commitment to hospital or community, and the growing over-indulgence of physicians in vacations, recreation, and "self-development."

The third category might include such things as "selling one's services" for whatever the market will bear, providing what the market demands and not necessarily what the community needs, patenting new procedures or keeping them secret from potential competitor-colleagues, looking at the investment of time, effort, and capital in medical education as justification for "making it back," or forgetting that medical knowledge is drawn from the cumulative experience of a multitude of patients, clinicians, and investigators.

Under the last category might be included referrals on the basis of friendship and reciprocity rather than skill, resisting consultations and second opinions as affronts to one's competence, placing the interest of the referring physician above those of the patients, looking the other way in the face of incompetence or even dishonesty in one's professional colleagues.

These and many other practices are defended today by sincere physicians and even encouraged in this era of competition, legalism, and self-indulgence. Some can be rationalized even in a deontological ethic. But it would be impossible to envision the physician committed to the virtues assenting to these practices. A virtue-based ethics simply does not fluctuate with what the dominant social mores will tolerate. It must interpret benevolence, beneficence, and responsibility in a way that reduces self-interest and enhances altruism. It is the only convincing answer the profession can give to the growing perception clearly manifest in the legal commentaries in the FTC ruling that medicine is nothing more than business and should be regulated as such.

A virtue-based ethic is inherently elitist, in the best sense, because its adherents demand more of themselves than the prevailing morality. It calls forth that extra measure of dedication that has made the best physicians in every era exemplars of what the human spirit can achieve. No matter to what depths a society may, virtuous persons will always be the beacons that light the way back to moral sensitivity; virtuous physicians are the beacons that show the way back to moral credibility for the whole profession.

Albert Jonsen, rightly I believe, diagnoses the central paradox in medicine as the tension between self-interest and altruism.[59] No amount of deft juggling of rights, duties, or principles will suffice to resolve that tension. We are all too good at rationalizing what we want to do so that personal gain can be converted from vice to virtue. Only a character formed by the virtues can feel the nausea of such intellectual hypocrisy.

To be sure, the twin themes of self-interest and altruism have been inextricably joined in the history of medicine. There have always been physicians who reject the virtues or, more often, claim them falsely. But, in addition, there have ben physicians, more often than the critics of medicine would allow, who have been truly virtuous both in intent and act. They have been, and remain, the leaven of the profession and the hope of all who are ill. They form the sea-wall that will not be eroded even by the powerful forces of commercialization, bureaucratization, and mechanization inevitable in modern medicine.

We cannot, need not, and indeed must not, wait for the medical analogue of MacIntyre's "new St. Benedict" to show us the way. There is no new concept of virtue waiting to be discovered that is peculiarly suited to the dilemmas of our own dark age. We must recapture the courage to speak of character, virtue, and perfection in living a good life. We must encourage those who are willing to dedicate themselves to a "higher standard of self effacement."[60]

We need the courage, too, to accept the obvious split in the profession between those who see and feel the altruistic imperatives in medicine, and those who do not. Those who at heart believe that the pursuit of private self-interest serves the public good are very different from those who believe in the restraint of self-interest. We forget that physicians since the beginnings of the profession have subscribed to different values and virtues. We need only recall that the Hippocratic Oath was the Oath of physicians of the Pythagorean school at a time when most Greek physicians followed essentially a craft ethic.[61] A perusal of the Hippocratic Corpus itself, which intersperses ethics and etiquette, will show how differently its treatises deal with fees, the care of incurable patients, and the business aspects of the craft.

The illusion that all physicians share a common devotion to a high-flown set of ethical principles has done damage to medicine by raising expectations some members of the profession could not, or will not, fulfill. Today, we must be more forthright about the differences in value commitment among physicians. Professional codes must be more explicit about the relationships between duties, rights, and virtues. Such explicitness encourages a more honest relationship between physicians and patients and removes the hypocrisy of verbal assent to a general code, to which an individual physician may not really subscribe. Explicitness enables patients to choose among physicians on the basis of their ethical commitments as well as their reputations for technical expertise.

Conceptual clarity will not assure virtuous behavior. Indeed, virtues are usually distorted if they are the subject of too conscious a design. But conceptual clarity will distinguish between motives and provide criteria for judging the moral commitment one can expect from the profession and from its individual members. I can also inspire those whose virtuous inclinations need re-enforcement in the current climate of commercialization of the healing relationship.

To this end the current resurgence of interest in virtue-based ethics is altogether salubrious. Linked to a theory of patient good and a theory of rights and duties, it could provide the needed groundwork for a reconstruction of professional medical ethics as the work matures. Perhaps even more progress can be made if we take Shakespeare's advice in *Hamlet*: "Assure the virtue if you have it not.... For use almost can change the stamp of nature."

CHAPTER NINE

TOWARD A VIRTUE-BASED NORMATIVE ETHICS FOR THE HEALTH PROFESSIONS

If he really does think there is no distinction between
Virtue and vice, why, sir, when he leaves our house,
Let us count our spoons.
Samuel Johnson

ABSTRACT

Virtue is the most perdurable concept in the history of ethics, which is understandable given the ineradicability of the moral agent in the events of the moral life. Historically, virtue enjoyed normative force as long as the philosophical anthropology and the metaphysics of the good that grounded virtue were viable. That grounding has eroded in both general and medical ethics. If virtue is to be restored to a normative status, its philosophical underpinnings must be reconstructed. Such reconstruction seems unlikely in general ethics, where the possibility of agreement on the good for humans is remote. However, it *is* a realistic possibility in the professional ethics of the health professions where agreement on the *telos* of the healing relationship is more likely to arise. Nevertheless, virtue-based ethics must be related conceptually and normatively to other ethical theories in a comprehensive moral philosophy of the health professions.

INTRODUCTION

In his highly influential work, *After Virtue,* Alasdair MacIntyre[1] details the decline of virtue-based ethics since the Enlightenment and the obstacles to its restoration absent a community of shared values to sustain it. In this essay I shall start with MacIntyre's conclusions and examine the possibility of a restoration of virtue-based ethics to normative status in ethics generally and, more specifically, in the ethics of medicine and the health professions.

Pellegrino, Edmund. "Toward a Virtue-Based Normative Ethics for the Health Care Professions". Kennedy Institute of Ethics Journal 5:3 (1995), 253-277.

I will argue: (1) that virtue-based ethics has lost its normative force because the moral philosophy on which it was based for so long is no longer intact in either general or professional ethics; (2) that, for a variety of reasons, the recovery of a common moral philosophy to sustain a normative theory of virtue ethics is too remote at the moment to be a viable possibility in general ethics; but (3) that virtue likely can be restored as a normative concept in the ethics of the health professions; and (4) that even in this limited realm, virtue cannot stand alone, but must be related to other ethical theories in a more comprehensive moral philosophy than currently exists.

This essay is divided into three parts: the first traces the origins, erosion, and present-day revival of the Classical-Medieval conception of virtue with particular emphasis on the reasons for its metamorphosis and decline; the second part provides a similar analysis of the concept of virtue in the ethics of medicine and the other health professions with an emphasis on the possibilities and requirements for its restoration as a normative concept; and the third part suggests how virtue-based ethics could be related to other major contemporary ethical theories in an integrated view of the four essential elements of the moral life, namely, agent, act, circumstance, and consequence.

ORIGIN, DECLINE, AND RESTORATION OF VIRTUE-BASED ETHICS

The Idea of Virtue Ethics

Virtue is the most ancient, durable, and ubiquitous concept in the history of ethical theory. This is so because one cannot completely separate the character of a moral agent from his or her acts, the nature of those acts, the circumstances under which they are performed, or their consequences. Virtue theories focus on the agent; on his or her intentions, dispositions, and motives; and on the kind of person the moral agent becomes, wishes to become, or ought to become as a result of his or her habitual disposition to act in certain ways. These phenomena are ineradicable elements of the moral life and any moral theory that ignores them fails to encompass the fullness and complexity of the challenge and struggle to be a good human being.

In a purely virtue-based ethic, the normative standard is the good person, the person upon whom one can rely habitually to be good and to do the good under all circumstances. This standard has been both the strength and the weakness of virtue-based ethics, the reason for its durability, but also for its fragility because of the circularity of its logic. The challenge is to provide a normative force for virtue outside of the circular logic that holds the right and the good to be what the virtuous person takes them to be while defining the virtuous person as the one who is and does what is right and good.

Every culture has a notion of the virtuous person—i.e., a paradigm person, real or idealized, who sets the standards of noble conduct for a culture and whose character traits exemplify the kind of person others in that culture ought to be or to emulate. These paradigm persons are celebrated in the myths and stories, poetry and ritual, of Non-Western and Western cultures. The moral values and characteristics of these virtuous persons are given formal expression in the philosophy and theology of each era and culture. They are formalized in varying degrees in the words of Plato and

Aristotle, the philosophy of Confucius[2] and Lao Tse,[3,4] the Hindu concept of Dharma,[5] and the humanism of African tribal cultures.[6] Often the paradigm figures, such as Jesus, Buddha, or Confucius, antedated the community of values that would sustain them. In fact, frequently, the community of values and beliefs was framed on the model and through the person and personality of the paradigm virtuous person. The intricacies and the primacy of the mutual relationship between paradigm virtuous persons and communities of values have yet to be explored in depth.

The Classical-Medieval Conception—Origins

In the Western culture, the most pervasive and enduring concept of virtue, the one most formally and fully developed, is found in the thought of Plato and Aristotle, supplemented by the Stoics and Epicureans,[7,8] and brought to full fruition by Thomas Aquinas. The fusion of those streams of thought became the Classical-Medieval synthesis that has shaped moral philosophy in the West for 2,500 years. Although it has gone through a variety of metamorphoses and decline over the centuries, the Classical-Medieval notion of virtue is re-emerging today among influential moral philosophers and is seeking its place among more recent normative ethical theories. This Classical-Medieval conception of virtue has also been the dominant one in the ethics of the health professions as professions. For this reason, it is the operative concept in this discussion of where to go "beyond virtue" in the wake of *After Virtue*.[9]

The Classical-Medieval synthesis has been the subject of intense scholarly exegesis for centuries. There is still much debate about various facets of the traditional notion of virtue—whether the virtues are one or many, how the doctrine of the mean (i.e., virtue as a mean state that lies between the extremes, the "vices," of excess and deficiency) applies to them, whether they can be in conflict, what "list" of virtues should prevail, and the like. An adequate discussion of these questions is beyond the confines of this essay, however. Rather, I have selected what I take to be the elements of the Classical-Medieval synthesis that are most important for a resuscitation of virtue-based ethics in the health professions—i.e., the idea of virtue (1) as excellence in traits of character, (2) as a trait oriented to ends and purposes (that is to say, teleologically), (3) as an excellence of reason not emotion, (4) as centered on practical judgment, and (5) as learned by practice.

In and through the character of Socrates, Plato first advanced the idea of virtue as *areté* —i.e., excellence in the knowledge of the good, which made for a good and happy life. On this view, knowledge of the good disposes one to the good life and to happiness. The search for one's own good is "the cornerstone of Socrates's moral philosophy"[10]; the virtue one possesses makes one good. Vice is the result of ignorance of the good. Throughout his dialogues, Plato developed a list of the virtues: fortitude (*Laches),* temperance (*Charmides),* justice (*Republic),* and wisdom, which with self-restraint (*sophrosyne*), characterized the virtuous person. This list has survived as a list of the cardinal virtues—i.e., those that might subsume, or be the basis for, the other virtues. Socrates asks, but never satisfactorily answers, the questions that are still asked: Are the virtues one or many? How are they acquired? Can they be taught?[11] (*Meno* 70a)

Aristotle retains the idea of excellence and adds a strong emphasis on the *telos*, the orientation of virtues to the ends and purposes of human activity. He defines virtue as "...the state of character which makes a person good and makes that person to do his or her work well..." (*Nicomachean Ethics* (*NE*) 1106a22-24*)*.[12] Thus, for Aristotle, the teleological orientation of virtue is two-fold—the fulfillment of the natural end of human life, namely happiness, and also the attainment of the end of human work. Aristotle links being a good person with doing well whatever one does and with achieving, to the greatest extent possible, the end of any human activity whether it be the conduct of the whole of one's life or the conduct of a particular work related to the role or roles one plays in everyday life.

On this view, virtue is a character trait under rational control. Virtue is not a "habit" in the sense of being an unconscious reflex. Rather it is a *habitus,* a predictable disposition to choose the good whenever confronted with a choice (*NE* 1105a27-33).[13] A virtuous person has knowledge of the good and chooses it for its own sake and from a firm character with regard to the passions (*NE* 1105b21-23).[14] The virtuous person must not only know the good but *be* good (*NE* 1102b26, 1148b18).[15] In contrast to Plato and Socrates, Aristotle takes account of emotion more clearly, but defines the virtuous person as one whose emotions are ordered by reason to the end of happiness.

Virtue is also practical in its orientation. For this reason, Aristotle's central virtue is *phronesis* or practical wisdom. Moral agents must consider what is appropriate to the occasion: "Virtue determines the end; practical wisdom makes us do what is conducive to the end" (*NE* 1145a5-6).[16] Thus, *phronesis* is the virtue that enables one to deliberate well in making moral judgments and to choose the means most suited to the end of the activity in which one is engaged. Practical wisdom is a "...true and reasoned capacity to act with regard to the things that are good or bad for men" (*NE* 1140b5).[17] *Phronesis* fuses the intellectual virtues, which have truth as their end—e.g., science, art, intuitive wisdom—with the moral virtues, which have the good as their end. The good person is the *phronimos*, the person of practical wisdom; the virtuous act is the act as it would be chosen by the *phronimos.*

Aristotle criticizes Plato's ethics as too general (*Politics* 1260a25)[18] and unmindful of the emotions (*Magna Moralia* 1182a20).[19] In keeping with his emphasis on the practical, Aristotle teaches that virtue is, itself, learned by practice. Thus, he answers in the affirmative one of the questions Meno put to Socrates (*Meno* 70a). By repeatedly acting in conformity with the ends of human life, as the man of practical wisdom would act, a person becomes habitually disposed to act virtuously. One can then depend on the virtuous person to act well in all circumstances.

Aristotle recognizes that certain things ought never be done—e.g., adultery, murder, and theft—and certain dispositions ought never be adopted—e.g., spite and envy (*NE* 1107a10-11).[20] With the exception of those acts and dispositions that do not allow of a mean, Aristotle does not lay down rules, duties, or principles. We must be "content" with the "...truth roughly and in outline..." (*NE* 1094b20).[21] Instead, in general, "...excellence is a state of choice lying in a mean related to us and in the way in which the man of practical wisdom would determine it" (*NE* 1107a1-3).[22]

Aristotle's mean is not just a mean between extremes; it is also the right amount for a given individual, determined not subjectively, but rationally as the man of practical wisdom would determine it.[23] The morally good is what the virtuous person does; the virtuous person is one who does what is morally good.

Thomas Aquinas,[24] in his great study of Christian theology and Greek philosophy, develops a virtue-based ethics that begins with the same elements as Aristotle's (*Summa Theologiae* (*ST*) II-II, 108: 2 and *ST* I-II, 119: 8-15).[25] He defines virtue very much as Aristotle does: "It belongs to human virtue to make a man and his work according to reason" (*ST* II-II, 108: 2).[26] He posits truth as the end of the natural intellectual virtues and the good of humans as the end of the natural moral virtues. However, drawing on Christian theology, Aquinas adds the theological virtues of faith, hope, and charity. These virtues dispose humans to attain their supernatural end—union with God in the beatific vision. The infused virtues orient humans to their ultimate end of union with God: faith orients to that end, hope enables the Christian to stay the course, and charity attaches the Christian to God (*ST* I-II, 119: 8-15).[27] Of the theological virtues, charity or love is the ordering virtue.[28]

For Aquinas, as for Aristotle, practical wisdom is a central virtue. Prudence is analogous to *phronesis.* Its function is the actualization of the other virtues in attainment of the goals of human life.[29] Not only does prudence link the intellectual and the moral virtues, as it does in Aristotle, but it also links those virtues to the theological virtues. Prudence is a "*recta ration agibilium,*" a right way of acting according to reason.[30] It disposes persons to choose means that most closely fit the *telos* of an act. Prudence is the virtue that sorts out the other virtues when they might be in conflict and provides practical judgment and discernment in complex circumstances thereby giving its possessor the capacity to select the means that will most closely approximate the end of a particular human activity.

The Classical-Medieval Conception—Decline

Both the Classical and the Medieval Christian conceptions of virtue were based on a clear moral epistemology and metaphysics. They were rooted in the conviction that there existed an objective moral order and a philosophy of human nature ascertainable by human reason, which, in turn, defined the *telos* for human activity. The virtues were traits that habitually disposed humans to act in accord with the ends of human nature—i.e., fulfillment in natural happiness for Socrates, Plato, and Aristotle and supernatural happiness in union with God for Aquinas. On this view, the virtues have normative force not because they are agreeable or admired but because they accord well with, and predispose to, the ends, the purposes, and the good of human beings as defined by an underlying metaphysics.

In the post-Medieval and post-Enlightenment periods up to the present, these metaphysical foundations for virtue ethics were seriously eroded by the confluence of a variety of forces. The possibility of a metaphysical definition of human nature or the good, the epistemological possibility of moral knowledge, and the possibility of a philosophical anthropology were all subjected to skepticism and denial. Beginning in the Enlightenment, theology, religious authority, and even reason were challenged as sources of morality. Aristotelian philosophy and the methods of scholasticism were especially suspect in science and theology. Hobbes and Locke replaced the Classical and Medieval philosophies of human nature with "realism" about the dubious nature of human motives and conduct; Hutcheson and Hume advanced moral psychology to counter the over-rationalization of Classical and Medieval ethics.[31] Virtues were replaced by a variety of competing concepts: rights for Locke, duty for Kant, moral sentiment for Hume and Smith, and consequences and utility for Bentham and Mill.[32,33]

From its inception, the concept of virtue had strong opponents who ridiculed it as a basis for morality. Glaucon, Ademantus, and, later, Thrasymachus, in Plato's *Republic* and Callicles in the *Gorgias* attacked the idea of virtue as unrealistic and vulnerable to submersion by power and self-interest. Later philosophers reinforced this anti-virtue bias. Machiavelli[34] maintained that the virtuous person was doomed in a world in which others were not virtuous; Mandeville[35] argued that vice was necessary for the survival of the economy and society; and Nietzsche thought virtue, especially the Christian virtues, was a mark of weakness unbecoming the Superman.[36,37] More recently, Ayn Rand,[38] voicing the implicit ethics of the marketplace, condemned the traditional conception of virtue as inimical to the ethos of success.

The concept of virtue survived these assaults in a revised form. As the philosophical foundations of the Classical-Medieval synthesis eroded, virtue was redefined in terms of the emergent newer schools of philosophy. For present purposes, only a few of the multitudinous revisions need be mentioned as examples: Hume[39] sees virtue as "...a quality of mind agreeable to, or approved by, everyone who considers or contemplates it." For Kant,[40] virtue is the coincidence of the rational will with every duty firmly settled in the character. For Bentham,[41] as one might expect of a utilitarian, a virtue is a trait that disposes its possessor to increase the quantity of happiness. Many other definitions followed, each framed in terms of an underlying philosophical system. The result was the eclipse of virtue as a normative concept by intuition, moral psychology, maxims, rules, and principles.

In the twentieth century, the revolution against a metaphysical or theological foundation for ethics came to full fruition. The history of this revolution is complicated beyond the scope of this paper. Suffice it to say that ethics turned to meta-analysis, to the dissection of the language of moral discourse, to the intuitive grasp of the good or of *prima facie* principles discoverable by morally mature persons, or to a variety of alternatives to principles, such as casuistry, hermeneutics, feminist psychology, care theory, or narrative. At present, these theories and a revitalized virtues-based ethics are in competition with each other. They share a repudiation of the philosophical and theological groundings that have traditionally given virtue-based ethics its normative thrust. Each of the theories holds one or another of the shards of the Classical-Medieval synthesis—i.e., of virtue-based ethics—without the philosophical cement to repair the damage done.

Virtue-Based Ethics—The Revival

Despite the convolutions in the concept of virtue wrought by a succession of philosophical systems, the ideas of virtue and the virtuous person were never erased.

Ethicists continued to confront the question of character of the agent. Principles, rules, maxims, intuitions, language analysis, and technical skill involving moral puzzles did not encompass the full complexity of the moral life. The central nature of the character of the moral agent could not totally be ignored.[42] As a result, several decades ago, a number of contemporary moral philosophers began to revive the idea of virtue and to seek a place for it in ethical theory.[43-48]

The philosophers who were most successful in doing so found it necessary first to revive, or at least to revise, the philosophical or theological substratum on which classical virtue theory had been built—either in Plato, Aristotle, Aquinas, or their commentators. It remains to be seen how successful these attempts to restore virtue will be in general ethical theory given the post-Modernist doubts about the utility of philosophical ethics or even of philosophy itself—especially in its current anti-foundationalist mind set.[49,50] It seems unlikely that a robust virtue ethics can be reconstructed since the probability of agreement on a conception of the good or the *telos* of human life is remote indeed. Such agreement is required, however, for any normative theory of virtue as "...a corrective to the tendency to act against the good,"[51] or any trait that ameliorates the human condition[52] or enhances evolutionary adaptation.[53,54]

MacIntyre has most successfully built on the Aristotelian notion of virtue and reformulated it in more contemporary terms, taking into account the erosion of the tradition and the moral consensus that gave the classical doctrine its normative strength. MacIntyre[55] builds his definition on three elements; he regards virtues as dispositions or acquired qualities that are: (1) necessary to achieve the good internal to practices,* (2) necessary to sustain communities in which individuals can seek a higher good as the good of their own lives, and (3) necessary to sustain traditions that provide necessary historical contexts for individual lives. Virtue, thus, is a character trait necessary to achievement of a good—a perfected excellence.[57] In this, MacIntyre adopts the teleological thrust of the Aristotelian definition of virtue and adds to it the sustaining force of a historical community of values.

This is not the place to evaluate MacIntyre's reformulation. However, he does make a genuine attempt to recapture some of the Aristotelian notion of virtue. MacIntyre[58] clearly recognizes the difficulties that his reformulation faces in the absence of a shared notion of the good or a community of values to sustain it. In a more Platonic vein, Iris Murdoch[59] also recognizes the need for and the difficulty of recovering a conception of the good as a foundation of moral life and of the virtues. Murdoch intimates strongly that the good has to confront religious reality as well, although she does not locate the good in formalized religious belief system. In this, she counts virtue as "...the most evident bridge between morality and religion."[60]

* MacIntyre defines a practice as: "...any coherent and complex form of socially established cooperative human activity through which goods internal to that form of activity are realized in the course of trying to achieve those standards of excellence which are appropriate to, and partially definitive of, that form of activity, with the result that human powers to achieve excellence, and human conceptions of the ends and goods involved, are systematically extended."[56]

In any case, the improbability of any recovery of the philosophical or theological substructures of virtue compounds the difficulties of a contemporary revival so far as general ethical theory is concerned. This is amply evident in the incommensurability of premises and methodologies characteristic of general theories of ethics. However, these impediments are less formidable in professional ethics, particularly in medicine and the other health professions. It is here that genuine possibilities for a restoration and reformulation of virtue ethics exist.

Difficulties Inherent in the Classical-Medieval Synthesis

Before turning to the possibility of restoring virtue ethics in the health professions, it may be well to examine the inherent difficulties of any virtue-based ethics as a normative theory. If virtue is to be restored to normative status, these difficulties must be acknowledged and addressed.

First is the circularity of justification to which I have already alluded, namely, that the good is that which the virtuous person does and the virtuous person is the person who does what is good for humans. Some grounding for virtue outside of this circular logic is necessary if the redundancy of this logic is to be avoided. Otherwise, virtue can become so intuitive and subjective as to be meaningless. What is virtue to one person's community is vice to another's. What some find "agreeable"—to use Hume's term—others find disagreeable with equal intensity.

In the Classical and Medieval construals of virtue, its grounding was in the ends and purposes derived from an underlying philosophical anthropology based in natural law. Within this anthropology, virtues could be defined, rejected, and even ordered with respect to one another. Their normative power arose not from their simple, intuitive affirmation as virtues but from the congruence of virtues with something more fundamental to which virtues and virtuous persons themselves conformed. This grounding is the antidote to the multiplicity of definitions and the proliferation of lists of the virtues—lists that sometimes grow to ridiculous proportions and include every imaginable agreeable trait form the most profound to the most trivial. Instrumental, moral, intellectual, and spiritual virtues become intermingled with "values," beliefs, preferences, tastes, and the like. Any characteristic agreeable to someone can be touted as a virtue.*

A second difficulty in virtue-based ethics is the paucity of the definitive action guidelines that give principles, rules, and maxims their force—at least in the abstract. A virtue-based ethics depends upon the grasp by the virtuous person of the good for humans in such a reliable way that, no matter what the act or the circumstances may be, that person will know how to attain the good. Such an open-ended guide to moral choice is sustainable only if there is, in fact, some agreement on the good for humans. A shared notion of the good gave focus to Aristotle's *Nicomachean Ethics* and *Eudemian Ethics,* to the Platonic dialogues, and to Aquinas's *Summa Theologiae.* But it is disagreement on the good that divides modern and contemporary ethical and

* Pincoffs expands Hume's notion of agreeableness into a bewildering list of likeable qualities that he considers virtuous.[61]

metaphysical theory. So much is this the case that many deem futile the pursuit of a definition of the good beyond intuition.[62] With many goods being equally defensible, there will be many interchangeable virtues and vices. The contemporary inclination of philosophy is to abandon the quest for the good, to define it by intuitive grasp only, or to deny its existence altogether.

Third is the difficulty of supererogation. The classical insistence on the virtues as excellence seems to demand too much. In a legalistically shaped society—one that, in addition, emphasizes individual choices and lifestyles—even the narrow idea of role-related responsibilities and duties is challenged. The only duty is not to infringe on the liberty of others. Everything else is beyond duty. In such a setting, virtue in the classical sense is too much to ask of individuals or communities and institutions.

Some would argue that the possession of virtues and the accompanying disposition to excellence is entirely fortuitous, the product of genetics, environment, or luck.[63,64] How, in justice, can we demand virtue from those who do not possess it innately? How do we attribute virtuous behavior to those who are genetically disposed to it? Is it not unfair to impose a demand for supererogation on those who are congenitally indisposed to even ordinary duties? Without the classical notion of virtue as an "excellence" consciously and rationally practiced, it may be difficult to see virtue as "virtuous."

Any viable normative account of virtue-based ethics must somehow engage these difficulties and objections. As I have already suggested, in our times at least, this is so formidable a task in general ethics that it likely is destined for failure. However, as I now hope to show, there is a reasonable possibility of satisfying the requirements for a normative virtue-based ethics in the more limited case of professional ethics.

VIRTUE-BASED ETHICS IN MEDICINE—HISTORY AND REVIVAL

Origins and Metamorphosis

The history of the concept of virtue in medical ethics follows in general outline the history of the origin and metamorphosis of virtue in general ethics that I have described. However, in medicine, virtue ethics resisted erosion for a longer period of time, and change, when it did come, did so over a period of twenty-five years, rather than the five or six centuries that it took in general ethics.

Therefore, in medical ethics, as in general ethics, virtue was the dominant normative theory for a long period of time. It is the basis for the Hippocratic Oath and the deontological books of the Hippocratic Corpus. In the Medieval world, as in the present, the Hippocratic ethic was joined with the ethics of the major world religions. For centuries, that ethic united physicians across cultural and national boundaries in a community of moral values based in the virtues of benevolence, respect for human life, and the vulnerability of the sick.

A quarter of a century ago, the dominance of virtue in medical ethics began to diminish for three reasons: First was the introduction of principle-based ethics,[65] which appealed to health professionals as being more definitive than virtue because of its concreteness and applicability to clinical decisions. Second, socio-political change toward participatory democracy, greater public education, distrust of authority, and the character failings of some physicians focused public attention on autonomy-based, contractual relationships rather than trust-based, covenantal ones. Third, and importantly, the religious and philosophical consensus that undergirded professional ethics, at least in the West, was challenged and weakened.[66]

Today, as a result, medical professional ethics is gradually being deconstructed as its conceptual substratum is progressively challenged. The Hippocratic Oath, the backbone of traditional medical professional ethics, is in danger of complete dissolution. It is already defunct in the minds of some very creditable ethicists[67]—done in by the societal pressures to substitute autonomy or social justice for beneficence and to relax the proscriptions against abortion, euthanasia, assisted suicide, breaches of confidentiality, and sexual relations with patients. In any gathering today, it would be difficult to find a commonly accepted set of precepts or virtues that should characterize the "good" physician.[68]

These changes are occurring in the domain of *professional* ethics—i.e., the domain of duties, obligations, and virtues entailed in the health professional's roles as a healer and as a participant in a special kind of relationship with a patient. Professional ethics centers on the generic obligations of the healing relationship, those common to physicians as physicians, nurses as nurses, and so on. Professional ethics is the realm of the ethics of the physician- or nurse-patient relationship. This realm is a domain distinct from the growing body of other ethical issues commonly subsumed under the rubric of "bioethics"—i.e., the issues of withholding or withdrawing life-support, euthanasia and assisted suicide, embryo research, organ and tissue transplantation, managed care, and the like; the whole panorama of new issues growing out of medical technological advances.

These are the "content" questions of bioethics—the questions that have become so problematic as a result of the loss of consensus about the meanings, purposes, and value of human life. Given the pluralism, the relativism, and the privatization of morals, there seems to be little hope for agreement on such questions at the moment. Recovery of a normative role for the virtue in such circumstances without agreement on the philosophical foundations for the virtues is quite remote. To recognize this fact is not to admit that moral truth is impossible or that virtue is no longer a viable concept, but only to suggest that a first, and more practical, step to confine consideration of a restoration of virtue-based ethics to professional ethics. Whether this opening later will extend into the realm of specific moral choices that are of such consuming interest in bioethics is unforeseeable at this time.

I will now address the reasons that professional ethics is a promising prospect for virtue ethics; what the requirements for a viable, normative ethics might be; and how those requirements might be satisfied.

The Restoration of Virtue in Professional Ethics

The Opportunity

There are several good reasons to suppose that a return to virtue is a reasonable probability in professional ethics. Paradoxically, some of the reasons arise from the deficiencies now being perceived in the dominant school of principle-based moral guidelines; others stem from the more limited scope of professional ethics within the larger field of bioethics.

First is the growing disquiet in the last decade with some of the limitations of principle-based ethics. Principles are thought to be too abstract, too removed from the contextual and experiential complexity of clinical decision making, and too conducive to an overly rationalistic, quasi-legalistic ethics that over-emphasizes quandaries and stifles compassion and moral creativity.[69,70]

Second is the criticism that *prima facie* principles need to be grounded in some more fundamental philosophical system to give them the normative weight they must carry. Such a foundation is needed to resolve conflict between and among principles in more than a pragmatic and functional way—perhaps even to give them a lexical ordering in specific situations, if not generally.

Third is the persistent appreciation that moral agents—i.e., personas acting—cannot be left out of moral judgments. This fact has hovered over general and medical ethics even in the period of its most radical change. The moral life is a life peculiar to the human species. The way in which principles, rules, caring, hermeneutics, casuistry, or any other alternative theory of ethics is conducted will depend on the kind of persons carrying out the moral acts and their analyses. Intention, moral psychology, and the "story" of the agent's life cannot be separated from the agent's moral behavior. To avoid looking at virtue and intentions and to assume that the only justification for moral acts lies in principles are thought by many to favor the right over the good.

These shortcomings in principle-based ethics are reinforced on the positive side by the nature of professional ethics. Unlike general ethics, professional ethics offers the possibility of some agreement on a *telos*—i.e., an end and a good. In a healing relationship between a health care professional and a patient, most would agree that the primary end must be the good of the patient. The healing relationship itself provides a phenomenological grounding for professional ethics that applies to all healers by virtue of the kind of activity that healing entails. In general ethics, on the other hand, at least at present, the analogous possibility for agreement on something so fundamental as the *telos*, end, or good of human life is so remote as to be practically unattainable.

The Necessary Ingredients

At a minimum, any normative theory of the ethics of the healing relationship based in virtue will require the following: (1) a theory of medicine to define the *telos*, the good of medicine as an activity; (2) a definition of virtue in terms of that theory; and (3) a set of virtues entailed by the theory to characterize the "good" health professional.

A *theory of medicine.* David Thomasma and I[71,72] have outlined a theory of medicine in some detail elsewhere. For the purposes of this essay, I will simply summarize that theory from which I will draw the *telos* and, thus, the virtues of the good physician or nurse.[73] The theory is grounded in three phenomena of the healing relationship, in the realities and actualities of the clinical encounter that establish medicine and nursing as particular kinds of human activity[74]: the fact of illness, the act of profession, and the act of medicine (healing).

The fact of illness. Persons become *patients* when they acknowledge that they are sufficiently concerned over a physical or psychological symptom to believe they need help. In this state, to varying degrees, they are anxious, dependent, in pain, disabled, and extremely vulnerable and exploitable. They are no longer free to pursue the things they want out of life without impediment. If they are to be helped, healed, and cared for, they must seek out a health professional, someone who possesses the knowledge to accomplish these ends for, and with, them.

The act of profession. To move from a state of health to a state of illness is an experiential and existential change in the way we perceive our humanity. In that vulnerable state of illness, the physician or nurse asks, "How may I help you?" Implicit in the question is the promise that the health professional possesses the knowledge needed to help and to heal and intends to use it in the interests of the patient and not at the expense of the patient's vulnerability. This "act of profession" is an act of implicit promise making that establishes a covenant of trust at the physician's or nurse's voluntary instigation. This self-imposed trust covenant imposes obligations on the professional from the moment it is made.

The act of healing. The promise made to the dependent patient directs the knowledge, techniques, and personal commitment of the physician or nurse to the *telos* of the relationship—helping and healing. The diagnostic, prognostic, and therapeutic acts—which are manipulative, judgmental, cognitive, and so on—must be directed to what is necessary to heal and to help *this* patient, to a technically correct and morally good decision and action. This is the immediate *telos* of the clinical encounter, which is, in turn, part of the ultimate *telos* of health care—the cultivation and restoration of health and the containment or cure of disease. To be sure, healing may occur outside of medicine and the health professions, but that which is specific to the health professions is the attainment of the *telos* of healing through the science and the art of medicine as a particular kind of human activity.

A Definition of Professional Virtue

The second ingredient of a virtue-based normative theory of medial ethics is a definition of virtue in terms of the *telos* of the clinical encounter. This encounter defines medicine as the kind of activity it is. A definition suited to professional activity would draw on the elements of virtue as defined by Aristotle and its adaptation to practices as defined by MacIntyre.

Drawing on these two sources, I define a virtue as a trait of character that disposes its possessor habitually to excellence of intent and performance with respect to the *telos* specific to human activity. Virtue gives to reason the power to discern and to will the motivation asymptotically to accomplish a moral end with perfection. For any profession, there will be a specific activity that, if executed well, makes the professional good or virtuous. Healing is the activity specific to nursing and medicine. Those dispositions that impart the capacity to heal well are the virtues of medicine, nursing, dentistry, and the like. They are the virtues "internal"—in MacIntyre's

(1981, p. 187) sense—to the practice. Possession of these internal virtues defines the good nurse or physician.

A List of Virtues

The third ingredient of a virtue-based normative theory of medical ethics is a list of virtues that will define the "good" physician, nurse, or other health professional. These are the virtues entailed by the phenomena of the relationship and the *telos* of medicine. They are the virtues essential to achieving the ends of medicine optimally and without which those ends would be frustrated or attained in less than optimal fashion.

Lists of virtues are notoriously difficult to compose. The following list is not meant to be inclusive of all the virtues necessary to healing. Rather, the virtues included are those most essential to the healing purposes of the clinical encounter. In that sense, they are "entailed" by the end of the healing relationship, that is, they are required if the end is to be attained. The virtues are not listed in order of preference. They reinforce each other so closely that to compromise one is to compromise the others. A lexical order among them would be difficult to defend.

Fidelity to Trust and Promise

This virtue is entailed by the ineradicability of trust in the patient-nurse or patient-physician relationship, the invitation of the professional to trust when the relationship is initiated, the importance of trust to healing, and the fact that, ultimately, the patient has no choice but to trust the professional.

Benevolence

This virtue intends the good of the patient. It is a *sine qua non* since the patient obviously seeks to be helped not harmed. Intending every act to be in the patient's interest is the gold standard of medical ethics.

Effacement of Self-Interest

Given the exploitability and vulnerability of patients, a certain degree of self-effacement is entailed since without it the patient can become merely a means to advance the physician's power, prestige, profit, or pleasure. In these days of managed and for-profit care, the need for effacement of self-interest is urgent if the patient is to be protected against exploitation.

Compassion and Caring

If the patient is to be healed in the fullest sense, the physician or nurse must have compassion—i.e., the health professional must be able to feel something of the patient's experience of the predicament of illness. Such feeling is essential to adjusting the treatment to the particularities of *this* patient's life story, time of life, and so forth. Compassion is the prelude to caring—to concern, empathy, and consideration for the patient's plight. On this view, caring in its several meanings[75] is more in the realm of virtue ethics than being an ethical theory of its own.

Intellectual Honesty

By virtue of the trust that health professionals enjoy and the power of knowledge and skill they exercise, physicians and nurses can be agents of great harm as well as great good. Acknowledging when one does not know something and being humble enough to admit ignorance is a virtue of healing. Knowing when to say "I do not know" is a virtue counseled by sources as different as the Babylonian Talmud and Galileo.

Justice

In the healing relationship per se, the virtue of commutative justice is implicit throughout. Commutative justice dictates that in interpersonal relationships what is owed to each is rendered to each and equals are treated equally. Taken as a principle, justice is blindfolded and applied strictly. But taking justice as a virtue in the healing relationship requires removing the blindfold and adjusting what is owed to the specific needs of the patient, even if those needs do not fit the definition of what is strictly owed.

Furthermore, when the physician is bound by a covenant of trust to *this* patient, distributive justice—what is owed to others in a more distant relationship to the physician—takes a lesser place. After all, the covenant, the promise to help, is made to an identifiable sick person, not to society at large nor to the managed care organization, nor even to other patients with similar needs. As I have argued elsewhere, this does not excuse the physician from societal justice outside of the covenant with a given patient here and now.[76]

Prudence

Practical wisdom, the virtue of deliberation and discernment, was central to Aristotle's virtue theory as *phronesis* and to Aquinas's as prudence. It is equally central to any theory of virtue in the health professions since any clinical decision of note requires prudent weighing of the alternatives in situations of uncertainty and stress. Knowing how to unscramble apparent conflict among the virtues, understanding their relationships to one another, and selecting the means by which to approximate most closely the *telos* of any particular healing relationship are essential tasks for the virtue of prudence in the health professions.

At a minimum, the foregoing seven virtues are entailed by the nature of the physician- or nurse-patient encounter. They can be supplemented by other virtues, but most others will be variants of these basic seven. One might argue that even the seven virtues could be reduced to benevolence, fidelity to trust, and prudence. Such a reduction begins to touch on Meno's question to Socrates about whether the virtues are one or many. In the end, however, it is less important to answer this question than to agree on a notion of the good for humans engaged in a healing relationship and on some list of virtues that are required to achieve the good within a community of healers (the profession) who can sustain that conception of the good.

VIRTUE CANNOT STAND ALONE

The schema of virtues for the health profession that I have outlined can give normative force to professional virtues, but, by itself, it is insufficient to constitute a comprehensive normative theory of ethics. The inherent difficulties of virtue as a normative concept are not, thereby, fully resolved. We may have gained insight into the kind of person the moral agent is, or is striving to become. We may also have given the verses—at least those pertinent to being a good professional—the philosophical foundation they require if they are to have normative form. Still needed, however, is a description of the way in which the ethics of the agent that is expressed in a virtue-based ethics relates to the ethics of the other elements of a moral event.

Granting the undeniable fact of moral agency, no matter what theory of ethics one follows, it remains to give an account of the nature of the act, the circumstances under which it takes place, and the consequences of the act. These are realities of "moral event," i.e., specific instances of moral conduct essential to moral judgment and justification. In the act, the circumstances, and the consequences lie those additional contextual complexities that the present upsurge of alternative theories of ethics seeks to encompass. Each alternative adds to our understanding of some important facet of moral judgment. Each illuminates the other theories as well. Like virtue theory, each is necessary, but not sufficient, as a normative theory.

Figure 1 depicts schematically how some families of ethical theories focus on different but interrelated elements in any moral event:

FIGURE 1. THE MORAL EVENT

	Agent	Act	Circumstance	Consequence
Theories	virtue	deontology	particularizing theories	teleology
Foci	character intention desire choice will accountability caring	right good duty rule maxim	caring for this person or group in this place, time, etc. narrative, culture, uniqueness of the person experience "situation ethics" casuistry	outcomes harms/goods pain/pleasure utility calculus

Virtue theories focus on the agent and his or her character as it is expressed in, and influenced by, intention, desire, choice, strength of will, and caring (in the sense of feeling for others). Accountability, innocence, and guilt are resultant of the interplay of these factors in the character of the agent. Many of these foci are in the realm of moral psychology. As such, they can impart understanding, but they are not ^normative. Moral psychology helps us to understand how and why a person might be the kind of person he or she *is*, but not the kind of person he or she *ought* to be.

Deontological theories focus on the act itself, on whether it is right and good—in keeping with some moral standard, i.e., a principle, rule, maxim, or duty, that is, itself, derived from an underlying moral philosophy. The agent is judged by whether, and to what degree, his or her moral conduct is in accord with a universalizable norm from which specific actions, rules, or guidelines are derived. The standard may be utility, beneficence, justice, or Kant's Categorical Imperative. Deontological theories have a normative force and a specificity not shared by concepts like virtue or caring. The specificity of principles is abstract, however. With deontological theories, there is always the difficulty of closing the gap between general moral rules and their application in particular moral events.

A whole family of theories are "particularizing" in the sense that they focus upon and emphasize the moral situation, the circumstances and the historical, cultural, and personal features that make each moral event unique. These are precisely the details on the other side of the gap that must be crossed in the application of principles or virtues. Some recent examples are: ethical theories based on narrative and story, lived experience, historico-cultural or genetic predispositions, caring for particular persons, casuistry, and hermeneutics. This family of theories fills in the rich detail of a moral event not capturable by virtue-based or deontological theories. Particularizing theories, like theories of moral psychology, are most valid for explanatory and heuristic purposes, but they are not per se normative. All particularizing theories suffer from being too closely enmeshed in concrete details to be normative—unless one is willing to accept situation ethics, and its conceptual liabilities, as a normative theory.

Finally, acts have consequences, and those consequences have moral force. If they produce harm, or more harm than good, they may be judged using a moral calculus of varying degrees of precision. The difficulties of such a calculus notwithstanding, consequences are ineradicable elements in any comprehensive normative theory. Like the other theories, consequences are linked to the circumstances and the nature of the acts in question. They are more or less independent of intentions—unless the character-damaging effects of immoral acts on the agent are taken into account as consequences.

In any case, what is evident is that full accounts of the moral life, particularly as it regards judgments of accountability and justification, require an integrated assessment of the four elements of a moral event—i.e., the agent, the act, the circumstance, and the consequence—in a relation to each other. Today's challenge is not how to demonstrate the superiority of one normative theory over the other, but rather how to relate each to the other in a matrix that does justice to each and assigns to each its proper normative force. The necessity of such an effort becomes clearer when one realizes that there are very few moralists who consistently use only one theory in their deliberations. Rather, it is a question of primacy of one theory over the others and of when one theory may be used in preference to another. If, instead of this primacy, attention is focused on the four elements of moral events, the challenge becomes one of the interrelationships between a variety of theories, each illuminating important facets of moral judgment.

I am not suggesting a feeble eclecticism, a cafeteria-style ethics, that would add a spoonful of virtue here, a principle there, and a dash of consequence in another place. Nor do I suggest a formless syncretism based in egregious compromises for the sake of a unity that enervates conflicting theories. Rather, the strength of each theory must be preserved, drawn upon, and placed in dynamic equilibrium with the others in order to accommodate the intricacy, variety, and particularity of human moral acts.

Here, as in the restoration of the normative force of virtue-based ethics, the possibility for some success is greater in the limited field of professional ethics, in which the good of the healing relationship is more easily definable than in general philosophy or in bioethics, where the nature of the good for humans is much more difficult to grasp.

CONCLUSION

The conceptual perambulations of moral philosophy over the centuries notwithstanding, virtue-based ethics continues to hover over ethical theory. This is because, being human endeavor, ethics cannot conveniently ignore the moral agent. But, if virtue ethics is to have normative force, it must break out of the circular logic that defines virtue as that which the virtuous person does and the virtuous person as one who acts virtuously. To break this circle, the concept of virtue must be defined in terms of some good, some *telos*, which the agent intends and acts to attain.

In the past, the *telos* was the good for human beings as derived form a philosophy of human nature. That *telos* and its foundation gave moral force to the virtues because of the virtues disposed a person to the good. In modern times, the philosophical notion of the good, and, consequently, of the virtues, has been seriously weakened. For a variety of reasons, there is little likelihood of recovering a common notion of the good, of the virtues, or of human nature. As a result, the recovery of normative force for virtue in general ethics is remote.

In professional ethics, however, the possibility is more realistic. Here, a definition of virtue, a theory of healing, and a list of virtues related to both are more clearly conceivable. But, even in this case, virtue-based ethics cannot stand by itself as a normative theory. It needs to be conceptually related to her ethical theories in a comprehensive, integrated moral philosophy of the health professions. The elaboration of such a moral philosophy is a daunting but necessary task for the philosophy and ethics of the health professions.

CHAPTER TEN

THE ANATOMY OF CLINICAL JUDGMENTS
Some Notes on Right Reason and Right Action

For it is uneducated not to have an eye for when it is necessary to look for proof and when this is not necessary.
Aristotle[4]

INTRODUCTION

Richard Cabot, one of the most celebrated of American diagnosticians, labeled his attempts to anatomize the process of differential diagnosis "a very dangerous topic—dangerous to the reputation of physicians for wisdom...Physicians are naturally reluctant on such matters, slow to put their thoughts to paper, and very suspicious of any attempts to tabulate their methods of reasoning."[1]

Sixty years later most clinicians remain reluctant and more than a little suspicious. Many still take refuge in the "art" and its exclusive mysteries, to resist formalization of their mental operations. In recent years, the "dangerous" subject has been boldly attacked by a few clinicians with unusual facility in the language of logic and statistics so that dissection of the tangle of science, art, and conjecture is now well underway.[2-7] They have been joined by statisticians, engineers, psychologists, and philosophers who are bringing the more sophisticated techniques of their disciplines to bear on this important and complex question.

Physicians and philosophers have puzzled for a long time over the nature of the physician's enterprise. Its dissection began with the Hippocratic physicians who first insisted on the primacy of observations of patients, refined by reason. They thus made medicine a natural science, separating it from both philosophy and religion with which it had so long been intimately associated.[8]

Intuitive, hieratic, artistic, and even magical elements of the physician's enterprise were not so easily removed, however. Celsus, the Roman Hippocrates, spoke of medicine as an "ars coniecturalis"; William Osler, the modern Hippocrates, deemed it "... a science of uncertainty and an art of probability." Medicine has yet to become a science comparable in method and explanatory power with the laboratory sciences—though this is the expressed aim of some of our contemporary thinkers.

The puzzlement continues today in the growing tension between the scientific-actuarial and the artist-intuitionist models of clinical judgment.[9] Each view tries earnestly to understand, and thus to improve, the clinical enterprise. One seeks to transform the conjectural elements into respectable science by formal analysis in terms of probabilistic logic or decision theory. Meanwhile, the other declares the nuances of clinical judgment to be an art, insusceptible to formal analysis, and improvable only by cultivation as one cultivates painting, music, or sculpture.

This essay undertakes nothing so pretentious as the resolution of what seems to be a polemically seductive polarity in viewpoints. It takes the view that: Clinical decisions can be made more rigorous logically, without reducing everything to algorithm and regression equations. While much of the process remains opaque and insusceptible to the extant methods of formal analysis, this need not forever be the case.

Much of the polarization between explanations of clinical judgment seems avoidable, if two significant features which have been neglected are sufficiently taken into account. These are: First, the overriding fact that the whole process is ordained to a specific practical end—a right action for a particular patient—and that this end must modulate each step leading to it in important ways. A value screen is thus, in a way, cast over the entire sequence. Second is the fact that no unitary explanation or logical method can encompass the several different reasoning modes and several kinds of evidence acceptable in answering the different kinds of questions the clinician must answer.

The aim of this paper is *not* to countermand the utility of scientific actuarial formulation, or offer in their stead a benignant eclecticism which allows equal place to the explicable and inexplicable, i.e., to the "science" and the "art" of clinical judgment. Rather, it hopes to locate more precisely the several reasoning modes useful at each of the sequential and simultaneous steps which eventuate ultimately in a clinical action. This localization constitutes the anatomy of clinical judgment, an essential foundation for further formalization of the process.

The complete process is a multi-step, end-oriented concatenation of decisions demanding different types of reasons and reasonings which will justify a particular course of action, for a particular patient, given that patient's particular existential situation at the time of the decision. Each step is shot through with uncertainties, some eradicable, some not. Selection of the "right" action requires optimization of these uncertainty states.

Inasmuch as the nature of the uncertainties varies, the logical instruments used to achieve optimization will vary also. Thus, the methods of deductive and inductive reasoning, of dialectic, ethics, and rhetoric are each appropriate to some step. Prudent and judicious action, rather than a true statement or scientific law, is the end to which the whole is directed. No one kind of evidence is universally applicable, and no single logical or epistemic mode suffices for all.

Customarily, discussion of clinical judgment ends at the establishment of the most probable diagnosis, or at best at the selection of a treatment. The third step—whether the treatment selected ought to be instituted, how, when, under what conditions—is usually not formally analyzed. Yet, one cannot speak legitimately of clinical judgment without seeing the whole process, particularly the way the end conditions the steps that precede it.

Four questions must be examined to sustain these assertions:

1. What is the character of the end of clinical judgment?
2. What questions must be answered in attaining that end?
3. How does the end project itself on each step, i.e., what kinds of reasons does it require?
4. What are the theoretical and practical implications of the proposed view of clinical judgment?

The answers bear to some extent on the difficult problem of a general theory of medicine. Such a theory must account for the full range of medical activity—seeking general laws of disease and treatment, but also taking specific actions in the interest of specific patients. Science, art, and the virtue of prudence infuse the several operations. But medicine justifies itself uniquely as medicine—as opposed to medicine as clinical or basic science, or as the art of performing medical acts—when it ends in a decision to act for, and in behalf of, a human who seeks to be healed.[10] To the extent that it identifies features which distinguish medicine from other human activities, the analysis of clinical judgment can contribute to the emerging structure of a theory of medicine.

WHAT IS THE END OF CLINICAL REASONING?

When a patient consults a physician, he/she does so with one specific purpose in mind: to be healed, to be restored and made whole, i.e., to be relieved of some noxious element in his/her physical or emotional life which the patient defines as dis-ease - a distortion of his/her accustomed perception of what is a satisfactory life. Usually some event has occurred—pain, lack of appetite, fatigue, trauma, a lump, spitting blood—some sign or symptom which exceeds a certain highly personalized threshold of tolerance in such fashion as to compromise, obstruct, or discolor the person's perception of him/herself and his/her health. At the point when this perception leads to the *need* to be healed, the person becomes a *patient.* This transition has two existential connotations crucial to this discussion. Becoming a patient is to become one who suffers (patior, pati), and simultaneously one to whom something is done, a recipient as distinguished from an agent (O.E.D.). The patient, then, is a suffering person who comes to the physician to have something done to assist his/her to regain hi/her former state or a more optimal one.

It is important to interject here that the term "patient" does not necessarily imply a passive restoration in which the physician is the sole agent. The patient ideally also participates in the restoration. He/she is seen as bearing a burden of illness which requires some action or decision mutually arrived at for cure to take place. The patient can yield his/her moral agency to the physician only by direct mandate. Only in the rarest circumstances will the physician legitimately be the patient's moral agent.[11,12]

The end of the medical encounter, and the process of clinical judgment through which it is achieved then, is restoration and healing—some corrective, remedial, or preventive action is directed at what the doctor and the patient perceive as a diminution of the patient's wholeness, each in his/her own fashion. The end is not a diagnosis, a scientific truth, testing an hypothesis or evaluating a treatment, though the knowledge derived therefrom enters into several states in making the decision to act.

The clinical decision comes at the end of a chain of deductive and inductive inferences, serially modified by recourse to "facts" and observations, usually themselves to some degree uncertain. Truth and certitude are, therefore, almost always problematic. Out of the uncertain conclusions of earlier syllogisms, a decision to act must be taken which has a different character from the conclusions that precede it. The conclusions of the earlier reasoning chains become premises for further reasoning. This is the normal condition of scientific reasoning—a cumulative and progressive series of hypotheses and conclusions, always open to further recourse to fact and experiment.

Each clinical decision is, however, a terminal and unique event in that it cannot remain forever open and it is not universalizable. It must close on the selection of one or a series of remedial actions—or none. The action chosen must be the "*right*" one for this patient. That is to say, it must be as congruent as possible with his/her particular clinical context, his/her values, and his/her sense of what is "worthwhile" or "good." What the physician and the patient seek together is a judicious decision, one which optimizes as many benefits and minimizes as many risks as the situation will allow. The definition of risk is highly personal, and it turns on the patient's estimate of a danger "worth" running. The end is, therefore, not a general statement of the probabilities, but a particular statement of what a particular patient *should* do.

The criteria of a right or good decision lie not in its certitude, rigor, logical or mathematical soundness, though the probability of a judicious action is enhanced greatly when these qualities inhere in the prior conclusions on which it is built. These qualities must be secured wherever possible, but they are not sufficient for a "right" decision. They can, on the view I am propounding, be displaced or modulated by the more complex criteria of a decision "good" for this patient—what among the many things that *can* be done *ought* to be done?

Clearly, value considerations and moral issues—for both the patient and the physician—can color the selection of the facts and reasons which justify placing one diagnosis over another, the justifications accepted for taking action, and the degree to which the physician persuaded or the patient assents to the final decision. The end must therefore be understood in all its fullness, because it projects itself so forcefully on the entire sequence.

The primary end of clinical judgment—a right healing action for a particular patient—imposes an atmosphere of prudence, over the whole process. Truth, for the practical intellect, is rightness with respect to human deeds, those dependent upon human will and intention. It differs thus from the truth of science which is a certain conformity with the reality it seeks to explain, and art, with the product it wishes to produce.

It is the end of medical judgment which also gives authenticity to the professions a physician makes—the he/she will use his/her knowledge and skill to "heal," according to the fullness of meaning of the word for his/her patient. Not to keep that end paramount is to make an inauthentic—indeed an immoral—profession. Medicine *qua* medicine is then more than a clinical or basic science applied to individual cases. It is a particularized knowledge of prudent healing actions, dependent upon scientific methods and art, but not synonymous with them.

Whatever formal analysis one favors—traditional syllogistics, the logic of probabilities, Bayesian conditional probabilities, decision analysis theory, information processing models, or judicial algorithms—each must account for the modulation and shaping imposed by the end. This would be so even if a high degree of certitude were possible at every step. Usually, however, we deal with varying "degrees of belief," and the judicious choice of actions becomes an even more critical and sensitive activity, difficult to formalize and formularize.

WHAT QUESTIONS MUST BE ADDRESSED AND WITH WHAT REASONING MODES?

When a person becomes a patient in the sense we have defined that state, a whole series of questions becomes crucial for him/her as a knowing and valuing being. What is wrong? Is it serious? What will it mean to me? Can it be cured, and by what means? Is the cure worthwhile? What will it cost? What *should* I do? These and corollary questions must be addressed if the process of clinical judgment is to be a complete and authentic medical judgment. They are reducible to three *generic* questions: *What can be wrong? What can be done? What should be done for this patient?* Let us look briefly at each question to see the kinds of reasoning relevant to each question, and what kinds of justifications are acceptable.

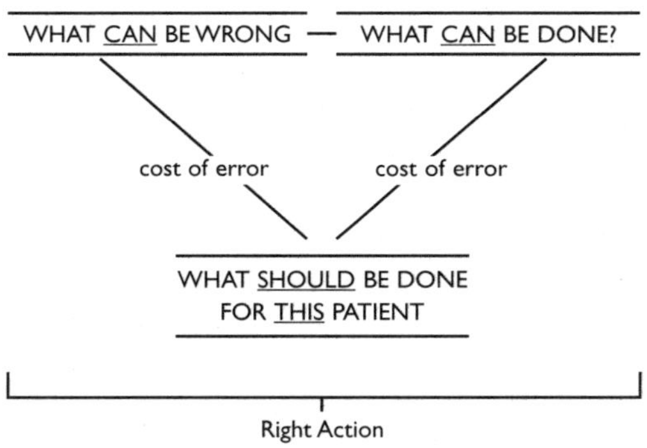

Fig. I

What can be wrong?

This is the diagnostic and classificatory question—the first part of the process and the one which has received the most vigorous theoretical examination. Given the signs and symptoms presented by this patient, what classificatory patterns fit best? Of the possible patterns, which is probable, and with what degree of certainty?

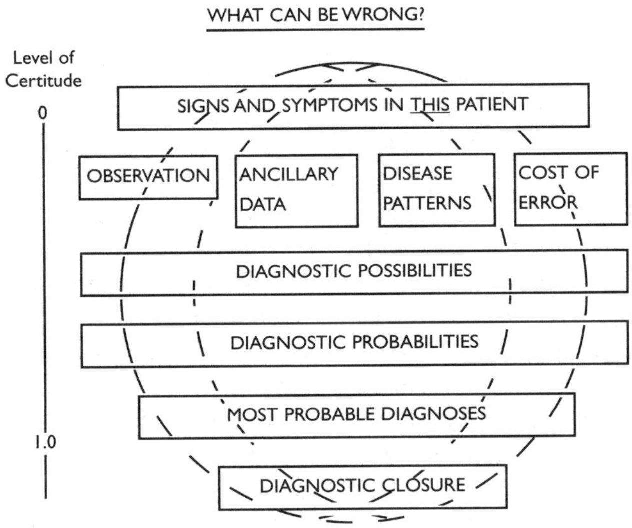

Fig. 2

This part of the process most closely fits the scientific paradigm and under ideal conditions can yield a diagnostic conclusion with a high degree of certitude—i.e., the error rate approaches zero. The conditions for such certitude must be stringent, however. The input data of signs and symptoms must be reliably observed, standardized and specified; the classificatory patterns must be equally reliably determined; the probabilities of different combinations of signs and symptoms must be derived from sufficient numbers and combinations of sets and subsets of signs and symptoms; laboratory and other ancillary data must be sensitive, accurate, specific, and precise. The rules of deductive or probabilistic logic must be followed rigorously.

In addition, a highly specific and sharply discriminating test is required—like a biopsy, fiber endoscopy, angiography, or an enzymatic or immunological determination. Where all these conditions are met, *diagnostic closure* can be obtained. This means that all essential criteria for a diagnosis have been met. The diagnosis could even meet the test of scientific "elegance" if it is arrived at with an economy of steps.

These rigorous conditions are only rarely satisfied in clinical reality. Bedside data are notoriously unstandardized and poorly quantified[13,14]; laboratory tests vary widely in sensitivity, specificity, reliability, and accuracy[15]; "Almost all data on the general incidence and prevalence of disease are inaccurate."[16] Even less secure are estimates of the cost of error of a clinical act so that the hopes of decision theorists to assign a numerical value to every nodal point in a decision tree are even less secure.[17-19] Finally, probability statements say something about the population of individuals sharing some common characteristic but they are weakest in their description of the actual state of any individual in that population.

Thus, even when the rules of probabilistic logic are rigorously applied the diagnostic conclusions are still open to question. They are, more often than not, tentative "working" diagnoses and have more the quality of opinions than scientific judgments.[20] Adding more empiric data may as easily compound an error as move the conclusion closer to the asymptote of a true statement. At some point adding more tests adds only marginally to certitude if at all.

Differential diagnosis consists then in the selection of some diagnosis as more probable, or more justifying of an action than others. At some point, every diagnosis must proceed without further recourse to empirical input. The strength of the case for each diagnostic claim must be assessable and put in some order of priority against the others. Why, for example, is this chest pain due to angina pectoris and not to the fifty or more other kinds of chest pain? The selection must be made when all the empiric data are "in," and further appeals to the empiric are either impossible or insufficient to bring us any closer to diagnostic closure. This part of the differential diagnostic process is not synonymous with application of the laws of statistical probability. Indeed, a critique of the statistical argument as one among other arguments is itself requisite.

The process of differential diagnosis is really most akin to the process of classical dialectic.[21] Each diagnostic possibility can be seen as a "claim"; the strength of arguments for, and against, each claim is evaluated; each position is clarified and set against its opposite; the inherent logical probity of each is delineated. Dialectical discourse properly conducted becomes an internal soliloquy in which the clinician examines his own conclusions critically, or tests them externally against his colleagues or consultants. No new truths are discovered this way, and the dialectic ends if an appeal to experience is possible. The process is therefore not "scientific" in either the classical or modern sense of science.

Differential diagnosis is usually addressed as synonymous with an assessment of relative probabilities. Yet part of the dialectical procedure is to examine the probity of the statistical method itself. When the facts are not determinative, we must establish which diagnostic claim has the strongest logical position. This is more akin to arguing a case in court than it is to proving a scientific hypothesis. The whole effort is to make one diagnosis sufficiently more cogent than the others so that it becomes a defensible basis for decisive action.

The dialectical process is especially important in science where it has been shown that psychologically the tendency is to prove rather than disprove one hypothesis.[22] New possibilities are often uncovered only by disproving an existing hypothesis entirely. Dialectical discourse assures an adversarial stance which challenges the tendency to settle too easily for a merely "workable" hypothesis.

The "old-fashioned" clinico-pathological conference was primarily an exercise in clinical dialectic. It has fallen into disrepute, yet it remains an invaluable way to teach the process of internal soliloquizing which enables the diagnostician to examine his own reasoning critically, when the possibility of adding more observations and tests is no longer open to him. Contemporary pedagogical opinion to the contrary, the dialectical discourse of a clinico-pathological exercise more closely approximates the clinical conditions of differential diagnosis than the scientific model of serial hypothesis testing.

In answering the first of the triad of questions that make up a clinical judgment, several different kinds of reasoning, and reasons, must be employed. To understand the pathophysiology of clinical manifestations, to define and apply a classificatory schema, "scientific" reasons are appropriate. To make general statements of probability for populations, statistical logic is needed. In differential diagnosis the rules of dialectic are the most pertinent. Uncertainty pervades every step of the diagnostic process from its epistemological assumptions to its logical operations. Each of several reasoning modes is suited to optimizing different forms of uncertainty. In the next section we shall see how the practical end modifies each of these modes at every step.

What can be done?

This is the therapeutic question. Having made some decision about the nature of the patient's problem, what kinds of actions could be taken to remove or ameliorate the probable disorder?

Here again, the process is in part, and under certain stringent conditions, scientific in character. When there is a verifiable data base on the course of the untreated disease, and its modification by drugs, surgery, diet, or other measure, the conditions for a scientific decision can be fulfilled. Equally indispensable is quantifiable and precise information about effectiveness and toxicity, since these must be weighed against each other before the decision is made. Under these conditions "closure" on a therapeutic action can approach certitude.

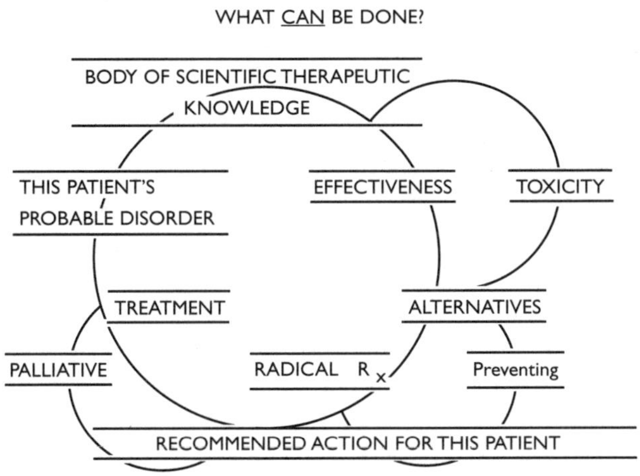

Fig. 3

The therapeutic decision is easy to make when there is a specific and highly effective treatment which demonstrably alters the natural history of the disease. Penicillin for pneumococcal pneumonia, isoniazide and PAS for tuberculous meningitis, vitamin B_{12} for pernicious anemia, or abdominal surgery for ruptured peptic ulcer are examples. In these instances, the action recommended can be scientifically validated, and it will in most instances take precedence over other considerations. The recommended procedure then becomes synonymous with right action; and little choice is open to patient or physician, though the patient may in extreme circumstances reject even this kind of advice.

Unfortunately, to a much larger degree than in diagnostic decisions, genuinely scientific information in therapeutics is scanty. The many pitfalls of therapeutic trials have been the subject of a vast literature. They are generally acknowledged to be among the most difficult experiments to design, control, carry out, and interpret.

Even the randomized clinical trial has come under fire recently.[23] Especially problematic are the large number of therapeutic maneuvers which are not *radical*—i.e., they do not eradicate the causal agent or the offending process. Their benefits, if any, are marginal and the ratio of risk to benefit often vacillates widely. One has only to recall the sad history of anticoagulants in myocardial infarction, the recent national dilemma about influenza vaccination, or the belated appreciation of the long-term vascular effects of oral contraceptives or antidiabetic agents.

Today, we must often decide whether to recommend complex, expensive, palliative procedures with unpleasant and dangerous side effects—as in chemotherapy for cancer. Data on effectiveness and toxicity are usually available in these circumstances, but the questions are a different order: Is the discomfort worthwhile for this patient? Is length of life more important to him or her than its quality? This kind of question must rest firmly on scientific data, but that is only the foundation for a discussion permeated by the physician's and the patient's value systems.

The therapeutic and prognostic domains may well be, as Feinstein opines, the truly unique elements of clinical science. They are also the least secure scientifically. We simply lack the long-term observations of carefully selected patients in sufficient numbers to warrant secure prognostications about the course of a particular disease in a particular patient. Without such data, it is impossible to ground effectiveness of any agent scientifically unless it is so radically effective that a few cases will suffice. If the untreated mortality is 100%, any change will indicate effectiveness, as it does in treating subacute bacterial endocarditis or tuberculous meningitis with specific antibiotics.

The choice of what action to recommend involves more questions of value, by far, than diagnosis. The closer we come to the end of the process of clinical judgment—the right action—the less useful and less available is the scientific model. Reasoning becomes, in smaller part, scientific and probabilistic, and in larger part, dialectical—arguing one alternative against another without recourse to new factual data.

What should be done for this patient?

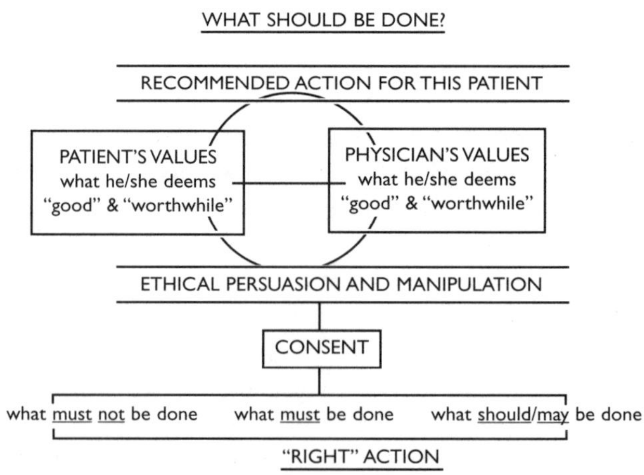

Fig. 4

Having decided what the probable diagnosis is, and what treatment can be expected to be most effective and least harmful, the final question in clinical judgment is whether the treatment *should* be used in this patient, and what alternatives can be offered. The right action—the best one for a given patient—is not always synonymous with the logically or scientifically deduced action. The amount and kind of information needed to secure a diagnosis may be quite different from that needed for decisive action. It is the task of the last stage of clinical judgment to make these distinctions with as much precision as possible.

Decisive action frequently involves the counterposition of what is good scientifically, what the physician *thinks* is good, and what the patient will accept as good. Scientific, personal, and professional values intersect each other and can be in conflict. The scientific evidence and the probability statements about diagnosis, prognosis, and treatment become arguments for or against a choice of alternatives—to do nothing, or, if something is to be done, what must be done, and what should be done.

If the patient exhibits the minimal criteria for an acute abdomen, signs of intracranial pressure, a stab wound of the heart, he/she *must* be operated upon; with severe blood loss, bacterial endocarditis, tuberculous meningitis, or diabetic coma proper, medical therapy *must* be instituted. On the other hand, a non-strangulated hernia, symptomatic gall stones, or mildly symptomatic benign prostatic hypertrophy are things that *should be* treated but may not be in the *must* category. Finally, hemorrhoids, varicose veins, or lipomata *may be* removed surgically; or mild hypertension, a cold, or sinusitis *may be* treated, but need not be.

When it comes to making the *right* decision—the *judicious* one for this patient—the categories of *must not, must, should,* and *may* can all shift, depending upon a myriad of factors in the patient's life situation and his/her notion of what he/she deems worthwhile. In the more obvious situation—like a Jehovah's Witness rejecting transfusion or a Christian Scientist rejecting surgery—the shift is to the *must not* category regardless of the canons of good science. In the more usual case, the categories into which a recommendation falls may shift several times in the course of the illness.

For one person, a lipoma, acne, or sebaceous cyst is something to be ignored; for another, it is a horrid blemish, so emotionally disabling that it demands removal. For this person *may becomes must.* For an elderly man or woman chemotherapy of disseminated cancer may mean a few months more of life, less pleasantly lived. For this patient, a *should* or *may* becomes a *must not.* For another person, the few extra months to do some essential things may make the rigor of treatment worthwhile. For still another, mild depression, anxiety, or headache is tolerable, and can be coped with without resort to daily medications; to another, as the twenty-four million Americans daily taking mood modifiers will attest, even slight anxiety must be treated.[24]

In making the "right" decision for an individual patient then, personal, social, economic, and psychological characteristics of the patient must be factored in. They clearly may modify, or even nullify, the scientifically cogent or logically consistent answers to the questions of what can be wrong? And what can be done? Here, where we are closest to the end, the *telos,* of the whole process, scientific modes of reasoning and scientific reasons are least pertinent, and indeed must be submitted to drastic revision in consideration of the patient's value choices.

The reasoning at this stage is mainly dialectical, ethical, and rhetorical. Physician and patient together must clarify the relationship of one recommendation with its opposite and weigh the reasons for each action. The ethical nature of the discourse at this point is obvious. Conflicts in the obligation of patient and physician to each other must be resolved before a "right" action can be settled upon. Where these conflicts are fundamental, the medical relationship may even be severed by either party, to be resumed with another physician.

Once the ethical and logical possibility and "strength" of arguments for one action over another are assessed by dialectic, then the reasoning becomes "rhetorical"—in the more classical sense of artful persuasion, of relating a dialectically established decision to prudent action, generating belief of another kind from scientific or logical cogency, belief that this particular action should be taken in preference to all others.[25]

We enter here the delicate realms of how much persuasion is ethically defensible, how vigorously the physician should pursue his/her own priority system. Does he/she believe the scientifically recommended action must take priority? Is he/she a therapeutic enthusiast who prefers to "do something" rather than nothing? Does he/she think people should be "strong" and ignore minor infirmity?

Likewise, the patient can use artful persuasion to modify the physician's scientific or dialectically secured recommendation to gain an action more congenial to his/her view of what is good. The patient's vulnerability can easily tip the resolution of conflict in the physician's favor. But these are subtle influences, as well, which can significantly shape the physician's final judgment.

The last question in the sequence then—what should be done?—the capstone question, as it were, which completes the whole structure, is the most prickly. Scientific and semi-scientific conclusions of varying degrees of certitude are examined under a light strongly tinged with moral hues. The accessibility of the questions to scientific modes of reasoning declines, as does the degree of certitude, as we move from determining what *is* wrong, to what *can* be done, to what *should* be done. The optimization of several kinds of uncertainty remains a central concern even when the conclusions are scientifically defensible.

The intermingling of several modes of reasoning—clinical scientific, probabilistic, dialectical, rhetorical, and ethical—does not suggest immunity from explicit statement nor deprecation of attempts to secure truly scientific conclusions. But it is warrant for setting limits on the utility of any of the current explanatory models—scientific, probabilistic, Bayesian, judicial simulation, decision analysis, inference, information, or catastrophe theories. Perhaps the fullest explication will come from some combination of these new theories and more classical modes of reasoning.

PROJECTION OF THE END OF RIGHT ACTION ON THE PROCESS OF CLINICAL JUDGMENT

We have seen that clinical judgment requires confrontation with three generic questions which end in a particular decisive action for a particular patient. Several interdependent reasoning modes are requisite and suitable to each question, and no one question is entirely isolable from the others. We are ready now to turn briefly to a more specific delineation of how the end of right action projects itself upon the way the questions are answered. We might accordingly label this section "clinical prudence" - or, medicine viewed as a virtue.

Whenever possible, the clinician will try to achieve diagnostic closure, i.e., satisfy all the stringent criteria for certitude in locating his/her patient precisely in a classificatory schema. This is the admirable aim of scientific medicine; it is the ideal taught in academic setting; the more it is achieved, the better foundation there will be for the decision to act, at least some uncertainty will be eliminated.

Many clinical realities can upset the orderly processes of diagnostic reasoning: the urgency of the patient's condition, the absence of a diagnostic set or algorithm which fits the presenting signs and symptoms closely enough, lack of specific tests to discriminate among probable diagnoses, incomplete or inconclusive probability estimates, limitations on data selection related to cost or geographic locale, unreliability of the patient as historian, and the dilemma of weighting the probability of a serious vs. nonserious, and treatable vs. nontreatable disorder, when none of these possibilities is definitely excludable.

Experienced clinicians deal with these commonly occurring inevitabilities with interpretative schemata, which enable them to act prudently on inadequate information and incomplete evidence. These schemata can be loosely regarded as rules of clinical prudence, empirically derived but certainly not mysterious sources of inspiration. We can examine a few of these.

Some Rules for Clinical Prudence

1. Act to optimize many benefits, minimize as many risks as possible.
2. The serious and treatable *must* not be missed; The non-serious and non-treatable *may* be missed.
3. Use the clinical Ockham's Razor: Don't multiply causes, diseases, tests or treatments without justifiable necessity.
4. "Rest" the case for any diagnosis or treatment with reluctance.
5. Clinical skepticism is the only guard against the tyranny of the "established" diagnosis, or ancillary data, and the findings of colleagues (lab, X-ray, etc.).
6. Maintain a high index of suspicion for uncommon manifestations of the common.
7. "Hoofbeats don't mean zebras," unless zebras are in the vicinity.
8. When the data are "in," continuing debate is the safeguard against error.
9. Recognize your own clinical style, prejudices, and beliefs about what is "good" for patients.
10. Be wary of hunches, intuitions, E.S.P.—gamble with your own fate, not the patient's.

For one thing, the clinician thinks not so much of meeting the criteria for diagnostic closure, but how much evidence is "enough" to take an optimizing action. Diagnostic closure for example in streptococcal pharyngitis might demand sore throat, plus cervical adenopathy, tonsifar exudate, and positive culture for Beta hemolytic streptococcus. The physician is justified in giving specific treatment with penicillin on any combination of these signs and symptoms and positive culture. But he/she usually acts presumptively—taking a culture, treating, and awaiting the culture to determine whether to continue or discontinue penicillin. If the patient, however, lives in a family or school in which streptococcal illness is frequent or currently present, the most minimal clinical sign may justify treatment even without culture.

Acute abdominal pain is another example. It may result from a wide variety of conditions all of which can present similar signs and symptoms. Examples are: ruptured peptic ulcer, appendicitis, twisted ovarian cyst, strangulated internal hernia, mesenteric adenitis, pancreatitis, cholecystitis. Some of these conditions require immediate surgery, some delayed surgery, some none at all, and in some surgery is positively dangerous. The surgeon looks not for definitive diagnosis but for the least signs of acute abdomen—spasm and rebound—which justify laparotomy. Only in this way can he/she assure that the treatable lesion is not missed. Each surgeon is allowed a certain number of normal appendices or negative explorations, provided he/she has *no* cases in which lifesaving surgery is missed.

In every branch of medicine, there are disorders for which specific and dramatic treatment or genuine cures exist. They must not be missed. They shape the diagnostic process very often out of proportion to their probability in a given case or in the general population. Some are rare like pheochromocytoma; some relatively rare like parathyroid adenoma; some are rare only in a particular locale like malaria or actinomycosis or blastomycosis. Still others were once common, but now infrequent, though still important like syphilis, malaria, or diphtheria.

The clinician's attention therefore may not be focused on getting all the information needed to fill out the most probable classificatory set in its entirety. Rather, more emphasis is placed on the information he needs to take decisive action, or to "rule out" the conditions which in the interest of the patient's safety must not be missed. The clinician must find justification for his/her actions, therefore, in terms of what is right and prudent for the patient. If a serious treatable disease cannot be adequately "ruled out," therapeutic trial may be used as a diagnostic maneuver, i.e., specific treatment is undertaken for the serious disorder, and diagnosis arrived at indirectly by observing the effect. Such a course of action may be taken justifiably even if the probability of a less serious, nontreatable disease is much higher.

A corollary principle, which to some extent balances the search for the treatable and serious, is the admonition "don't look for zebras when you hear hoofbeats." This is a precaution against accepting the rare and esoteric even if the symptom complex is suggestive. Obviously, one cannot justify missing the more common, or losing the more unusual manifestations of a common disorder in the search for the curable but esoteric. Of course, on the African plain, hoofbeats do mean zebras and not palomino ponies or quarterhorses.

Equally influential is the clinician's Ockham's razor—"plurality of causes and diseases is not to be assumed without necessity." Clinicians, particularly in the clinicopathological conference, are conditioned to seek unitary explanations of signs and symptoms. This is another of the organizing principles which become part of the projective schema used by clinicians to select, screen, and weigh data and to justify their decision. The same advice is salutary in therapeutics—the rule of therapeutic parsimony states that treatments must not be multiplied without necessity.

Another rule of prudence is the cultivation of a "high index of suspicion"—another quasi-rational way to cope with uncertainties and avoid "missing" something. Clinicians who follow this rule are unusually sensitive to the most minimal criteria for a diagnosis. They use that sensitivity to open up previously unsuspected possibilities or challenge what appears to be a more firmly established diagnosis.

Indeed, the most dangerous ground for clinical judgment is often not in making a new diagnosis, but in maintaining an index of suspicion high enough to challenge what appears to be an established diagnosis. Physicians, like all humans, tend to rest their cases if no contrary position challenges it. They become locked into or even enamored of the patient's classification, which can render them unresponsive to the most obvious signals of a new disorder, or an original diagnostic mistake. The more prestigious the original diagnostician or institution and/or the more respect one has for the colleague who has made the diagnosis, the more seductive is this error.

Skepticism is, as Santayana so mordantly said, the "chastity of the intellect"—and an indispensable attribute of the prudent clinician is an untiring skepticism about every aspect of a diagnosis or treatment. Perhaps the greatest failing of the contemporary clinician is an overadulation for laboratory and x-ray data fed in by specialists, whose techniques grow more arcane and also more potent daily. Far too often, a right action is justified by the uncritical acceptance of a chemical determination, a biopsy, or an x-ray examination.

I do not intend to provide here a complete primer of clinical prudence. These few principles derived from experience illustrate how the intensity of the clinician's concentration on the end—a good decision for his/her patient—provides a projective schema which shapes every step on his way.[26]

Projective schemata are, of course, individualized and personalized. They summate what a particular physician holds to be "good" medicine. Which rules of thumb are selected, why, and how, are fascinating questions still very much open to logical and psychological examination. A whole series of attitudes of mind, logical and epistemological assumptions, are combined to make up a clinician's diagnostic and therapeutic "style," just as genuinely as the way word and phrase are used to make up a writer's style. The clinician's "style" is really a statement of the reasons he/she will accept as justification for a particular action, for setting aside certain probabilities, or for earnestly persuading a patient to take one course rather than another, equally earnestly propounded by his/her colleagues.

Are these not the elements of the "art" of medicine, and are they not closed to precise analysis, the way the style of Horace or Camus is closed? I think not. I agree with Claude Bernard's comment in warning against sole reliance on clinical instinct and clinical sense.

> Everyone knows in fact that habit may give a kind of empirical knowledge of things sufficient to guide practitioners, even though they may not always be able to account for it at first. But what I

> blame is willfully staying in this empirical state and not trying to get out of it.[27]

Each clinician's rules of prudence need more precise statement. Many are held in common by all good clinicians. Their utility or fallacy can and must be better studied. Most theoreticians have concentrated on the *normative* aspects of clinical judgment. We need to know more about the descriptive nature of the process—who uses what justifications, and how do they benefit or imperil the outcome for the patient? How much difference in mortality, disability, side effects, costs is there between a good and a poor decision maker?

Some physicians are therapeutic enthusiasts. They treat more often than not; they require less justification for using a medication than parsimonious therapists, who insist on demonstrable evidence of effectiveness and frown on the use of placebos or chemical coping for minor disorders. How much of "style" is simply peer conformity, personal intolerance of ambiguity, and obsessive compulsion to "prove" the diagnosis, or satisfy some idealized notion of what constitutes clinical "science"? Much of the cost of medical care, and even its outcome and satisfaction for the patient can turn on how the clinician plays the "game" of clinical judgment.

The psychological components in different reasoning styles are coming under closer investigation.[28,29] We also need more extensive empirical descriptions of the reasoning habits of "good" and "bad" clinicians. What is the effect on outcome of different habits of reasoning? Which ones are crucial, which incidental, and which positively deleterious? In this era of concern for the quality of care, answers to these questions cannot be avoided for very long.

There remain, to be sure, certain features of clinical judgment which for the moment seem closed to explicit analysis. Clinicians have their undeniable moments of sudden insight and discovery. Some clinicians are more consistently accurate in their insights than others. What does happen at that precise moment when the clinician decides that there is "enough" information to "make" a diagnosis or "take" a decisive action? Or, when a set of signs and symptoms suddenly "assembles" itself into a new classificatory pattern? Or, when a patient's clinical features suddenly "fit" a previously described pattern; or, when the precise datum which will answer a puzzling question is suddenly identified?

There is no reason to suspect that clinical diagnosis is unique in this regard. The phenomena of "insight" and "discovery" are common to scientific and nonscientific endeavors. Polanyi and Lonergan have attempted to describe the deep epistemological structures and relationships which permit the leap from the obvious and the known to the previously unknown. Polanyi holds that scientific knowledge is never wholly explicit but resides in tacit understanding which provides the belief which makes thinking about a truth possible. Lonergan links belief to immanently generated knowledge. Polanyi's "discovery" and Lonergan's "insight" are likened by their authors to the "Eureka" of Archimedes.[30]

To what extent these epistemological notions can account for the obscure features of clinical reasoning is problematic. What must be avoided is the easy appeal to some special illumination peculiar to clinicians. To resort to terms like "art" or intuition is to impede explication of a socially significant process. Whatever name we use to subsume the indefinable elements in the process, the effort to explicate them further is a moral as well as intellectual responsibility.

This warning against subjectivism is consistent with a major thesis of this essay—that the nature of the end projects itself on the steps leading up to it. Everything in medicine ultimately is judged by its end—the healing of a patient—even those steps we think most immune to pre-logical or subjective interpretation like pattern definition and recognition. In defining a disease pattern, for example, we must choose among an infinite set of properties—signs, symptoms, tests, etc. That resultant pattern is useful only if it includes a finite and manageable number of characteristics. In making the finite selection we apply a test of utility, related to the purpose of the pattern definition. That purpose is making a "right" decision for a particular patient.

In pattern recognition, the selection is similarly shaped by the end. We seek sufficient congruence with the pattern characteristic of the more serious or the more treatable disorder. We select in favor of patterns which optimize the decision for the patient even though they may be less defensible by the rules of logic or probability.

Statisticians, logicians, and engineers can help the clinician to apply criteria of validity to the characters he/she selects and to manipulate the sets once they are defined. But these aids are of limited use without definition of the purpose for which the classificatory set is to be used. Sokal, a pioneer in mathematical taxonomy, recognizes that in medicine we may limit ourselves to fewer characters than might be taxonomically desirable because we want those most pertinent to decisive action for a patient.[31]

Projective schemata shaped to the practical end of decision making are to a significant degree subjective. But they do not provide warrant for a wholly subjectivist interpretation of clinical judgments. The schemata can themselves become objects of critical scrutiny. We can in fact often judge whether a clinical diagnosis, treatment, or decision is the right one by the outcome for the patient. The test of reality is always there in medicine, and it sharpens and corrects the projective schema, and the values assigned in each of the more formal inferential steps. It is as Ernan McMillin said of the interpretive schemata of science which contemporary philosophers of science have adduced to counter the ultra-objectivism of logical positivism.

> But what must be emphasized is that the skills of interpretation that help bridge the gap between the formalism of inference and the subjectivism of sheer personal assertion are themselves continually responsive to the demands of the objective order.[32]

In medicine we have more immediate and dramatic verificatory possibilities than in many other sciences (death, recovery, disability, complication, dissatisfaction). We can aim realistically therefore to reduce to a minimum the residuum of indefinable elements in each step of the process of arriving at clinical action. This applies even to the more subtle nuances in style which distinguish superior from merely average clinicians.

SOME THEORETICAL AND PRACTICAL IMPLICATIONS

Clinical judgment is what physicians do that most clearly distinguishes their enterprise from other human activities. If there is to be theory of medicine therefore, an understanding of clinical judgment must be a central element—though certainly not the whole of such a theory.

This essay has argued two major theses which bear on a theory of medicine: that clinical judgment is justified and defined by its end—a decisive action for a human in distress and that different kinds of reasons, and reasonings, are appropriate to the formulation of a "right" end.

There are several important implications for a theory of medicine or at least its prolegomenon as well as medical education. Only two of these will be examined briefly: 1) Is medicine a science, art, or virtue or all three; 2) What information should a physician have?

Medicine—science, art or virtue?

Sober has, in this conference, summarized the arguments on both sides of the art-science controversy and they need no repetition.[33] He firmly identifies clinical reasoning with scientific reasoning. On the view we have proposed there is no question that significant parts of the process do fit both the classical and modern descriptions of a science.

Deductive, inductive, and retroductive inference are used to evaluate, interpret, and explain clinical observations. Hypotheses are tested by further observation, experiment, and measurement, and reliability, accuracy, and standardization of data are sought, if not always achieved. These criteria of the scientific method are most clearly pursued in making the diagnosis and selecting and evaluating treatments. Medicine is even more convincingly a science when it seeks explanations of clinical phenomena, in theories and mechanisms of disease. Medicine then fits Einstein's definition of science as:

> ...the century-old endeavor to bring together by means of systematic thought, the perceptible phenomena of this world into as thoroughgoing an association as possible. To put it boldly, it is the attempt at the posterior reconstruction of existence by the process of conceptualization.[34]

But the principal aim of medicine, its distinguishing feature, is not the explanation of clinical phenomena, useful as this may be in raising the clinician's enterprise above empiricism and technicism. Explanations in Einstein's sense are the proper business of the sciences basic to medicine, but they are not synonymous with medicine. Medicine exists as medicine only when it engages in the full range of activities which constitute clinical judgment and which lead to decisive action in the interest of a particular patient.

In its complete expression as medicine, the clinician's enterprise embraces non-scientific as well as scientific reasons and justifications. This essay alludes to the dialectical nature of differential diagnosis, the ethical construction in deciding what is "good" for the patient, and the rhetorical dimensions in the mutual persuasion essential to a decision taken jointly by patient and physician. These latter are skills traditionally imparted by the liberal arts and humanities. They may be exercised in medicine on data validated by scientific method. While dependent upon the reliability of these data, medicine is not identical with the means whereby they are validated.

Is medicine then in any sense an art? Not as the term is used in the current art-science controversy. We have argued that clinical judgments must not be assigned to realms of the intuitive and ineffable which find their source in a presumed special intellectual light possessed by clinicians. I would prefer to reserve the word art in medicine to the perfection of the things done by the physician—the craftsmanship without which the decisions taken would be improperly, unsafely, or clumsily done. The art of medicine lies in the degree of perfection each clinician exhibits in history taking, physical examination, performance of manipulative techniques like surgery and various diagnostic maneuvers—the work done.

These must not be mindless activities. They are a tekne in the classical sense—knowing what to do, how to do it, and why one does it. Art and tekne were synonymous in Aristole and both involve reasoning, "...art is identical with a state of capacity to make, involving a true course of reasoning."[35] Aquinas, extending the Aristotelian notion, called art a *recta ratio factibilium*, thus distinguishing it from science, a *recta ratio speculabilium* and prudence, a *recta ratio agibilium.* The undeviating determination of the work to be done (art) is distinguished from the undeviating determination of what is to be known (science) and the undeviating determination of the act to be done (prudence).[36,37]

If we carry this distinction a trifle further medicine becomes not only science and art, but also the virtue of practical wisdom—"...a true and reasoned state of capacity to act with regard to the things that are good or bad for man."[38] Aquinas expanded the Aristotelian concept somewhat. He argued that, while art gives the capacity to reproduce a good work it does not assure that the product will be used for a good end. That remains to the virtue of prudence—"Consequently, prudence which is right reason about things to be done, requires that a man be rightly disposed with regards to ends."[39]

In this sense then, medicine is both art and virtue. It is art since it is certainly concerned with the perfection of what it does—with the skills needed to make logically secure clinical decisions and to do the procedures decided upon. But it is also a virtue since it must make "right" choices about the ends and purposes for which the decisions and actions are produced. Medicine must not only perform well but act well, it must choose what should be done to heal a particular patient whose good is the true end of the whole activity.

Medicine is then all three—science, art, and virtue synergistically and integrally united in the clinician's daily activities. To disarticulate one member of this triad from the others is to dismember medicine—the essential feature of which is the special relationship each holds to the other. When this happens one becomes a scientist, an artist, or a practitioner, but not a physician. Clearly, any unitarian formalization of the clinician's activity is bound to be misleading, and to define a part of what constitutes medicine but not the whole of it.

What should a physician know?

I have explored elsewhere the many meanings of the term medical humanism—which can so easily become a slogan for whatever version of intellectual or practical activities we wish to justify.[40] Here it is only necessary to reiterate that medical humanism is both a cognitive and compassionate response to the person of the patient. It embraces humanism as a set of cognitive skills largely derived from the humanities and these are integral to the conception of medicine as science, art, and virtue. Humane medicine—indeed moral medicine—requires that the physician understand the distinctions between these intellectual and practical activities, the kinds of reasons each may adduce, their limitations when applied to each other's realms, the different sources of their methodology, and the different subject matter appropriate to each.

If there is any merit in these proposals, they should be reflected in what it is physicians are expected to know. If medicine is a science, and art, and a virtue (in the classical sense)—medical students will need a more explicit education in the non-scientific components of clinical judgment. The skills required for sound dialectical, ethical, and rhetorical reasoning modes must be more explicitly incorporated into professional education—especially in the clinical contexts within which decisions for patients are being made. The liberal arts, and the humanities, even though they might have been presented in pre-medical studies, need vigorous refurbishment in medical education where it will become more obvious to the student the he *needs* the liberal attitudes of mind to function fully as a physician.

The liberal arts have a legitimate place in medicine, not as gentle accoutrements and genteel embellishments of the medical "art," or even to make the physician an educated man. Rather, they are as essential to fulfilling the clinician's responsibility for prudent and right decisions as the skills and knowledge of the sciences basic to medicine.

These are very good reasons for reinfusing the liberal arts into medical education in addition to, but not necessarily to replace, the liberal education in the universities. Premedical education is shallowly rooted for a variety of reasons: The pressure for admission to medical school converts non-scientific subjects into obstacles to be endured rather than essentials to an educated life. Similarly, the humanities may have become too specialized themselves to fulfill their functions as instruments of the liberal arts. Appreciation of the humanities may come more slowly than in the sciences - usually only after the young physician has had some experience of the moral nature of so many of his decisions. Then, the intellectual constraints of a life dedicated only to professional studies are only belatedly perceived. For all these reasons, the liberal arts and humanities are today being taught as part of a medical education in a significant number of schools.[41]

The full implications of the anatomy of clinical judgment for the philosophy of medicine cannot be examined further in this essay. Clearly a theory of medicine must account for this, the physician's most characteristic activity. Hippocrates was partially right to make medicine a natural science; Celsus to call it a conjectural art, and Osler, a science of uncertainty. Any theory of medicine must accommodate all these elements and in the special way demanded by the need to make particular decisions for particular patients. A theory of right thinking, right doing, and right acting must then be related to each other. The theory of medicine must also be shaped by the end to which all medical activity points—a right healing action—for that is what defines medicine uniquely.

> It is a simple fact but almost universally ignored in modern thought that when one loses sight of the end of one's thought and action, the thought and action waver between fanaticism and futility.[42]

III

The Nature of and Education for Humane Clinical Practice and Humane Clinical Research

In these writings, the reader will taste the breadth of Dr. Pellegrino's erudition and the inclusiveness of his thinking about the health care team and the legitimate role of the patient in the health care enterprise.

CHAPTER ELEVEN

EDUCATING THE HUMANIST PHYSICIAN
An Ancient Ideal Reconsidered

> *We must understand what man is, for he is the subject matter of the science of medicine for whom it is promulgated. To understand him is to understand the world, for he is similar to the world in his construction. He is the microcosm, the microcosm in miniature.*
> *The Caraka Samhita*[1]

In the growing litany of criticism to which our profession is increasingly exposed, there is one that in many ways is more painful than all the rest. It is the assertion that physicians are no longer humanists and that medicine is no longer a learned profession. Our technical proficiency is extolled, but in its application we are said to be insensitive to human values. We are, in short, presumed to be wanting as educated men and as responsive human beings.

The assertion is painful because there is some truth in it. Moreover, it comes from those who experience our behavior - our students and our patients. And, in truth, our art is indeed in danger of being engulfed by its technological apparatus. But most painful of all, the assertion strikes at the reality that alone gives authenticity to our profession - our unique charge to answer the appeal of a sick and anxious person for help that is both competent and considerate.

The criticism is especially poignant for medical educators, at whose door much of the responsibility is laid. We are told that we neglect the teaching of human values and the *art* of medicine; that in our zeal for science we ignore liberal studies; and, most telling of all, that the patient care we provide in our teaching hospitals and clinics is itself dehumanizing.

Even our friendlier critics are alarmed by the recent trend to shorten medical education. They fear that our haste will further erode the liberal education of future physicians and thus accentuate the dehumanization of the student and the depersonalization of the patient. These anxieties reach crucial dimensions when viewed against the context of the erosion of personal elements inherent in medicine's increasing institutionalization and specialization.

The terms *humanism, compassion,* and *liberal education* are all shibboleths easily employed to advance one's own political, social, or educational ideologies. Without some clear display of the anatomy of these concepts, physicians will only respond with defensive denial, while their critics will yield to enraptured denunciations. As always, the patient will be victimized by an exchange of diatribes, rebuttals, and contumely. Worst of all, we will miss the opportunity to reexamine these terms and redefine them in their contemporary setting.

There is indeed a genuine and urgent dilemma. Society has the right to require that physicians be competent, that they practice with consideration for the integrity of the person, and that some of them also be educated men who can place medicine in its proper relationship to culture and society.

Medicine enjoys a unique position among disciplines - as a humane science whose technology must ever be person-oriented. Its practitioners are, therefore, under an extraordinary mandate to live, and work within a humanistic frame. What does it mean to educate a humanist physician in contemporary society?

To answer this, we must first examine more closely what we mean today by this ancient ideal. The term *humanist* is too often appended to the term *physician* in an intuitive and altogether imprecise fashion. I suggest that the ideal encompasses two essential but distinct sets of components - one affective and one cognitive. These differ markedly in content; the one does not guarantee the other. In the best examples they are complementary, but they may also be in conflict. Each requires a different mode of learning and teaching.

The failure to make these distinctions leads to pretension, on the one hand, or unfilled expectations, on the other. In either case, the concept loses credibility, and this must be prevented in these times when medicine faces unprecedented demands on all its humane components.

THE PHYSICIAN AS HUMANIST—A BIMODAL CONCEPT

So much feeling surrounds the idea of the physician as a humanist that it is somewhat precarious to attempt a clarification, for clarification requires a dissection of the major components of the idea of humanism. Thus, we run a risk of generating an antinomy where ideally none should exist. Nonetheless, much confusion will arise if we fail to comprehend fully the differences in the two concepts that are inextricably associated with any discussion of humanism - medical or otherwise.

Two concepts of the idea of humanism were recognized by Aulus Gellius, the second-century grammarian, when he spoke of the meaning of the word *humanitas*, from which "humanism" was later derived. He distinguished *humanitas*—education and training in the "good" arts - from a "good" feeling toward all men. *Humanitas* is more properly subsumed under the Greek term *paideia* - an educational and cognitive ideal; and the "good" feeling - what we would call compassion - is more akin to the Greek concept of *philanthropia*.[2]

Following Aulus Gellius, we can discern the same two ideals when embodied in the term *humanism in medicine.* One, the cognitive, deals with the physician as a man, a cultural being possessing ideas, values, and modes of expression in word and art. The other, the affective, concerns the feeling of the physician for the person-as-patient experiencing the existential trials of illness. Together, these ideals enable the physician to understand his science and also to identify with the humanity of those he serves.

These two ideals must further be built on a firm basis of technical competence. Without clinical craftsmanship, the physician-humanist is without authenticity. Incompetence is inhumane because it betrays the trust the patient places in the physician's capacity to help and not to harm. Throughout this essay, I shall assume that education in clinical competence always proceeds, *pari passu,* with the affective and cognitive elements of humanism, our major concern.

The Complete Physician is one who is capable in all three dimensions: he is a competent practitioner: he is compassionate; and he is an educated man. To use the classical terminology, he combines *techné* with *philanthropia* and *paideia.* Few men can perform with perfection, or even adequately, at all three levels. We must repress the tendency to apotheosize our profession by expecting all physicians to excel in all three. No educational formula, ancient or modern, can make of everyone who studies medicine the renaissance men or polymaths some vainly hope for.[3] A more realistic educational goal is to open the possibility for all students and practitioners to live in some measure at each of these three levels. Competence and compassion are clearly requisites for each physician if he is to meet his social responsibilities adequately. The extent to which he must also be an educated man is more variable and less intimately related to his social utility.

THE AFFECTIVE COMPONENTS

Compassion: Its Meaning and Erosion–Of the two components of humanism, the affective is more frequently mentioned by today's critics of medicine. They decry the lack of compassion they perceive in the care of patients. Compassion is most often equated with humanness and even with humanism. What do we mean by compassion as an affective attribute of the humanist physician?

Com-passion means co-suffering, the capacity and the willingness of the physician somehow to share in the pain and anguish of those who seek help from him. It connotes some understanding of what sickness means to another person, together with a readiness to help and to see the situation as the patient does. Compassion demands that the physician be so disposed that his every action and word will be rooted in respect for the person he is serving. Compassion is reflected in a disposition to "feel" along with the patient. When it is genuine, compassion is unmistakably sensed by the patient and it cannot be feigned. It is not to be confused with pity, condescension, or paternalism. Clearly, compassion is an affective and behavioral characteristic that bears little relationship to a cognitive appreciation of any of the humanities. Nor is it altogether synonymous with the political or activist bias of many students and young physicians, however well-motivated they may be, to help the socially and economically disenfranchised members of our society.

Potent influences in modern medicine and society now conspire to erode and even extinguish compassion. Among the most influential are our fascination with technology, gadgets, and instruments; the inherent depersonalizing influences of our highly institutionalized social structures; the replacement of care by individuals with care by the "team"; the thrust of a scientific medical education that focuses on man-the-object-of-study; and, finally, a medical education that itself is fraught with rigidities and does little to help the student develop his own humanity.

Can the affective components of humanism - the *philanthropia* of Gellius - be assured in the education of physicians? Formal education would appear to be of limited value, since humanness and compassion are not disciplines to be learned in classrooms. Indeed, whenever we study man, even his affective and behavioral components, we must in some sense make him an object and distort him. This is true even of those disciplines, like the social sciences and the humanities, that look at the conscious and imaginative dimensions of man's existence. They may help us to understand humanity abstractly, but not to behave compassionately. We must remember with Jung that "the patient is there to be treated and not to verify a theory."[4]

Compassion In the Student-Teacher Relationship–Before the student can begin to feel the plight of his patient as that of a person seeking help, he must develop a fuller insight into his own developing humanity. The affective education of the student starts with the means most significant for him - the humanization of his medical experience. By dealing in a personalized and compassionate way with the special circumstances into which a medical education places young people, the teacher may forestall that subtle erosion of sensitivities that is a genuine danger of too much immersion in the study of man as an object of science.

The student-teacher relationship has many similarities to the patient-physician relationship. In both circumstances, one person is seeking help from another who is presumably wiser and has power over the petitioner. Both student and patient must face personal challenges in emotionally trying situations. When the teacher helps the student in a compassionate and understanding way, he illustrates how the student can in turn give the same understanding to the patient, who is dependent on his humanness as the student is dependent on the teacher's.

The rigidity of current curricula and testing methods, as well as the trial-by-ordeal proclivities of some faculty members, are perceived by many students as "dehumanizing." This experience erodes their own capacities for humane relationships with patients. Granting a certain inevitable hyperbole in such assertions, the only effective way to inoculate compassion is to practice it. In each of their contacts with students, patients, and even with experimental animals, the faculty must exhibit genuine care. The clinician-teacher has truly awesome responsibilities here. One careless action at the bedside will undo hours of lecturing about the dignity of patients. Conversely, one act of kindness and consideration will make compassion a reality and an authentic experience. Student disaffection is often a masked appeal for models they can sincerely imitate.

There are some obvious critical incidents in the life of a medical student that can have a profound effect on his emotional maturation as a person. The way the faculty handles his responses to these experiences may determine whether or not the student later approaches his own patients humanely. Some of the nodal points at which a student may need help in dealing with his own feelings are the first encounter with the cadaver or with the helplessly ill or dying patient, the death of his "own" first patient, identifying with young patients who are seriously ill or disabled, and trying to help patients seeking assistance in the vast, impersonalized, hurried, and often physically depressing circumstances prevalent in too many large teaching hospitals.

Opportunities must be provided for students to express their feelings of conflict and anxiety with many of these potentially shattering experiences. Some personal adaptation must be effected that avoids rejection of self or profession, on the one hand, or too ready acceptance of the inevitability of an impersonal attitude, on the other. A judicious and interested faculty can encourage students to persist in gaining competence while simultaneously working to make the care of patients more humane. Even the well-intentioned student may be tempted to subvert the effort required to attain competence by self-righteous attacks on the "system" and the human failing of the clinical faculty.

Compassion and the Patient–Humanness and compassion in dealing with patients, the focal point of our concern, is not easily measurable. Yet, there are some rather simple behavioral criteria that can be monitored specifically as a beginning effort in any attempt to see whether at least the rudiments of humanness and consideration are being exhibited. Clinical faculty and students might repeatedly ask themselves a series of very simple questions that arise in every patient-physician encounter.

First, do we teach students to satisfy the fundamental questions every person who is ill and anxious brings to the physician? The patient wants to know: What's wrong? How did he get that way? Is it serious? Can you cure it? What will it cost in money and loss of dignity? What are you going to do? Will it hurt? These are simple questions, but to an alarming degree, patients may see many doctors, have many tests, pay many bills, and not receive answers to these simple questions.

The issuance of a diagnosis and a standardized explanation may be convenient for the physician or all that his time will permit. Yet, this can be the first step in making the patient an object and not a person. Each patient wants answers to all these questions put into the context of *his* life. This is more than individual treatment, which merely means treatment as a unit. Personal treatment, instead, gets at the uniqueness of the person behind the unit. Or, as Thomas Merton said so sagely, "The person must be rescued from the individual."[5] Physicians who have neither the time nor inclination for this degree of personalization are bound by the first rule of humanness to see that other members of the health care team are permitted to answer the personal questions that lie at the root of the patient's plea for help.

Second, can we accept the patient for what he is and not what we think he should be? The German novelist Hermann Hesse puts it well: "No man has ever been entirely and completely himself. Yet each one strives to become that - one in an awkward, the other in an intelligent way."[6] To be compassionate, we must accept each person's striving - the ignorant and the intelligent, the successes, the failures, the poor, the wise, the weak, the strong, and even the evil ones. All must receive our expression of willingness to help. This is impossible unless we continue to grow as persons ourselves. "If the doctor wants to help a human being, he must be able to accept him as he is. And he can do this in reality only when he has already seen and accepted himself as he is."[7] We can never feel with another person when we pass superior judgment, only when we see our own frailties as well as his.

Third, do we handle our authority in a humane way that respects the life values of the patient? The health professional is always in danger of extending his authority in technical matters over the patient's system of beliefs and values. Dag Hammarskjöld articulated the unique responsibility of those in authority thus: "Your position never gives you the right to command. It only imposes on you the duty of so living your life that others can receive your orders without being humiliated."[8] This is sound advice, to which we must attend whether we deal with patients, students, or our own professional colleagues. It has an important corollary: We must not "put down" the patient when he detects our uncertainties and even our errors. To be humane, we must ever be ready, as Galileo said, "to pronounce that wise, ingenious, and modest statement - 'I do not know.'

Compassion, practiced in these terms in each individual patient transaction, is the irreducible base for mitigating the inherent dehumanizing tendencies of today's highly institutionalized and technologically oriented patterns of patient care.[9] The student's distress with deficiencies in our present system is meaningless unless he realizes he can remedy them by humanizing his own relationships with the patients he is privileged to examine and help.

Compassion and "Humanistic" Psychology–Recently, a variety of means derived from "humanistic" psychology have been introduced to improve the experiential-affective elements of learning. Carl Rogers has called for the use of the encounter group involving faculty and students in an attempt to forge a better unity between cognitive and affective learning. He has urged a reappraisal of all education from this point of view and has already initiated a series of encounter sessions for medical educators for this purpose. Other measures, like psychodrama and psychosynthesis, are sure to be explored in an effort to remedy the defects in affective learning among medical faculty, students, and practitioners.

The success of such measures will be difficult to evaluate. For some, they will no doubt leave a lasting impression; others will reject them. For many, a transient experience of limited value will probably occur. We must avoid the conclusion that the only way to learn the affective components of humane medicine lies in any particular psychological mode. There is as much danger of psychologic overkill in medical education as there is of scientific overkill. We cannot ignore the capacity of at least some students to become empathetic, humane, and sensitive practitioners without necessarily dissecting their emotional lives to this fine degree.

Little of a lasting nature will be achieved until the affective components in the student's learning become the conscious concern of the majority of clinical teachers. To limit this concern, and the teaching that goes with it, to those whose specialties are in psychology or the behavioral sciences is to create a pedagogic ghetto that many students and faculty will eschew.

Before they can be evaluated properly, the newer psychologic techniques must be continuing experiences for teachers and students in their own institutions. One possible achievement, as judged by my conversations with those who have attended the Rogers sessions, is a reduction in the emotional overtones that seriously impede discussions of even the cognitive elements in medical education. If encounter sessions encourage a more reasonable dialogue in the cognitive domain, they will be well worth the effort.

Affective experiences and behavioral enhancements of humane attitudes by newer psychological techniques are promising, but the affective elements in the patient-physician transaction must also be studies in an intellectually rigorous fashion. The Spanish medical philosopher Pedro Lain Entralgo has undertaken a comprehensive analysis of this subject.[10] His work is an excellent starting point for those who wish to approach the subject cognitively. Ideally, the affective training of both student and teacher should be united with the cognitive examination of the affective components in the personal relationships of patient and physician, student and teacher, and student and patient.

THE COGNITIVE COMPONENTS

The Domain of Liberal Studies–Medical students today are, commendably, most concerned with the affective components. They exalt them, perhaps too readily, over the cognitive in their zeal to remedy some of the more obvious depersonalizing tendencies in medical education and practice. In the past, we have run the danger of suppressing the human values in medicine by an over-adulation of its rational and scientific elements. We will not serve mankind any the better if we now yield to the dominance of romanticism, intuition, and introspection propounded by some under the heading of medical humanism.

As a cognitive entity, humanism has a complex history, which Kristeller and others have attempted to clarify.[11] It originated in the nineteenth century with Niethammer as *humanismus*, an ideal of the classical and liberal forms of education to be set against the vocational and scientific then gaining ground in education. *Humanism* itself derives from the word *umanista* used in the Italian universities of the Renaissance to designate the teachers of the humanities - those studies included in the *studia humanitatis*, the language and literature of Rome and, to a lesser extent, of Greece.

In this older sense, humanism is a literary and educational ideal, one that has lost much ground in today's universities. But almost from the outset, the term became identified with a certain set of values that set man as the central focus of concern - belief in the dignity and worth of the person, the democratic process, and human rationality. These values, as Edel has emphasized, are not a philosophical system sui generis, but rather what he terms a "philosophical strain" or "a corrective process, the guardian of a human balance against seeing man as more than a man or less than a man."[12] This "strain" is expressed in an extreme form in the religion of man proposed by Auguste Comte. More commonly, it is a bias found in many philosophical systems. Thus, we can speak of Christian, Marxist, atheistic, or scientific humanism. The humanist strain deals with values, and it is thus quite different in cognitive content from the more classical form of literary humanism.

Classical and Literary Humanism. Let us first examine the cognitive elements in traditional or literary humanism. This ideal was best exemplified in the lives of such physician-scholars as Linacre, Caius, and their modern counterpart, Sir William

Osler. Gilbert Murray said of Osler, in nominating him for the presidency of the Classical Association, that

> he stands for a type of culture which the Classical Association does not wish to see die out of this world - the culture of a man who, while devoting himself to his special science, keeps nevertheless a broad basis of interest in letters of all kinds.[13]

Osler is essentially the physician as educated man, combining superb clinical talents, scientific perspective, and human concern with the capacity to excel in those skills that traditionally have been identified with a liberal education - the ability to think, write, and speak with clarity, taste, persuasiveness, and moral sensitivity. As Else has pointed out, language was the principal means through which these goals were attained.[14] These were the skills which freed man, "liberated" him, and made him human.

The cognitive skills thus subsumed in this sense of humanism were those that uniquely belong to man - the capacity to speak, write, reason, invent, create the beautiful, and judge it. Traditionally, they were taught by formal study of the disciplines of languages, literature, history, philosophy, and especially as exemplified in the writings of the Roman and Greek classics.

Education of this type is no longer a common denominator for professional people. Indeed, it is regarded by some as elitist and even antithetical to the major social responsibilities of physicians. It is, moreover, an education increasingly difficult to obtain by reason of today's crisis in the humanities. This crisis is the culmination of several factors: a decline in the teaching of the classical languages in which literary humanism is based; transformation of the humanities into technical specialties; and a decided shift in cultural ambience toward the nonliterary and more intuitive modes of communication and expression.

Genuine literary humanism has always been a rare accomplishment for physicians as for other men. Some medical educators and practitioners still persist in the hope that some formula can be found enabling us to produce physicians who are educated men in this sense, and this is essential if medicine is to be humanized. The cognitive elements of classical humanism are undeniably important for physicians as professionals; even more so if physicians are to transcend the confines of even so broad a discipline as medicine. It is as Berenson said of the Italian painters of the Renaissance, "Painting therefore offers but a partial and not always the most adequate manifestation of their personality, and we feel the artist as greater than his work, and the man as soaring above the artist."[15] The cognitive elements in literary humanism can enable the physician to "soar above" his profession.

Not many students today perceive the value of a rigorous education in the cognitive elements of traditional humanism. Some will perceive them later in life, when medicine itself becomes so routinized as to verge on boredom.

Others, perhaps the majority, will never perceive the life-enhancing qualities of traditional humanistic study. What, then, is a realistic future for the cognitive skills and knowledge supposedly imparted by liberal studies in the education of physicians?

Humanities in Medicine: Approach for Today–We cannot permit the possibility of contact with traditional humanism to decay completely. Too much of man's capacity for a life of satisfaction is contained within it. We owe every student at least the opportunity for contact with liberal studies at some point in his education. But today we are required to offer this opportunity in a variety of ways not limited to the premedical years.

Some students will continue to follow the patter of a professional education built on a prior base in the liberal arts. For the majority, the most effective teaching of humanistic studies will occur within the context of medical education itself. Here, the student's motivation and goal directedness will help to focus the cognitive features of the humanities. The medical context is rich in possibilities for explicating the essential cognitive skills unique to humane and liberal studies. The pedagogic aim in the pre-degree years is to uncover the student's interest in these skills and, in the years of continuing education, to reinforce them in his own experiences as a person dealing with other persons in the medical transaction.

This mode of teaching the cognitive components of humanism will require special adaptations of *what* is to be taught, *how* it is taught, and *who* teaches it. At this time, a variety of approaches is being tried in a dozen or so medical institutions attempting to infuse humanistic elements into the corpus of medical education. Two recent institutes on this subject, under the auspices of the Society for Health and Human Values, summarize these current experiments.[16] While these reports indicate a wide range of approaches, some conclusions seem quite clear.

First, what is to be learned? There is no one discipline or combination of disciplines that will assure acquisition of the requisite intellectual skills. Instead, what we must seek is to inculcate that knowledge an educated man must have to distinguish him from his colleagues who are merely competent. Professor Wayne Booth succinctly summarizes these skills as learning how to think critically for ourselves, how to experience beauty for ourselves, and to make our own choices among possible actions.[17] These are the skills that make a man free - the "liberal arts." If he possesses them he is no longer subservient to the thoughts, actions, or esthetics of those who can examine these matters critically. Neither the sciences nor the humanities can encompass these skills entirely. Each can contribute to their development. The traditional emphasis on the literary content of the humanities must be expanded to include some of what the scientist now contributes to our cultural milieu.

Second, how shall these skills be taught? To be most effective with the goal-oriented medical student, the cognitive skills should be taught within the framework of a medical education - indeed, as an integral part of that education. Medicine is admirably suited to this purpose. It abounds in experiential data about the human condition and illustrates easily the concrete importance of the cognitive skills of humanism in clinical decision-making, the lack of which, in my opinion, is one of the major defects of clinical medicine today. Medicine is also the focal point for much of our most recent and important knowledge of man and his behavior.

Teaching in such a context necessarily proceeds from the concrete, personal, and immediate to the abstract, general, and more ultimate concerns of mankind. It demands use of the case method and seminar rather than the lecture and reading assignment. It centers on personal involvement by the student with the specific concerns of his patient and thus gains a relevance scarcely equalled in other types of teaching.

These teaching modes are quite unfamiliar to the usual teacher of the humanities, and this brings us to our last question: Who shall teach? Certain special characteristics are demanded of the teacher who essays to teach the cognitive skills of humanism in the medical setting. He must be an able and secure scholar in his own discipline; he must be committed to communicating that discipline to medical students and physicians; and he must be willing to enter serious and continuing dialogue with the medical culture, while bringing his special viewpoint to bear on the phenomena of the medical experience.

Not many bona fide humanists are prepared for this sort of teaching. Hopefully, more of them will see challenges and benefits for their own studies in an intimate exchange with medicine. If current interest among medical educators grows, we will need to educate some humanists specifically for the engagement with medicine. There is some danger at present, as with any new field as yet unproven intellectually, that the field may fall to the willing and eager rather than to the most competent teachers.

Clearly, the cognitive components of traditional humanism embracing its literary elements and its intellectual attitudes are important in the education of the physician-humanist. To be effective and useful in today's university and with today's student requires a mode of teaching and a faculty with characteristics different from those that prevail in the universities' departments of humanities at present.[18,19]

The Domain of Values–There is another domain of cognitive knowledge that is contained in the concept of the humanist-physician, and that is the domain of values as objects of serious study in medical education. We cannot provide medical care within a humanist frame without a knowledge of the intersections in values that occur at every stage of the medical transaction. The meanings of these intersections for the patient, the physician, and society bear directly on the outcome of medical management. Medical teaching now requires the infusion of a perception of the value questions as a correlative device, much in the spirit of the humanistic strain alluded to by Edel.[12]

At every step in the medical encounter, human values are set against each other: those of the patient with those of the physician, those of society with those of the individual, and those of the physician as scientist and teacher with those of the physician as healer. Each person and each community is identified by commitment to a certain configuration of beliefs, choices, and priorities about the things believed to be important. These values have meanings quite specific for each person and each community, and these meanings must be understood by anyone who presumes to treat either the person or the community.

We now live in an era in which the ancient and long-standing image of the physician as a benign authoritarian is intolerable to most educated people. Patients have the right to make choices among alternative modes of management in keeping with the values they conceive to be most important to them. The physician must understand the basis of the patient's value choices, respect them, and work within their confines much more sensitively than ever before. In a matter so personal as health, the imposition of one person's values over another's - even of the physician's over the patient's - is moral injustice.

Practitioners, students, and faculty members, therefore, need a formal knowledge of the meaning of values and the varieties of systems within which values are expressed. They need especially to understand the genesis of their own value systems and to recognize the gap that inevitably develops between the values of the professional and those of the society within which a profession may function.

Physicians do not reflect very often on the values peculiar to the process of professionalization through which they pass. Nor are they and their teachers sufficiently conscious of the imprint made by the prevailing mode of medical education and its traditional orientation on their own value systems. These values very soon become the prelogical foundations for the physician's behavior, for his normative ethics, and for his apodictive statements on what is good for the patient and society.

The significance of an orientation to values as objects of more serious study and experience in medical education is very much heightened by the new problems of individual and social ethics which derive from the enhanced capabilities of modern biomedical science.[20] The physician's stance with reference to abortion, euthanasia, human experimentation, genetic manipulation, behavioral control, and a variety of other urgent and dramatic new issues in medical practice is based in a set of values the foundations of which he rarely examines critically.

It is impossible to confront these and other new questions in the ethics of health care without a reconceptualization of the foundations of medical ethics. Such a restructuring of traditional normative and deontological ethics is dependent on a reconceptualization of the values on which traditional and contemporary ethics systems are based. Value questions underlie the legal, political, and social mechanisms for decision-making in the public as well as the most private matters of medical and health care.

Medical axiology is an underdeveloped - indeed, almost nonexistent - discipline at this time. It can be taught at several levels - at the fundamental level of value theory, then at the applied level of clinical decision-making, and finally at the community level of public policy-making. Integration of knowledge from a variety of disciplines is requisite if a true medical axiology is to emerge. Law, ethics, political science, philosophy, and social and cultural anthropology are intermingled in any critical inquiry into the value questions in health care.

"Medical" axiology, like "medical" philosophy, "medical" history, or "medical" sociology, demands an interdigitation of principles from the humanities and the social sciences with concrete experiential data derived from specific clinical situations in which value questions influence the outcome for human beings seeking help. A whole new set of questions of very great human concern is emanating from the emerging dialogue between medicine and biology, on the one hand, and various of the humanities and social sciences, on the other.

These questions at the interzone between medicine and the other university disciplines have not been explored in depth. Yet, even at this early stage, they must be taught and exemplified in medical education. The content and the methods requisite to teaching at the junctions of medicine, the humanities, and the social sciences are just beginning to receive explicit attention.[16] No success-assured formula is available for wide application. The impatient student who hopes to humanize medicine overnight through some curricular thaumaturgy is sure to be disappointed.

In the immediate future, we face a tense period in our attempts to develop a more humanistic frame for medical education. On the one hand, our knowledge of human values is rudimentary and needs deepening. On the other, we face the urgency and the high expectations of all who hope for elimination of the deficiencies in our present modes of learning. Faculties in medicine and in the traditional disciplines must undergo significant attitudinal adjustments before these nascent studies can flourish. Concomitantly, they must also develop the intellectual rigor without which they cannot survive in the medical curriculum.

Nevertheless, the formal teaching of human values, at all levels of medical education, offers a sound mechanism for liberalizing and humanizing the student's technical and professional learning. The study of values may well provide a more realistic and a more widely applicable avenue for liberal education for today's medical students than the cognitive elements of traditional or literary humanism. Without deprecating the latter, it seems more likely that the study of human values will open a more attractive road toward attainment of those attitudes of mind formerly associated with the best in traditional humanistic studies.

It goes without saying that learning the cognitive domain of human values will be totally ineffectual if it is not accompanied by affective learning and by explicit example in the behavior of the faculty, especially its clinical members. In the realm of values, the humanistic strain is attainable only where the patient is in fact treated with full dignity as a man, enabled to participate democratically in decisions that affect his being, and approached with tolerance for his fallibility and that of his physician.

THE IDEAL RESYNTHESIZED

For the purposes of clarification of the goals of his education, we have intentionally disassembled the ideal of the humanist-physician. This disassembly enables us to understand the full spectrum of meanings within the ideal and to denote educational goals specifically designed to explicate each of the integral components of humanism. By so doing, we can avoid diffusing our educational goals over a vague territory more emotionally than rationally defined. More important, our dissection may perhaps permit a resynthesis of the ideal in terms more consistent with the motivations of today's students and the contemporary responsibilities of the profession.

The ideal humanist-physician would fuse all elements - the affective and the cognitive domains we have described - the whole built on a base of technical competence. Professional education, then, has as its goal the making of a competent clinical craftsman; affective learning has the goal of making a humane and compassionate practitioner; and the cognitive elements of humanism, modified in the two ways I have suggested, should make for an educated practitioner. These three levels in the life of the physician should interpenetrate and reinforce each other. Very few persons will ever experience excellence in all dimensions, but recognition of the full expression of the ideal establishes a bench mark against which the degree of an individual's humanistic education can be assessed.

Medicine enjoys a special position among the disciplines. It centers on man in all his dimensions and shares some part of his reality with the humanities, the social sciences, and the experimental sciences. Pursued to its fullest expression, medicine can be truly humanizing, for its object of study and concern is man.

John Ciardi's recent exposition of the concept of esthetic wisdom is apposite: "the sum total of all the great artist becomes in his life's exposure to his medium. The artist's environment," he adds, "is not the world but the world as his medium reveals it."[21]

I submit that medicine, like the arts, also provides a kind of human experience that makes it a special medium for revealing the world. It too, can yield an esthetic wisdom of its own special object, man. Medicine taught in a humanistic frame prepares the student for its humane practice. Practice in a humanistic frame reveals even more about the microcosm, as Caraka perceived in the quotation that opened this essay.

CHAPTER TWELVE

THE CARING ETHIC
The Relation of Physician to Patient

This symposium deals with the most fundamental topic in medical ethics today: the relationship between the person who is ill and those who profess to heal him—physicians, nurses, the family, the minister, and the social worker. My assignment is to focus on the ethical aspects of this relationship which have become so complicated in recent decades. I will base my comments not so much on the application of specific ethical principles regarding the rights of patients or the humane aspects of what it is to be ill and what it is to be healed. I want, in short, to concentrate more on the caring than the curing aspects of the relationship, and on the moral obligations subsumed in the notion of caring.

I make this distinction because in those two words *cure* and *care*, the recent history of medicine is capsulized. The dominant notion in medicine for most of its history has been caring, even when the physician may have thought he was curing. It is only with the introduction of truly scientific means of therapeutics that cure has become possible in any real sense. As a result, the caring aspects of the healing relationship have come to be neglected, and even denigrated.

What is the relationship between caring and curing? What are the moral obligations of healers—physicians, nurses, all who come into direct hands-on contact with sick people?

It is interesting to note at the outset that both words *curing* and *caring* have the same Latin root: *curo, curare*—"to cure," "to take care of," "to take trouble," and later "to treat" medically and surgically, to "heal" or "restore" to health. For the greater part

 "The Caring Ethic: The Relation of Physician to Patient". In: Anne H. Bishop and John R. Scudder, Jr. (ed.). *Caring, Curing, Coping: Nurse, Physician, Patient Relationships.* Tuscaloosa, Alabama: University of Alabama Press; 1985: pp. 8-30.

of medical history these various senses of curing and caring were essentially one. It is only with the beginnings of truly scientific and therapeutically effective, discrete therapies that the possibility of cure without care has existed.

The word *cure* is now used by many health professionals in a radical sense: to refer to the eradication of the cause of an illness or disease—to the radical interruption, and reversal, of the natural history of a disorder. The result of a "cure" is to restore a patient to at least the state he or she was in before the onset of illness and, possibly, to an even better state of functioning. The possibility of "cure," in this sense, turns on the availability of scientific medicine: truly effective therapeutic modalities which make it possible to cure without caring.

Specific, radical, and effective cures—in the technical sense—have been acquired in greatest profusion during the lifetime of physicians who entered the profession following World War II. Here and there, largely through empirical good fortune, some truly effective cures existed before that time (cinchona bark for malaria, foxglove for heart failure, mercury for syphilis), and some were discovered by scientific investigation earlier in this century (insulin, liver extract, sulfonamides). But the golden era of specific therapy has just begun, and its promises are still to be fully apprehended. We are now in the era of synthesis of natural and manmade agents, designed to attack the molecular and cellular sources of disease. We can invade any body cavity to excise, reconstruct, or transplant diseased organs and tissues. Radical cure and restoration—not amelioration or disease containment—have become realistic and legitimate goals of medicine.

It is easy, and perhaps some think it desirable, to forget that the greatest part of the history of medicine was based in a different conception of cure, associated with care of the ill and sick. To be sure, the extensive pharmacopoeias of the Chinese, Indian, and Roman physicians implied curative powers. Fortuitously, some items in them *did* cure; but most were worthless or even dangerous. Cure, if it occurred, resulted largely from the body's self-healing powers and the physician's compassion, caring, encouragement, and emotional support.

The ancient grounding of medicine in care and compassion is now challenged by a biomedical model which defines medicine simply as applied biology. On this approach, the primary function of medicine is to cure, and this requires the physician be primarily a scientist. This model still includes containment of illness, by slowing down its progress and amelioration of its symptoms, but it focuses on *things* to do for a particular disease that are measurably effective.

In response to this narrow definition, some advocate a broader approach that adds the sociological and psychological aspects of illness. Others would expand this further to a "holistic" approach, adding the religious and spiritual dimensions of illness to the bio-psycho-social model. These expanded concepts of medicine are limited by the impossibility that all physicians can acquire the requisite understandings and sensitivities the biopsychosocial model demands. Also, such a model tends to absorb all the health professions into medicine, expanding its pretensions beyond all reasonable hope of fulfillment.

In this essay, I wish to examine what we mean by "caring" and the necessity of a clear concept of the totality of its meaning as a basis for reformulation of professional ethics. I will concentrate on professional medical ethics, largely to avoid the presumption, not unknown to physicians, of prescribing for other health professionals. I believe, however, that we are all joined in a common task of healing, helping, and caring and that the same moral obligations bind us all in those endeavors.

There are at least four senses in which the word *care* can be understood in the health professions.

The first sense is care as compassion—being concerned for another person; feeling or sharing something of his or her experience of illness and pain; being touched by the plight of another person. To care in this sense is to see the person who is ill, and at the center of our ministrations, as more than the object of our ministrations; as a fellow human whose experiences we cannot penetrate fully but which we can be touched by because we share the same humanity.

The second sense of caring is doing for others what they cannot do for themselves. This entails assisting them with all the activity of daily living that is compromised by illness: feeding, bathing, clothing, meeting personal needs—physical, social, and emotional. Physicians do little or none of this kind of care. Nurses do much more, but far less than they used to do. The large part of this kind of care is given by nurses' aides in today's "team nursing."

The third sense of caring is to take care of the medical problem—to invite the patient to transfer responsibility and anxiety about what is wrong, and what can and should be done, to the physician or nurse. This implies assurance that the latter will direct all appropriate knowledge and skill to the "problem" the patient presents, to intervene in the natural history of the disease.

The fourth sense of caring is to "take care": to carry out all the necessary procedures, personal and technical, with conscientious attention to detail with perfection. This is a corollary of the third sense of care, but its emphasis is on the craftsmanship of medicine. Together the third and fourth senses are what most physicians subsume under the rubric of *competence.*

These four senses of care are not separable in optimal clinical practice. Nonetheless, in reality, they are often separated, and even placed in opposition to each other. Or all four senses are reduced to one, to the exclusion of each.

For example, the biomedical model of the physician-patient relationship places emphasis on technical competence and conscientiousness, relegating the first two senses—which are more effective than technical—to other health professionals. On the other hand, the expansionist models of medicine—the holistic or biopsychosocial—embrace all dimensions of care, blurring the distinctions between them. Partitioning or conflating the four senses of care poses dangers to patients, because it either neglects one aspect or presumes to do too much.

It is essential that each sense of caring be recognized for its contribution to the healing relationship. Each must be placed in its proper place in an order of priorities determined by the needs of a particular patient. Care is of one piece. The challenge to health professionals is to attend to each sense of care, and thus relate one to the other, so that they enhance the healing relationship for each patient.

In the ideal healing relationship (patient-physician, patient-nurse), each health professional would attend to each dimension of care in every ministration. When this is not possible, as in contemporary care, the four senses of caring must be provided by conscious partitioning of functions among members of the medical or health care team. The moment we make such divisions we must appreciate that the unity of care is threatened. Special attention must then be exerted so that no aspect of caring is neglected, because no member of the health care team accepts the responsibility or sees it as proper to his or her professional tasks or status.

Integral care—that is to say, care that satisfies the four senses I have defined—is a moral obligation of health professionals. It is not an option they can exercise and interpret in terms of some idiosyncratic definition of professional responsibility. The moral obligation arises out of the special human relationship that binds one who is ill to one who offers to help.

To assess whether the curing or caring model is foundational for medical practice, it is necessary to examine the three fundamental elements of the physician-patient relationship. The first element is the person who is ill and needs and seeks help. The second element is the act of profession—the promise the healer makes when he or she enters into the relationship with the person who is ill. The third element is the act of medicine or the act of healing. The following discussion of these three elements should make it clear that although curing and caring are essential parts of medical practice, caring "founds" that practice.

What is the meaning of being ill? Most people regard themselves as in a state of health, but this state cannot be determined absolutely. Despite all recent attempts to define health, no better functional definition has been given than by Galen, who defined health as that state in which we feel able to do the things we wish to do with minimum pain or discomfort. This means that you can feel you are in a state of health, and not feel ill, even though you have a disease. Indeed, many of us have disease within us, yet are able to do the things we want to do with minimum discomfort and disability. When something happens that shakes us out of this feeling of being in a healthy balance, it prompts us to seek help.

That balance is upset by a symptom: a pain in the chest, finding a lump, loss of appetite, morning nausea, dizziness on bending over—you name it. When such symptoms are perceived as a change in the function of our whole organism, they become sufficient to lead us to seek help. We become *patients* when we need help bearing a problem, a pain, a concern, an anxiety. It makes no difference whether a problem is emotional or physical; when we seek professional help, we become patients, and in becoming patents we enter a new existential state, of dependency and vulnerability. In this state, called *illness*, the body becomes the center of our concern because it is an impediment to, rather than a willing instrument for, the things we want to do.

The second element in the patient-physician relationship is the act of profession. When a patient enters a physician's office, the physician will say "What can I do for you?" or "How can I help you?" This is an act of profession, rather than a greeting, because within our social structure the physician is "ordained" as the one to whom the ill come for help. The physician's offer to help contains two implicit promises. First, the physician is competent and possesses the knowledge you need; second, he or she promises to use that knowledge in your interest.

The relationship of a vulnerable human (in the state of illness) with another human who has declared and professed that he or she is competent to heal is different from a commercial or legal relationship. A commercial relationship is based on mutual self-interest; a legal relationship is based on contract. A patient-physician relationship is based on profession and trust. Patients must trust the physician because illness has disabled them, has forced them to face the fragility of personal existence and placed them in a vulnerable state where they are dependent on another human being. This extreme vulnerability requires that the physician's relationship to the patient be based not on mutual self-interest, or contract, but on profession.

The gap between the patient's illness and the physician's profession is closed in the act of medicine, the third element. This moment of clinical truth is the decision on what to do. Medicine does not come into existence until a decision is made about a particular human being in a particular life-context, here and now. Medicine, science, the biological sciences are preparatory for the moment of clinical truth, in which the physician and patient, together, decide what ought to be done.

What ought to be done has two elements: the *right* decision and the *good* decision. By "right" decision I mean that it must be technically correct, must use the best scientific knowledge. Therefore, science is fundamental to all kinds of medicine. Medical science can determine what is physically wrong, what can be done about it, and what is likely to be the outcome; but it cannot tell what ought to be done for the *good* of a particular patient. If you follow the cure model, the biomedical model, then what is medically good—what is medically indicated, what is scientifically correct—becomes what is good for the patient.

But reflect for a moment and you'll see that the two are not the same. The good decision must also fit the particular person's concept of the good life and the way he or she wants to live. The good decision must fit the patient's value systems, belief systems, and (if present) religious and spiritual convictions. In short, a good decision to the extent that it is humanly possible, must take into account how the scientifically indicated fits into the particular values, beliefs, and convictions which define the patient as person.

All physicians face the conflict between a technically right curing decision and the patient's conception of a good decision. For example, this conflict often arises in treatment of a Jehovah's Witness, who can be cured of certain acute situations with a blood transfusion; but the Jehovah's Witness has religious convictions which, for him or her, preclude that possibility. The right decision technically is not the good decision, because it violates the promise that the physician will use his competence for the good of the person who is ill and vulnerable. A person in a vulnerable state is in an unequal relationship, in which another has control of his or her life at that moment. Obligations are greatest on the one who has this power in the healing relationship, because he or she has voluntarily professed to work for the good of this particular patient.

Cure in the radical sense is not the only aim of medicine. The end of medicine, in the philosophical sense, is a right and good healing decision for a particular human being. A medically right decision might be to resuscitate a critically ill patient in hope that time would eventually lead to cure. Or if a patient had said no ("I'm not willing to pay the price of continuing to suffer; I am ready to face death; I am ready to begin the day of my dying"), the right decision and the good decision would be in conflict. What we have then, at the moment of clinical truth, is an intersection of value systems which is the central and focal problem of medical ethics.

Today, the moment of clinical truth at the intersection of value systems must be faced without the traditional security of a noble, unfailing, universally honored code of ethics. The recent revision of the AMA Code, as well as the Hippocratic Oath and the many codes derived from it, are useful, but they are inadequate for the most crucial ethical question of our day: How do we assure that moral choices, among and between persons whose values and ethical systems may vary widely, can be made in a morally defensible way? How do we preserve our personal moral accountability in a pluralistic society, and assure our patients that we will respect them as moral agents?

Without deprecating various codes, we must recognize that they have lost some of their force because they suppose a homogeneity of philosophical and theological values that is no longer the case. With so many differences at so many fundamental levels, is medical ethics doomed to atomization? I do not believe so. Despite the greater complexity of clinical decisions in a democratic and pluralistic society, the realities of being ill and being healed (or cared for) have not and will not change fundamentally.

To care for a patient in the full and integral sense I have outlined requires a reconstruction of medical ethics, one that attends to the concept of care in its broadest sense and, indeed, makes caring a moral obligation. There are three requirements for a reconstruction of medical ethics that, I believe, are capable of confronting some of the dilemmas of today's clinical decisions and professional ethics. They define the conditions for an effective reconstruction of the edifice of medical ethics:

1. Such an ethic must be approached in a modular fashion.
2. It must incorporate a clear notion of the "good" of the patient.
3. It must refurbish the concept of profession.

We have long been accustomed to thinking of medical ethics in terms of a uniform code or as a single set of self-contained, self-justifying principles. The erosion of a common philosophical and theological belief system makes this concept no longer tenable. Instead, a complete medical ethics consists of four modular components, closely linked and interdependent, to be sure, yet separable in actual ethical discourse and moral choice.

The first module consists of the positions we take on specific ethical issues of the day: euthanasia, abortion, terminating treatment, living wills, artificial insemination—any of the multitude of new questions that technological capability puts before us. Much of the strife of ethical discourse and decision arises from opposing positions on these issues. Most people simply assert their positions as "right" and "good," and reject argumentation that exposes the sources of their opinions.

The second module contains the philosophical sources upon which the positions in the first module are based. These are in three large categories: (1) the theory of ethics to which we subscribe: deontological, utilitarian, contractarian, consequentialist, or teleological; (2) the construal we place on the fundamental ethical principles of truth-telling, promise-keeping, beneficence, nonmaleficence, justice, and the like; and (3) our concept of the nature, destiny, and worth of human existence.

The third module comprises our theological and religious beliefs: what we think about God, our duties to Him, and the ultimate destiny and meaning of human existence. Believers and nonbelievers alike take positive or negative positions on these questions which seriously affect their moral choices.

The fourth module is less well developed than the other three. Unlike them, it is not substantive in content, but deals with the ethics of the process of interpersonal moral decision making. It comprises our positions on such things as patient participation, strong and weak paternalism, libertarianism, protecting the autonomy and moral agency of the patient, telling the truth, manipulating consent, and handling conflicts between the interacting parties (physicians, other members of the health professions, patients, and their families). This module should aim at assuring a morally defensible transaction between persons who may differ widely on the substantive ethical issues, yet must enter a medical transaction with each other. This is the ethics of a moral relationship between physicians and patients, irrespective of their positions on specific medical-moral questions.

Out of the interaction between these four modules of medical ethics we arrive at what we think is right and good in a particular clinical situation. A complete and mature medical morality requires us to be clear about our positions in each module. Only then can we understand the basis for our actions, and where and at what level we disagree or agree with patients (and others) in clinical decisions.

It is unlikely that we will ever again enjoy wide agreement on the philosophical or theological sources of our medical morality. It is therefore unlikely that we can achieve general agreement on specific clinical-moral decisions. If any common principles are possible, they will probably be deducible only in the fourth component, in a procedural ethics which respects the obligations of each person to be faithful to his or her belief systems.

Development of this fourth module is our most urgent need in medical ethics in a democratic society. The Hippocratic corpus says very little about the process of making decisions. If anything, it is strongly paternalistic, and even warns against sharing information with the patient. The most recent revision of the AMA Code is silent on this subject, though it is treated under the heading of consent in "Opinions of the Judicial Council." On the whole the most vexing questions about who decides and how are still left largely to individual interpretation.

This deficiency is no longer acceptable. Patients and their families want to know how we will make our decisions, who will have the final say, and how we will handle potential conflicts. Also, they will increasingly want to know our position on the major medical-moral questions. This is becoming a major issue on the agenda of medical ethics.

"GOOD OF THE PATIENT" CONCEPT

Any ethics of the process of clinical decision must begin with a clear notion of the good of the patient. This is a complex notion, to which it is easy to give superficial assent. All too often, it is little more than a rhetorical device. It is rarely carefully analyzed, yet it is the final criterion of whether a decision is morally sound. It is therefore the unifying theme of all medical ethics, and particularly of any ethics of moral choice and decision making.

The good of the patient is a compound notion, with at least three components which can sometimes be in conflict with each other. A morally good clinical decision should attend to all three senses of patient good and resolve conflicts among them.

Biomedical Good. This is the good a medical intervention can offer by modifying the natural history of disease in a patient. It can be cure, prevention or containment of disease, amelioration of symptoms, or prolongation of life. It is the good aimed at by the doctor's craftsmanship and the result of scientifically correct decisions about what can be done and carrying it out safely, competently, and with minimal discomfort. An intervention that can effectively alter the natural history of the disease is "medically indicated." For the purpose of this discussion, *biomedical good* is synonymous with *medical indication.*

Characteristically, physicians make two errors with respect to medical indications. The first is to reduce the whole of patient good to medical indication. This leads to the fallacy of the medical imperative: if any good can be achieved by a procedure, that procedure must be done. On this view, medical ethics is reduced to doing whatever is medically indicated; and any other sense of the good of the patient is ignored.

The second error is to mix quality-of-life assessments with medical indications. On this view a treatment or procedure is judged not only by what it can do to change the natural history of a disease, but by the kind of life that results in a particular patient. On this view, some external observer's opinion—the physician's—of the worth-whileness of another person's life is used to deny treatment. This is an unjustifiable mingling of categories of judgment. Whether someone's life is worth living is not measurable by medical means, and therefore it is not the doctor's prerogative to determine. The physician should define, as accurately and objectively as possible, what kind of life might result from treatment, so that the patient (or surrogate) can determine whether it is worth living. This determination should not, of course, be colored by nonmedical value judgments in arriving at medical indication.

Patient's Concept of His/Her Own Good. A biomedically good decision is scientifically correct, but is not automatically a good decision from the patient's point of view. It must be placed within the context of the patient's life situation and value system. It must square with what the patient thinks is "worthwhile," given the circumstances and choices forced by illness. Only the patient can weigh the probable medical benefits of treatment against pain, disability, and loss of dignity that those benefits may "cost" him or against some ultimate good such as his concept of his own spiritual destiny. Only the patient (or proxy) can determine whether the quality of life predicted by the physician is worthwhile. The range of satisfactions of the sick and disabled is narrowed, but what is left may still be savored by the patient.

When the patient is competent, he can himself ascertain what is in his "best interests." When he is not, his surrogates must ascertain, as closely as possible, what the patient would have taken to be his best interests, were he able to make the choice himself.

The patient's interest, defined this way, is necessarily subjective and relative. It is the patient's best estimate of what he thinks is good for him, and we cannot know what it is until we ask the patient. This does not deny the fact that some objects of patient interest might be inferred incorrectly, or might conflict with biomedical good or with what others may deem to be in the patient's interest.

The Good of the Patient as a Person. The third sense of "patient good" is the good most proper to being a human. Philosophers argue endlessly about what constitutes the distinguishing feature of being human: freedom, rationality, consciousness, capacity for language, art, or culture. Without trying to settle these debates, it would be hard to deny that one observable feature unique to humans is the capacity to make choices, to set up a life plan, and to determine one's goals for a satisfactory life (among the many possible ways to conduct a human life).

The good that is proper to humans *as* humans is that which fulfills our potentialities as individuals of a rational nature, capable of choice. To be treated as humans is to be accorded the dignity of choosing what we believe to be good and to be accountable for our wrong choices. We cannot exercise our humanity fully unless we are free to make our own mistakes.

The good that is peculiar to being human is the freedom to express our humanity in a choice which is our own. That choice may be right or wrong: what a reasonable person might or might not do. It might, or might not, square with the doctor's concept of good. That it is the patient's good does not make it good in an absolute sense, but we violate a greater good if we do not allow a person to choose.

SOCIAL GOOD

As the cumulative effects of individual medical decision alter the world's demography and high technology consumes an ever larger percentage of our resources, the good of society comes more and more into conflict with the good of the patient. The economic and social costs of prolonging lives of infants, as well as the aged and disabled, are intruding themselves into clinical decisions. A growing body of critics takes physicians to task for exalting individual patient good over that of society. Yet that is the commitment the patient expects.

Are we justified in violating that trust, without changing the explicit promise we make to help the patient? Can physicians be agents of social and fiscal good, and still serve the three senses of patient good which I have described? In the years immediately ahead, this will be perhaps the most vexing dilemma the physician will face.

ETHICS OF THE PROCESS OF CLINICAL MORAL CHOICE

The possibilities of conflict between these various components of "the good of the patient" underscore the need for a careful definition of *which* good we mean in defending a specific clinical decision. It also implies some ranking of these various senses of patient good. This is a subject of its own, and I can only suggest an order.

The highest sense of the good of competent patients is that which preserves their capacity to act in a fully human way—that is, to express and act on their perception of their own good. That good is owed all patients, simply because they are human. If a patient is not competent a surrogate or proxy is expected to ascertain what choice the patient *would* have made. A patient's freedom to choose is limited only when it poses a direct, immediate, and discernible harm to another person, or if fulfilling the patient's perception of good would violate the physician's conscience. The physician is a moral agent, as well as the patient, and cannot be expected to cooperate in what the physician considers to be wrong.

Patients' conceptions of their own good, which rank right behind their good as a human person, take precedence over biomedical good or medical indications. To force medical good on a patient, or to accomplish it by deception or manipulation for the "patient's good," is to violate a patient's good as a human being, and as an agent entitled to make moral choices.

Biomedical good and medical indications are therefore lowest in the hierarchy of senses in which we can interpret the good of the patient. Beneficial as they might be, they do not justify violation of the higher good of the patient as a human being to express his or her choices and to determine the specific nature of what is in their "best interests."

An ethics of the process of clinical moral choices, therefore, obligates the physician to respect the several dimensions of the good of the patient and to keep them distinct and in proper order when they are in conflict. Some of these obligations are as follows.

In all decisions, the physician has the responsibility for an objective assessment of biomedical good—that is, how the proposed treatment will change the short- and long-term prognosis and history of the disease. That assessment must be objective, scientifically sound, and free of "quality of life" criteria. In this way, patients or their surrogates are enabled to determine accurately what is in the patients' best interests.

Assessment of the good to be achieved by a medical intervention should be presented to the patient (or surrogate) as sensitively and clearly as possible. It must be fitted to the patient's educational, cultural, linguistic, and ethnic background. The physician has an obligation to assist the patient to make as cogent a choice as possible—and without coercion or deception.

After they have been properly, and sensitively, informed, patients may ask the physician to make the decision for them; and the physician then has a mandate to do so. Such a mandate is very different from automatically assuming that "the doctor knows what's best" for the patient and from taking a strangely paternalistic role from the outset.

With an incompetent (or never-competent) patient, the physician should accord the same freedom of choice to surrogates. He has the additional, difficult obligation to be sure that a surrogate is competent to make the decision and that the surrogate is acting in the best interests of the patient.

The process is greatly complicated in the case of infants, where the family's wishes and its quality-of-life determinants may color a decision. But the physician's concern must be the infant, for the infant is the patient, *not* the family. With the never-competent patient, there is no way to ascertain what the patient would see as his or her interests. Therefore medical good—the probability of improving the patient's functioning or comfort—assumes a more dominant place than with the competent or once-competent patient.

When serious moral disagreements between physicians or surrogates occur, and especially in the case of infants, recourse should be had to a judicious, uninvolved, deliberative group—a consultant, an ethics committee, a court-appointed guardian. If all this fails, court intervention may be necessary—but this is not the way to determine what is morally right. It is an inferior way of determining which decision is to be made and to be sure that *some* decision is made that protects legal rights.

The best clinical decisions are those in which medical good, the patient's interests, and the freedom to choose are congruent; and in many cases they are. Most often, differences can be "negotiated" if they are approached in trust, without deception, and with sensitivity. The quality of the relationship between patients, families, and medical attendants will often be the deciding factor, rather than rules of procedure or moral algorithms.

Unfortunately, the "trust relationship" required for so momentous a decision as, let us say, a no-code order is becoming ever more difficult in contemporary medical care. Team care, multiple consultations, rotations of house staff, institutionalization, stress at the moment of decision—all complicate the relationship. In public and teaching hospitals there is often no one with a sustained relationship with the patient who can serve as a personal physician in the delicate process of making moral choices. This is an intolerable impediment to ethical patient care in the complicated nexus of today's clinical decisions and the reconstruction that medical ethics will demand.

An ethics of moral decision making must include respect for the moral agencies and the moral accountability of all health professionals who interact in the clinical decision. The physician may have technical, and even legal, authority to perform certain acts; the nurse and social worker, authority to perform others; but no one has moral authority over another. Thus all members of medical and health care teams are morally accountable to themselves and to their patients. Each promises to help and to act in the patient's best interests.

There will be times when orders cannot be followed because the moral principles of some team members are violated. At other times, if a serious transgression of our obligations to patients occurs, "whistle-blowing," with all its painful consequences, may be necessary. Physicians need far more awareness of and sensitivity to potentialities for moral conflicts with other health professions, and they must learn to deal with such conflicts in a way which respects the moral agencies of their colleagues.

REFURBISHING THE IDEAL OF A PROFESSION

Our act of profession is the promise we make every time we offer to help a sick person. It declares implicitly, to the patient and family, that we are competent, that we will use our competency in the interests of the patient, and that we can be trusted not to abuse the privileges our promise entails in helping to manage some of the most significant events in a person's life. It allows us, in the patients' interests, to learn all their weaknesses and foibles, to probe, palpate, price, and incise their bodies—a degree of intimacy that one does not accord strangers.

No idea has been more debased than the idea of a profession. Today, anyone who undertakes an activity full time, for pay, or with high skill—anyone with special competency or knowledge, anyone with a college degree or credential, anyone who performs some needed service—can call himself a "professional." The list ranges from athletics to astrophysics, from carpentry to salesmanship, from medicine to mortuary science, from pipefitting to politics. Whoever is not an amateur, dilettante, hobbyist, or apprentice is accorded the title "professional."

I have no quarrel with recognition of anyone who pursues excellence in performance, particularly in this age of slovenly craftsmanship. Nor do I wish to preserve the term "professional" for some elite purpose. True elitism is not born of titles anyway, but of the voluntary self-imposition of higher-than-ordinary standards.

Nonetheless, we must not forget that our act of profession as healers is a declaration of commitment—an act of consecration (to use Cushing's word) to a way of life that is not ordinary. It is a promise that we will not place our own interests first, that we will not exploit the vulnerability of those we serve, that we will honor the trust that illness forces upon those who are ill. This necessity for a higher standard impelled Plato to use medicine as his paradigm of the ethical employment of knowledge. Medicine was for him a *tekné*—a craft and art, to be sure, but significantly different from all the others.

Later, in the first century A.D., when the word *profession* was first used by Scribonius Largus, it was tied to a special promise to help humanity and to place it above one's own interests. This has always been the doctor's special promise, his common devotion, and the source for his ethical obligations. When medicine lacks this ethical dimension, it becomes not just a business, trade, or technique, but a betrayal of trust that demeans both the physician and the patient, and leads to angry and satirical attacks on physicians in the world's literature. Pomposity, callousness, and cupidity are common human failings, but they elicit special rancor in physicians because our severest critics expect better of us.

The most corrosive force is still abuse by physicians of the trust that the nature of their duties demands. We must *merit* the trust our act of profession invites. If we do not rise to those obligations, we can hardly protest when we are satirized, treated as trades- or businessmen, and regulated as such. Moral credibility is ours to establish and ours to lose. We cannot blame the FTC, Congress, the media, or the moral standards of society.

The nature of the acts we are expected to perform, together with the trust they demand, form the basis of our professional morality. They are binding on health professionals, even if their philosophical and theological principles differ widely. Only we can determine whether our act of profession is a solemn promise, a contract, a commodity transaction, or a business deal. How we "translate" our act of profession tells more about us than all our rhetoric or codes of ethics.

Our moral choices are more difficult, more subtle, and more controversial than those our profession faced previously. We must make them without the heritage of shared values that could unify medical ethics. Our task is not to abandon hope in medical ethics but to undertake what Camus called "the most difficult task of all, to reconsider everything from the ground up, so as to shape a living society inside a dying society."

That task is not demolition of the edifice of medical morality, but its reconstruction along three lines: (1) replacement of a monolithic with a modular structure for medical ethics, with special emphasis on the ethics of making moral choices in clinical decisions;

(2) clarification of what we mean when we speak of the "good" of the patient, and setting priority among the several senses in which that term may be taken; and (3) refurbishing the traditional ideal of a profession as truly a "consecration" of our expertise.

The reconstruction I have suggested calls upon all of us in the health professions to attend to the full spectrum of meanings of the word *care.* Care is the moral base upon which our professional obligations, our ethics, are to be re-formed. Caring, instead of a narrow concept, becomes synonymous with what we are all about, each in our own way. It is also the "common devotion" of all health professionals—the overriding consideration that should bind us in an enterprise that transcends the self-interests of our individual professions.

CHAPTER THIRTEEN

THE BOOK OF JOB

> *How wonderful were your scriptures! How profound! We see their surface and it attracts us like children. And yet, O God, their depth is stupendous. We shudder to peer into them, for they inspire in us both the awe of reverence and the thrill of love.*
> *St.Augustine,* The Confessions

INTRODUCTION: JOB, THE PARADIGM OF SUFFERING

Literary masterworks survive, not because they resolve some universal human dilemma, but precisely because they do not. Their special appeal lies in the fact that they confront the mystery of human existence; they do so in exalted language that evokes the tremendum of religious experience; and they offer multiple levels of interpretation and meaning. They leave the fundamental questions tantalizingly unanswered, but also tantalizingly alive for every era to ponder. All lasting works center on the question of man to which, as Karl Rahner has said, "...there is no answer." Job is preeminently such a book.

Job confronts the enigma of human suffering directly, poignantly, and in sublime poetic language. It leaves us deeply disquieted, but never indifferent. Job has been read in a multitude of ways: as a paradigm of patience; a test of righteousness; a proof that good may come from evil; and evidence of the meaninglessness of human existence; a proof of God's indifference, or His moral ambivalence. Some conclude that the answer to Job's question is abandonment to God's will; others, the rejection of God as a cosmic sadist; and others that human, not divine, love is the only reality upon which we can rely. Whatever the interpretation, all ages have recognized that the Book of Job describes an inescapable human experience, one that each of us ultimately must confront and to which we must fashion a personal response.

Paul Claudel, the French poet-diplomat, after 50 years of struggling with the meaning of the Book of Job, concluded that, "it is the most sublime, the most poignant, the most daring, and at the same time the most disappointing...and the most offensive of the books of the Bible." As an enigma, its closest competitor is that other strangely fascinating piece of Wisdom literature, the Book of Ecclesiastes.

Even a partial list of the luminaries who, like Claudel, puzzled over Job's intriguing text, is overwhelming in length and intellectual power. Among the *saints* we find Jerome, Chrysostom, and Gregory, the latter devoting four entire books of meditation to Job's dilemma. Among the *theologians* we can count Luther, Kierkegaard, Buber, Danielou, and Calvin. The latter was moved to devote 159 sermons to Job. The *philosophers* include Maimonides, Spinoza, Hobbes, Kant, Nietzsche, Royce, Paul Weiss, and Walter Kaufman. 'The *writers* include Lamartine, Voltaire, D. H. Lawrence, and Robert Frost. Archibald MacLeish cast Job as a modern businessman. William Blake illustrated the Book of Job with his mystical engravings.

If to this partial list, we add all those who have wrestled with the theme of human suffering and its meaning, we would embrace much of the world's great literature - from the folk tales of Ancient Egypt and the Middle East, through Sophocles, Aeschylus, and Euripides, to Marcus Aurelius, St. Augustine, Dante, Shakespeare, and Goethe to Dostoyevski, De Unamuno, Camus, Kafka, John Gardner, and Samuel Beckett. No serious writer or thinker has been able to ignore Job's anguish, his questions and his desperate need for answers. Can we believe in God with the mysteries of evil and justice unanswered? Does suffering have meaning? Does meaning itself exist? All art ultimately must touch these questions, or remain forever ephemeral and on the surface of life.

What can a physician add to what has already been so copiously and perceptively written about Job? I am neither an exegete, biblical scholar, philosopher, theologian, or literary critic. I cannot discourse on the metaphysical compatibility of evil with the existence of a good and just God. Nor can I add anything to the learned debates about the provenance, authorship, chronology, unity, linguistics, or poetic merits of the text.

My own fascination with the text of Job is as a paradigm of human suffering - physical and spiritual. As such, it speaks to the physician who meets Job daily in the suffering of his patients. He is under a moral imperative to comprehend that experience as best he can. Without that comprehension the physician cannot fully help or heal. Without it, he cannot prepare for the inevitable experience of his own suffering.

What I can offer is one physician's meditation on Job, on what the text reveals of the nature of suffering, its impact on the human spirit, and the things we must understand to help each other in the presence of illness and misfortune. I shall concentrate on the human experience of Job, his friends' efforts to console him, and the insights we can gain from Job's dialogues with his friends. I will comment on what this rich text reveals to doctors, nurses, patients, and pastoral counselors, and all of us. Job is a text we must study if we are to be healers rather than wounders of the sick and the afflicted.

I know even these aims are not modest. But, at least, I hope to avoid the intellectual and spiritual arrogance of another physician who commented on Job's text. In his *Answer to Job,* the physician-psychologist, Carl Jung, humbly promised to meditate on the text "....as a layman, and a physician who had been privileged to see deeply into the psychic depth of many people." Instead of keeping that promise, however, Jung had the audacity to put God on the analytic couch. He found God entrapped in a Manichean emotional conflict, caught between His good and evil natures. God, according to Jung, was guilt-ridden because He violated the Covenant in His treatment of Job. Jung also psychoanalyzed Christ, Ezekiel, and St. John and reinterpreted the doctrine of the Assumption! Jung achieved a level of hubris unparalleled even in a profession not particularly noted for its humility! While I may not, by the nature of my task, avoid pretentiousness entirely, I think I can avoid Jung's own Super-Jehovah complex.

OUTLINE OF THE BOOK

The line of Job's story is of the utmost simplicity. It has what Northrop Frye has called a "U" shape. Job starts out prosperous; he is smitten by calamities; Job is restored to his former status. Within that simple line lies one of the most profound metaphysical and spiritual odysseys in all of literature.

The story of Job was originally probably limited to Chapters 1, 2, and 42, what are now the prologue and epilogue. The intervening poetic portion is a later addition to the "story."

The book of Job opens in heaven where we learn that Job, a prosperous and righteous desert chieftain in the land of Uz, is beloved by God for his piety and faithfulness. Satan is scandalized by such a paragon of virtue and challenges God's trust in Job. Job's piety, Satan says, is nothing but well disguised self-interest. Satan taunts God, "Just reach out and strike what he has, and he will curse you to your face."(1:11) God is so confident of Job's righteousness that he turns Job over to Satan's power, at first exempting only Job's person from harm.

Job is visited by a series of calamities. He loses all his flocks. His home is destroyed and all his children killed. Yet, Job remains faithful. "Yahweh gave, and Yahweh took away. Blessed be Yahweh's name."(1:21) But Satan is still not satisfied. He challenges God further, "reach out and strike him. Touch his bone and flesh and he will curse you to your face"(2:5). God, still confident of Job's righteousness, hands him over to Satan's power "only spare his life,"(2:6) He says to Satan. Job is now afflicted with a terrible skin disease and reduced to a pitiful state, seated on an ash heap, scraping himself with a potsherd. So dismal is his predicament that Job's wife tells him to curse God and die. Job refuses, saying, "Shall we accept good from God and not accept evil?"(2:10)

At this point, the story changes from prose to the most powerful kind of poetry. Job is visited by three friends. At first, when they see the state to which he has fallen, they grieve silently with him for seven days and nights. Job then delivers a soliloquy lamenting his fate, cursing the day of his birth and yearning for death to release him from his suffering.

His three friends can no longer contain their silence. Each delivers several cycles of speeches to which Job replies. Each speaker sets forth, in various ways, the traditional teaching that evil is the wages of sin. They imply, at first indirectly, and then by direct accusation, that Job or his children have sinned in some way or they would not be punished by a just and good God. Job vehemently denies their accusations and vigorously protests his friends' rationalizations. He refuses to confess to transgressions he has not committed. Job challenges God's righteousness. He prays fervently for someone to hear his case - some neutral judge - whom he can confront face-to-face. If only he could present his case, the injustice of his sufferings would be clear.

Job's debate with his friends ends in stalemate and Job soliloquizes again, protesting his innocence. He recites the code of righteous behavior by which he has lived his whole life. He pleads again for God to answer him. Now a new counselor, named Elihu, enters the debate. He is a young and arrogant man who castigates Job's three friends for their ineffectiveness in arguing with Job. He launches into his own long tirade against Job's protestations of innocence - using the same arguments as the others, but more vehemently and more accusingly.

Finally, God does speak directly to Job, out of a whirlwind. He does not answer Job in Job's terms. Instead, in magnificent verse, He hurls a series of ironic questions at Job. God questions Job's fitness to understand even the simplest mysteries of His creation. Yet these, wondrous as they are, are far from exhausting God's power. Job is mistaken to think that God or the moral order of His universe, can be understood in human terms or measured by man. God challenges Job, "will the contender with Shaddai yield? He who reproves God, let him answer for it."(30:2)

Job is overwhelmed. He has had the confrontation he begged for, but not as he could possibly have imagined. Job admits he is of small account, "Lo I am small, how can I answer you?"(40:4), and resolves to speak no more. But the Lord continues His challenges. Would Job dare to condemn God, that he might justify himself?(40:8) God continues His rhapsody on the mysteries of the cosmos which man cannot understand, including the existence of evil. At no point does the Lord use any of the conventional explanations so laboriously and confidently argued by Job's friends.

Job has now had wish. He has seen the Almighty with his own eyes. He abases himself before God and repents for the folly of daring to be God's critic. He no longer asks for reason, but for compassion: "I had heard of you by hearsay, but now my eyes have seen you. So, I recant and repent in dust and ashes."(42:5-6) The book ends in a prose epilogue in which God chastises Eliphaz, one of Job's friends: "My anger burns against you and your two friends for you have not spoken the truth of me as Job did."(42:7-8)

Job's friends must offer sacrifice, but they will not be forgiven unless Job prays for them. Job's prosperity is restored several-fold; his honor is regained, he lives a long life, and dies in peace.

THE ODYSSEY OF JOB'S SUFFERING

In his preface to *Prometheus Unbound,* Shelley warns about the nontransposability of prose and poetry and his abhorrence for didacticism in poetry. All attempts to extract explicit meanings or morals from poetry as exalted as Job's run the risk of puerility. It is what Job's poetry evokes in each of us about the human experience of suffering that draws us irresistibly. We can see Job in ourselves, or families, friends, and our patients. In Job's dialogue with his friends, we recognize our own attempts to help and to give some rational grounding to suffering. We feel Job's anger, protestations, and puzzlement, his sense of injustice and alienation. Everywhere they greet us:

in every hospital, home for the aged and retarded, in the hospices, the prisons, in the victims of the Holocaust, and in every oppressed land. The sheer massiveness of human misery and the inevitability that we, too, will suffer, hover silently over even the most prosperous of us.

The physician sees all of this up close in the inhabitants of that city of suffering - the hospital he traverses daily. He sees how illness shocks, shatters, and estranges. He cannot help being pulled into the sufferer's experience if he is truly a healer and not simply a tinker of diseased organs and disabled bodies. To be sure, the physician must practice detachment - but he must practice a compassionate detachment. He must have a capacity to step back from Job's ills and anguish, to diagnose them accurately so as to treat them rationally. But, if he is also to help, he must confront, with his patients, the deeper anguish that transcends the pain and the physical ravages of the disease.

Illness and sickness create the deepest suffering and the most severe test of life's meaning. Recall that neither God nor Satan regarded Job as fully tested until his "flesh and bone" were touched. Job suffered the loss of all he cherished. While Job lamented his losses loudly and pitifully, he sank into the deepest depths of his despair and resentment only when God permitted Satan to afflict him with a frightful skin disease. It is after this that Job began to hurl his sharpest blasphemies, questions, accusations, and bitterness at God.

Once personal illness is added to Job's other burdens, he is like the Psalmist "on the brink of Sheol," "a man bereft of strength."(Psalm 88)* He oscillates between abjectly begging for the death and pleading for restoration of his health. He accuses the very God from Whom he demands justice. Over and over again, Job asks, as does every afflicted human. Why? Why me? Why now? Why not all the unrighteous who prosper and live long lives? "What have I done to you, man watcher? Why have you made me your target? Why am I a burden to you?"(7:20) But Job gets no answer, even after he confronts God eye-to-eye. The mystery of suffering must remain a mystery; it is beyond human rationality. Job learns that no human has a claim on God. No human can presume to be a critic of the cosmic order. Job is finally overwhelmed and reconciled, not by a reasonable explanation, but by a religious experience. He is struck by awe and fear of the Lord and painfully learns the lesson of the psalmist of Psalm 111, or in Job's own words: "Behold the fear of the Lord, that is wisdom. To turn from evil is understanding."(28:8)

For the physician, Job is the incarnation of his own patient with whom the physician goes through the experience of suffering. Illness is a special assault on the whole person - as much on the spirit as on the body. Suffering is more than physiological pain. Pain and painless disease, alike, beget anguish because they contract the possibilities of human existence. The horizons of what may be hoped for are foreshortened. The afflicted is, in Job's words, one..."Whose way is hidden, whom God has fenced about."(3:23) Sickness is the unfailing evidence of our ultimate and ineradicable finitude - the sign of the fragility of personal existence. It exposes unequivocally the vulnerability, dependence, expendability, and exploitability always lurking just beneath the surface of human life. It terrifies the one who is ill, and those who attend him or are dear to him.

* Text of the Jerusalem Bible

The one who is sick can no longer define and pursue his own goals. The purposes of his life are predetermined by the disease. It takes center-stage. Sickness makes the body and the mind the enemy of the self; it obtunds all plans. It forces a confrontation with the numinous: "Why do you rear man at all? Or pay any mind to him? Inspect him every morning? Test him every moment?"(7:17-18) How shall I respond, what shall I say, how shall I live? The answers must be our own if we are to remain persons. Men and women can endure extreme pain and suffering when there is hope, or explanation. Without these, the suffering person faces the terrible possibility of a dissolution of his entire being.

Suffering demands that endurance and dying be personal enterprises. It unmercifully exposes our freedom to fashion a personal response. In that freedom lies the paradoxical possibility of healing even the dying patient. Unlike Job, we must respond without seeing God eye-to-eye, without directly confronting His ineffability. To embrace or reject suffering, to make it our own experience and not become its passive object, is the final test of that autonomy we hold so dear when we are healthy.

WIDE RANGE OF RESPONSES

Physicians, families, and friends must be prepared for a wide, unpredictable, and often shocking range of responses to Job's questions posed by the sick person they love, and think they know. Is suffering a punishment for sin, or is it a preventive? Is it a means of atonement and reconciliation? Or is it, as the Stoics said, an inexorable, inexplicable law of nature, useless to resist? Is suffering evidence, as some Existentialists would have it, of God's indifference or the meaninglessness of meaning itself? Is it the way of salvation as Christ taught? Or is it, as Nietzsche insisted, that the whole idea of salvation itself is the result of the Christian's "inability to let suffering be senseless." Is the sufferer, like Kafka's protagonist, accused of an unspecified crime by an accuser he will never meet? Is he, like Oedipus, suffering because of a curse on his family, or like Prometheus, for opposing God's will, like Lear or Macbeth, for a defect of character, or like Jason and Medea, for an excess of hubris?

The whole complex, contradictory, and vacillating nexus of rationalizations of suffering is incarnated in each sick and suffering human. And it is into this tangled nexus that the physician and others must enter. In the modern world, suffering is not very often accepted, simply and submissively, as God's will, as Job first accepted it. Rather, modern man resists openly the affront to pride and self-esteem, which misfortune, disease, and death represent. Job himself was not entirely the model of steadfast faith and patience which St. James makes him out to be. (5:11)

Job's text teaches us how to discern the many ways in which humans react to suffering. We must comprehend the range of those responses if we are to help, and not exacerbate the suffering. Despite Shelley's abhorrence for the didactic, we must yet look at the more mundane practical lessons Job's human predicament can teach all of us.

We note, for example, that Job's friends spent a week with him in silence. Considering their later clumsy attempts to console him, this was perhaps the best thing they did. Their presence was a genuine act of empathy. It is the first step we, too, must take - to *be* with the sick, to listen to their soliloquies, to say just enough to show we are there, and to allow their hurt to show itself. A receptive silence, one that communicates compassionate concern without pitying, allows the patient to vent his resentment and anger to another person.

But, like Job, the patient is, in reality, speaking to God. There is, in us, a deep impulse to vent our sufferings. We who attend the sick are privileged witnesses to those struggles. The sick person sooner or later knows that there may be no answer to his questions. What he needs is our understanding that the struggle is a personal, deeply spiritual, and perilous one. Often we help most if we help least - if we listen in silence, as Job's friends did at first.

Like them, we cannot remain forever silent. Inevitably we must enter the experiences of illness and suffering in *this* person. But we must do so without shock, surprise, or moralizing. We must not allow our sensibilities to be offended by what we hear in the patient's soliloquy. Above all, we must avoid trying to win an argument: "But what does your arguing prove?"(6:25) Like Job's counselors, in our zeal for explanation we run the risk of becoming not friends, but accusers, usurping God's prerogatives of judgment.

We cannot rightfully expect that God will speak directly to us as He did to Job. Yet we must not forget that Job himself, even before he had his confrontation with God, knew that he could not win his case against God. "But how can man be acquitted before God? If He deigned to litigate with him, could he answer Him one in a thousand?"(9: 2-3) The inescapable fact is that Job cannot argue his case against God nor can Job's friends presume to argue God's case against Job.

Most offensive to Job, and to any suffering or sick person, are condescension and presumption. Let us listen to Job's own words to his friends:

> I know as much as you know
> I am not inferior to you
> Rather would I speak with Shaddai
> I wish to remonstrate with God
> But you are daubers of deceit,
> Quack healers all of you
> I wish you would keep strictly silent
> That would be wisdom in you, (13:2-5)

We need to appreciate, too, that the experience of illness is not penetrable by others and none of us can know how we will respond. Thus, Job says to his friends:

> Will it be well when he probes you?
> Can you trick him as men are tricked? (13:9)

> Will not his fear overwhelm you? (13:11)

> Your maxims are ashen aphorisms
> Defenses of clay your defenses.
> Be silent before me that I may speak. (13:12-13)

God Himself agreed with Job and castigated Job's friends just as severely for not speaking truly. He preferred Job's honest protestations to the pious hypocrisy of his friends who dared to argue God's case against Job. If we are to avoid the same condemnation, we must listen carefully to Job's words when we are in the presence of our suffering patients, families, or friends.

Job, like his counterparts in every age, asks repeatedly for our compassionate listening, not moralizing speeches:

> Pity me, Pity me, Oh my friends.
> For the hand of God has struck me.
> Why do you pursue me like God? (19:21-22)
>
> Hear my word attentively,
> Let this be the solace you give.
> Bear with me, let me speak,
> When I have spoken, mock on. (21:2-3)

Over and over again, Job beseeches his friends to hear him out, to understand his plight, to feel compassion for his predicament, but not to preach to him.

In some of the most forceful words in all literature, Job speaks for all the suffering in all the ages. We are all tempted to play the roles of Bildad, Zophar, and Eliphaz, and some of us, even the more arrogant role of Elihu. Job is blunt in his condemnation of their theologizing. He speaks eloquently for all those patient sufferers who, out of deference, do not tell us to "shut up" as Job so forthrightly told his friends.

We must be prepared, therefore, if we would help, to hear outpourings of rage, doubt, uncertainty, despair, hope, and numbness all intermingled. They will come from believers and non-believers alike. So estimable a Christian as C. S. Lewis, in the depth of this own grief at the loss of his wife, went so far as to say:

> The conclusion I dread is not 'So there's no god after all' but 'so this is what God's really like. Deceive yourself no longer.' How often had bitter resentment been stifled through sheer terror, and an act of love - in every sense an act - put on to hide the operation? (Lewis went even further:) Is it rational to believe in a bad God? Any way in a God so bad as all that? The cosmic sadist?

We are shocked by such language, coming as it does from a committed Christian. Remember that C. S. Lewis, before his own grief, wrote one of the most coherent and rational treatises on the metaphysical and theological problem of evil. Even so fine an intellect could be crushed by the actual presence of suffering.

But Lewis's odyssey, like Job's, finally led him to reconciliation: "and so, with God, I have gradually been coming to feel that the door is no longer shut and bolted. Was it my own frantic need that slammed it in my face?" We who would help must be humble before such anguished cries. We must stay with the sufferer as he descends the limb of his despair and his hurt. We must hope, and pray, and listen, as he struggles to reascend the other limb of the same "U" that Job traversed. We presume too much if we think our logic can give meaning to suffering before the sick man, like Job, has met God in the crucible of his suffering. Meaning does not come from syllogisms.

We must remember again and again, that God chastised Job's friends for their pietistic formulae. God suffered Job's sharp rebukes. God alone understood the full depths of Job's anguish. We cannot forget that Christ Himself in those last moments of His own anguish, uttered those forever chilling words:

> When the sixth hour came, there was darkness over all the earth until the ninth hour; Jesus cried out with a loud voice, 'My God, My God, why has thou forsaken me?' (Mark 15:35)

Even Christ, Who knew the Father and His purposes, felt the human experience of abandonment in His darkest hour of suffering.

Job reminds us, too, that we cannot fully comprehend another's suffering. We cannot hope to understand why *this* person responds *this* way. It is easy when we are well to preach and criticize:

> I have heard plenty of this;
> Galling comforters are you all
> Have windy words no limit?
> What moves you to prattle on?
> I, too, could talk like you.
> If you were in my place.
> I could harangue you with words,
> Could shake my head at you. (16:2-4)

Pierre Wolff, in an arresting but profound little book entitled *May I Hate God,* probes the depths of feelings we may expect from those who suffer. He warns that hatred can overcome reason but that hate is itself a sign of residual love. We cannot hate that to which we are indifferent. Job's friends accuse him of blasphemy. But as Wolff points out, behind Job's seeming blasphemy there was more love than in the sterile, hypocritical piety of Job's friends. Indifference is a form of murder, because it erases a person from our consciousness. Indifference is what most wounds the sick in today's hospitals at the hand of competent but detached health professionals.

Job was not indifferent to God as a Stoic or existentialist might be. Nor was God indifferent to Job. He confronted Job eye-to-eye. He thundered at him. He did so because in Job's anger He detected love. And for his part, Job detected God's love for him even while he had to learn the impossibility of ever fully understanding evil.

ABIDE COMPLAINTS, RESENTMENTS

We must abide the sufferer's complaints and resentments because the need to express them is a cry for help. All health professionals have an obligation to help the sick person to express these feelings in his own way. This is the first step toward healing the wounded humanity of the sufferer. Somehow we must help him heal his relationship with God, the cosmos, and his own humanity. Allowing the sufferer to reveal the content of his suffering is to respect his dignity as a person. It is one way to negate the alienation from the human community which the sick person so desperately feels.

Whoever opens himself to the revelations of the inner self of another assumes moral obligations. Too often, the patient stifles his anguish for fear of ridicule and rejection. We must never belittle the sentiments of the sick, or take advantage of their vulnerability. To use that vulnerability to convert, or to proselytize, is to usurp the place of God with Whom the only meaningful confrontation can occur. That is what Job's friends did, to the disgust of both God and Job.

This does not mean that we must be altogether mute, that we are not to offer spiritual consolation, or help the sufferer find meanings in his sufferings. We can respond to his probings, share our own faith and convictions and our own questionings and prayers with him. What he needs most is our compassion - a conviction that we genuinely feel something of his predicament, that we understand its uniqueness and impenetrability. This impenetrability does not dissolve the common bond of humanity between us. It is this bond that ties us to all suffering humankind.

If we, too, have suffered affliction, we must beware of using the sick person as an excuse to exhibit it, to impress him with our experience, or to assuage our own anguish. Some of the more zealous organized efforts to help others to "deal with" their grief can trample on the uniqueness and privacy of the experience. There is no "approved" way to suffer, grieve, or die. But whatever way fits the patient, he can be helped if we listen, meditate his questions with him, avoid reproach, and avoid trying to win a debate.

Some of the sufferer's troubles will be self-generated to be sure: the result of his own acts or attitudes to suffering itself. Nonetheless, we do best if we hear out the patient's lament and absorb some of his hostility and resentment. To do so is not to praise or agree with it. This is a bogus brand of compassion, cheaply bought and cheaply given, more suited to mutual self-satisfaction than genuinely helping.

Often the patient has a profound need to lash out in frustration at someone or something. Often, it is those nearby - the doctor, nurse, or family - on whom the hostility is displaced. C. S. Lewis put it this way:

> All that stuff about the cosmic sadist is not so much an expression of thought as of hatred. I was getting the only pleasure a man in anguish can get, the pleasure of hitting back.

Physicians and others who receive these lashings must understand their origin, must absorb some of the hostility, and must not strike back. To strike back, or to avoid the patient is to neglect a prime moral imperative of the professional healer.

Many of the complaints we hear today about the aloofness, inhumaneness, and indifference of modern medicine arise from the neglect by physicians and nurses of the vivid lessons Job teaches. Much of the current emphasis on "humanism" in medical education derives from a need to inculcate some measure of compassion in the physician's education. Without compassion, the physician's competence can be damaging or simply self-serving. Job's text is an indispensable *vade mecum* for those who presume to help and heal the sick and the suffering.

We can speak of healing even if the patient is beyond our help scientifically. Reflecting on Job's experience, it was not death he feared so much as abandonment, the injustice he saw in his afflictions, the lack of a chance to make his case heard, to confront his God, to be able to abjure the indifference of the cosmos to his plight. Limited as our powers may be, the true healer is committed to helping the patient to reassemble his life to the extent possible even in fatal illness. We may not be able to reexpand the contracted horizon of possibilities, but we can help the afflicted person make his own response in his own way, and, thus, restore some of the wholeness of his person lost in the assault of illness.

For those who have a religious faith, hope can be restored, not necessarily in recovery, but in reassembling some meaning to life that lies in the possibilities of a personal response to suffering. Even in naturalistic terms, suffering is not without value to the sufferer and those around him. No one has understood this better than Miguel de Unamuno. Only a few quotes from his *Tragic Sense of Life* will suffice:

> Suffering is the substance of life and the root of personality for only suffering makes us persons. (224)

> Suffering is a spiritual matter and the most immediate revelation of consciousness, and it may be that our body was not given to us except as a means of suffering. Whoever has never suffered much or little has no consciousness of himself. (231)

> For in truth, human beings love each other spiritually only when they have suffered the same sorrow, when they have ploughed the stony earth joined together by the mutual yoke of a common grief. It is then that they know one another and feel for and feel with one another in their common anguish and pity one another and love one another. (149)

Miguel de Unamuno's profound insights into human suffering reveal the possibilities of personal growth inherent in anguish. His observations are first steps to the deeper understanding that comes from religious faith. I have not attempted to deal at this level because others have done so eloquently. I have confined myself to a meditation as a physician. But as a believing Roman Catholic Christian, I see the existential predicament of the suffering human, as Job did, as primarily a spiritual and religious experience. Pope John Paul II, in his beautiful apostolic letter, *On Human Suffering,* has summarized what the Christian faith teaches about suffering and healing to those who profess it.

Job's text can be read on many levels. Only one has occupied me here: the text's sublime evocation of one human being's encounter with the most universal experience of all - suffering and illness. No matter what progress medicine may make, how long it may extend our lives, or how carefree our existence may become, the experience of suffering will remain, and will not deviate much from Job's account.

Job's text will always inspire, instruct, and intrigue every age to come. For the physician and the nurse, it is an indispensable textbook. But it is a book for all of us, especially today when we equate the experiences of illness and healing with a commodity transaction or an experiment in applied biology, or the fixing of a piece of machinery or an opportunity for medical entrepreneurship. Suffering and illness are extravagant contradictions to our Promethean aspirations. We see those who succumb to them as a scandal. So we sequester them in hospitals and nursing homes; we complain about how much they cost us and how much they demand of our time and energy. We urge them to die sooner, or we deny them life entirely when they are malformed before or after birth.

Our age needs to ponder the Book of Job so as to regain its bearings, to understand that the sick and suffering have a moral claim on us. For the doctor and nurse, Job remains the text par excellence which teaches what suffering is about. For the rest of us, it is the reminder of the confrontation we cannot escape, the confrontation which paradoxically, as Unamuno said, "…is the substance of life and the root of personality for only suffering makes us persons."

Job is, and will remain, the book we must all eventually live. It comes as close as any book to what Carlyle called it, "the greatest book ever written with pen." But the Book of Job is part of a greater book - the book which transcends literature and aesthetics and whose "very nature" it is to "affront, perplex, and astonish the human mind." (Merton1)

Job is one of the oldest parts of the Bible. Early on, God issued His powerful challenge to our demands for justice. Centuries later, He challenged us again. Paul Claudel puts it this way:

> We have reached Gethsemane. This is not the story of a rich proprietor's loss of his estates, of a family's loss of its children and of bone and flesh being seized upon by a blind and ignorant enemy. This Gethsemane, where God was made man. God took upon Himself all the horror of mankind. Behold old Job! You asked for Justice and here He is in answer to your plea. You asked Him to appear as an equal. He has done that. What have you to say? (Claudel 9)

For some of us, this is the answer to Job's and our own odyssey through anguish to the fulfillment prophesied by Isaiah, "He was bruised for our iniquities and the chastisement of our peace was upon him and with his stripes we are healed." (53:5)

For others, the mystery remains. The magnificence of Job is not that we can question it for answers, but that it questions us, and poses the right question. For the physician, Job is his patient and himself. Sickness is the event that forces the question upon modern man. How will we respond? How will we help others, and ourselves, when the inevitable overtakes us?

CHAPTER FOURTEEN

BENEFICENCE, SCIENTIFIC AUTONOMY, AND SELF-INTEREST: Ethical Dilemmas in Clinical Research

INTRODUCTION

The ethics of clinical research may be viewed from three different perspectives: the process of acquiring new knowledge, the moral use of the knowledge acquired, and the ethics of the investigator seeking this knowledge.

The ethics of the process of human investigation has been the focus of attention ever since the Nuremberg trials exposed the atrocities perpetrated by Nazi physicians on their experimental subjects. The ethics of process emphasizes informed consent, institutional review boards, and legal regulation of human experimentation. The moral use of the knowledge gained by clinical investigation has also received wide discussion on subjects such as fetal tissue transplantation, reproductive technology, the artificial heart, and human gene therapy. Much less attention has been given to the third perspective, the personal morality of the clinical investigator. Yet, the clinical investigator is the ultimate safeguard of the experimental human subject. The investigator designs the experiment, prepares the protocol for peer review, obtains the necessary consent, interprets the results, and monitors the safety of the experiment.

This third perspective on the ethics of clinical research is the focus of this essay. This perspective is often neglected, it is central to the moral quality of human investigations, and it is of special significance in, for example, pediatric research, where the vulnerability of the infant or child imposes graver responsibilities on the investigator than in the case with adults, who can give informed consent or refusal.

The essence of the moral dilemma faced by all clinical investigators is the potential conflict between the investigator's roles as scientist, physician, and private individual. Each role is dominated by a different value: for science, it is truth; for medicine, it is beneficence toward the patient; and for the investigator as an individual, it is self-interest. Each value, along with its subsidiary set of standards and procedures, is legitimate in its own right. But when these values come into competition, as they may in clinical research, serious moral dilemmas result.

How investigators deal with these value conflicts ultimately determines the safety of the patient. This, in turn, determines the degree to which society will permit or restrict the scientific autonomy necessary for valid research. However, no matter how rigidly human experimentation is regulated, the ethical sensitivity of the investigator remains an integral part of the moral equation.

I will examine this moral sensitivity under three headings: the covenantal nature of clinical investigation; the difference in the value systems of the investigator's concurrent roles as scientist, physician, and individual; and the resolution of potential conflicts through application of the ordering principle of "Autonomy in trust."

THE COVENANTAL NATURE OF CLINICAL RESEARCH

Clinical research is an invasion of the integrity and privacy of the person who is the research subject. This invasion necessarily places the person at some risk for a result that, by the very nature of research, must be problematic. Nothing in the nature of science or its internal need for freedom and autonomy constitutes an autonomous moral right to engage in human experimentation. Rather, clinical research is a privilege accorded the investigator by social consensus. Society permits experimentation with humans because of the benefits that the whole society, as well as the experimental subject, may gain from new medical knowledge. The clinical investigator thus enters a covenant with society when he or she accepts the privilege of experimentation involving fellow human beings.

In addition, the investigator is also party to a covenant with the experimental subject. For the potential good of others, of medical science in general, or of the subject, physicians persuade a patient to become simultaneously a patient and a subject. By the act, the good of the patient, which should be primary in the purely therapeutic encounter, is now diluted by another good - the knowledge to be gained by experimental manipulation of the patient's care. The patient is, therefore, knowingly put at some risk for the sake of an uncertain good. By consenting to participate in a research protocol, the subject trustingly yields up some personal moral claims to safety in return for a potential good for him or herself or others. The patient-subject thus has a moral claim on the investigator's fidelity to respect the implied promise that the investigator will judiciously balance the patient's interests and those of the scientific protocol.

These two covenants - one with society and one with the experimental subject - form the basis for the moral obligations specific to clinical investigation. Although these covenants arise in a trust relationship that institutional review boards and research regulations can help safeguard, their subtler nuances cannot be spelled out in such regulations. Rather, like the therapeutic relationship, they rest ultimately on the character and moral integrity of the investigator.

Society permits human experimentation under carefully circumscribed conditions because it is the only way medical knowledge can be verified for use in the amelioration and cure of human disease. In vitro studies, animal models, and computer simulations can go only so far. Ultimately, the new drug or surgical procedure must be tested in human subjects. To be faithful to both covenants - with the patient and with society - these tests must, in the first instance, be scientifically sound. A research plan that lacks scientific integrity places human subjects at risk needlessly and irresponsibly and does violence to society's and the subject's legitimate expectations of science and scientists.

We acknowledge the importance of the canons of good science; however, we must also appreciate that clinical medicine is not itself a science. It possesses a set of values that differ from those of science in fundamental ways.

VALUE SYSTEMS

The Values of Science

The end of scientific endeavor is truth, i.e., knowledge as a good for its own sake. This is the ordering value in science. To achieve this end, science must be free to examine any question and use any method suited to answer the questions it poses. It must design those questions rigorously and examine them experimentally for their verifiability and falsifiability. Observations must be accurate, honestly reported, objectively interpreted, subjected to peer review, and shared openly with colleagues and the world at large.

These values and standards imply a certain degree of objectivization of the subject under study. But in clinical investigations, the "object" of study remains a human being - either a healthy volunteer or a sick person. Here, and in the case of most animals in general, the canons of science may conflict with another set of values - those that define the endeavor of medicine.

The Values of Medicine

In contradistinction to science, whose ordering value is truth, the ordering value of medicine is beneficence. Medical knowledge is sought for a specific end: the healing, helping, and curing of human beings. The good of the patient is the primary end of medicine. To achieve this end, medical knowledge must be particularized to meet the needs of this patient in this clinical situation. Its aim is not, like the aim of science, the discovery of generalized concepts, theories, or laws about human physiognomy or disease.

In addition, medical knowledge must be applied compassionately and sensitively to the uniqueness of the predicament of illness in this person, a predicament that is not wholly penetrable by the physician. Truth telling and confidentiality are mandatory if fidelity to the trust that patients must place in doctors is to be preserved. In those critical moments when a clinical decision is made, the character of the physician remains the patient's ultimate safeguard for which no contact, however carefully constructed, can fully substitute. Whatever agreement is made with the patient must inevitably be channeled through and carried out by another person - the physician.

Medicine is, therefore, not primarily science, although it uses science. In medicine, truth must be sought and applied for the good of the patient. It is not an end in itself.

Medical truth, unlike scientific truth, services the value of beneficence. This inescapable fact not only gives a moral complexity to the activity of the physician who engages in clinical investigations but also limits the scientific autonomy of clinical investigators.

The Investigator's Self-Interests

In addition to the inherent tension between the values of science and medicine, there is a third set of values that further complicates the ethics of clinical research. These values derive from motives and impulses of self-interest that are normal to human beings but may, under the special circumstances of clinical research, present moral hazards.

Like other humans, the clinical scientists desire to advance their own career, improve their income, and experience the satisfaction of peer approval and public recognition. These motives may result in an excessive drive to compete, to be the "first" to report results, to win the Nobel prize, or simply to enjoy the personal satisfaction of an elegant experimental design elegantly carried out. Whatever its source, unrestrained self-interest can blunt moral sensitivity and can lead to conscious or unconscious violations of the covenants between physician and society and between physician and research subject that permit clinical research in the first place.

For example, self-interest may erode the high standard of moral sensitivity that should guide experiments with especially vulnerable groups: the aged, the hopelessly ill, the retarded, the infant with multiple defects, the fetus, the patient with HIV infection, the embryo, or that new fictive entity, the "preembryo." In addition, researchers may justify their compromise of informed consent by citing the benefits to society, other patients, or the eventual cure of a serious disease. When does the investigator step over the line between a truly informed consent and telling just enough to keep the subject from being scared off? No formula can spell this out in advance. No set of regulations can fully protect even the well-educated, fully competent subject. How much more vulnerable are the poorly educated, the sick, or the parents of a desperately or hopelessly ill child or infant?

For the physician-scientist, the moral obligations of the investigator are much heavier than the legal. A legally adequate consent form may not be morally valid. A morally valid consent aims at true "con-sent," an agreeing together in which both parties enter a relationship based on mutual trust and the expectations of fidelity to that trust. Obviously, there must be written consent forms, and they must be examined and approved by peers and institutional review boards. However, the moral integrity of the investigator who obtains the consent is what assures the moral validity of the consent procedure. The investigator decides how much to tell the patient or family, what facts to emphasize, which to withhold, and how to present them.

Institutional pride or hubris is a further corrosive influence. The institution's drive to be "first" is a mixed motive; it can be effective is raising institutional morale and productivity, but it is also capable of submerging moral imperatives on grounds of exigency and "survival." In competition with other hospitals or universities, institutional pride can desensitize an institutional review board to certain dubious projects and can lead to unrealistic reliance on the character of a staff member who is nationally prominent or politically powerful.

The intellectual hubris of the investigator plays its part too. It tempts the academic physician-investigator to arrogate the privilege of scientific autonomy to him or herself. The public, it is argued, cannot possibly comprehend the importance of scientific research or judge the details of a particular experiment. In the long run, it is further argued, the good of all will be better served if we place our trust in the integrity of the scientist's judgment.

Even if we grant that the majority of clinical investigators are honorable people, the dangers of this line of reasoning are obvious. Experience sadly teaches that there is no necessary correlation between academic prestige or intellectual acuity and moral behavior. In a matter as complex and finely balanced as clinical research, the general public may be more perceptive of the moral dilemmas than is the most "enlightened" scientist. We need only recall the recent egregious examples of fraudulent research in prestigious institutions to support this statement.

Personal profit has, in recent years, come to rival prestige and career advancement as a motivating factor in scientific investigation. Pharmaceutical companies are understandably eager to have their products evaluated in humans by the most renowned institutions and investigators. To this end, for-profit companies have expanded the ways in which they can provide financial incentives. They may assume a potion of the investigator's salary, provide certain "fringe" benefits, such as travel and accommodations at deluxe resorts for "research" meetings, offer consulting fees, give gifts of various kinds, or promise a share in the profits from the products being tested.

The matter is further complicated when the healthcare industry enters long-term contractual arrangements with a university to support research. The usual proviso is that a company will support research facilities and personnel in return for privileged access and a share in the patenting rights to the products developed. These industry-university compacts are especially attractive today when governmental and philanthropic sources of research funding are insufficient. Some of our most prestigious universities have entered into what may well turn out to be Faustian compacts. Eventually, many of them will be forced to pay their part of the bargain, especially if corporate profits fall to unacceptable levels or the "investment" in research turns out to be insufficiently productive financially.

Freedom of access and the sharing of research results have, traditionally, been values of science. In many of the contractual arrangements between investigators and pharmaceutical companies, there are provisos that recognize the investigator's right to publish in peer-reviewed journals. Still, in business one does not alert one's competitors to a new product before it is ready for marketing. Just how strongly such negative incentives to data sharing actually operate is difficult to say. Investigators, for fear of losing long-term research support, might consciously or unconsciously withhold information about new discoveries until the time to release it is commercially propitious.

These are a few examples of the kinds of conflicts of interest that pose a potential danger to experimental subjects. They can compromise beneficence, the central value in medicine, and can pose a threat to the values of science. The objectivity, accuracy, and reliability of observations and data interpretation that science requires can be destroyed subtly by financial incentives and by institutional and personal pride. In many cases, if investigators do not produce papers in quantity and if their results are not definitive or are contrary to the interests of those who support them, the emoluments and rewards will stop. Thus, both scientific probity and subject safety may become victims of self-interest.

Physician and Scientist—Can One Be Both?

The unique personal conflict in clinical research, and the one least soluble by simple measures, is the conflict of identity investigators must inevitably experience between their roles as scientists, interested in fact and data collection, and their roles as physicians, interested in care and cure. Physician-investigators must perforce be committed simultaneously to the values of science and the values of medicine. Even if they can avoid the temptation of self-interest noted above, they face the difficult task of balancing and ordering the values of truth and beneficence against each other.

This problem was recognized several decades ago by Otto Guttentag, who considered it serious enough to suggest that the physician caring for the patient might be other than the physician conducting the experiment. The issue Guttentag raised is far from settled and can manifest itself at almost every point in any clinical experiment, especially in randomized clinical trials. It has never been squarely faced.

One example of this conflict is in getting consent for a patient's entry into a study. The patient's major concern is understandably for the most effective treatment of his or her disease. A patient who suffers from a chronic or fatal disease for which there is not treatment or only a dubious one is vulnerable to any promise of help. Under these circumstances, an experimental protocol raises expectations that all is not lost.

It becomes very difficult for patients to separate the physician-scientist role from that of physician-healer. For patients, these roles are personified in all the physicians taking care of them. The physician can easily obtain consent to an experimental protocol simply by emphasizing the hope of cure and down-playing the risk and experimental nature of the treatment. Even the built-in uncertainties of the randomized clinical trial can escape the patient's consciousness under these circumstances. Selective hearing is a powerful device that helps the patient sustain hope when the illness is incurable. The investigator must guard against taking advantage of this normal tendency in such people.

After consent has been obtained, the physician-investigator's role can become even more ambiguous. As the patient's physician, he or she would be impelled to intervene at the first sign of danger by modifying or discontinuing the protocol. As scientist, he or she would be bound to persist in the protocol until the statistical evidence for harm or benefit was conclusive. Discontinuing the experiment too soon results in frustration of scientific obligations; waiting too long results in frustration of obligations as the patient's doctor.

When the study involves a double-blind procedure, there are further problems. If physicians do not know whether their patients are on a placebo or a potent, impotent, or toxic medication, they will have difficulty interpreting whether changes in the clinical course are a result of the disease or a therapeutic or toxic effect of the agent being tested. As investigators, they must remain "blind" until it is statistically clear that the patient is suffering from an aberrant or beneficial effect of the treatment. As personal physicians, they would need to break the code at the first suspicion of harm.

Another difficulty arises when the treatment under study is an improvement over an accepted and reasonably effective standard treatment, e.g., testing the efficacy of a new drug for rheumatoid arthritis, angina pectoris, or hypertension. Here, the experimental design might include a control group, a group on standard medication, and a group on the new medication. If assignment to these groups is randomized, a patient might, for a time, be deprived of standard treatment and placed on a new, untried, and possibly ineffective treatment or on a placebo. Again, the physician-as-scientist must adhere to the protocol. On the other hand the physician-as-caregiver who gives priority to beneficence over scientific truth might not think the associated risks of a procedure justifiable for a particular patient.

There are many other circumstances that put the physician's roles as caregiver and as scientist into conflict. These role conflicts need more careful scrutiny. They do not constitute absolute impediments to clinical research, but they underscore the need for investigators to be self-critical and to recognize when the values they must observe as physicians are in conflict with the canons of science or self-interest.

SCIENTIFIC "AUTONOMY IN TRUST"

The moral dangers inherent in clinical research can never be removed entirely. Human experimentation is a necessity if new treatments are to be discovered and validated. The regulatory measures already in force have done much to place legal, social, and institutional constraints on clinical research. However, not enough emphasis has been placed on the special nature of the freedom and autonomy the clinical investigator enjoys. One way the needs of good science can be balanced against the needs of the patient-as-subject is through a consideration of the concept of "autonomy in trust" - the recognition of a moral order of priority that will resolve conflicts as they arise.

The intellectual autonomy of the scientist is autonomy held in trust. By "autonomy in trust," I mean the conscious acknowledgment by investigators that they are allowed freedom to pursue rigorous scientific goals in human experimentation only if the welfare of the patient is always respected as primary and superior to the values of science and self-interest. This concept implies that scientist-physicians will always regard beneficence as the guiding principle, even to the point of effacing their own self-interest or nullifying the scientific validity of their work. The autonomy necessary to good science is morally tenable if it is seen as held in trust for the good of the patient.

No quantitative formula can set forth explicitly the limits within which autonomy in trust should operate. Instead, investigators must develop a sensitivity to the privilege of doing research involving humans. That privilege is fragile and requires constant awareness not only of the intersections among the three value systems but of the priority of the well-being of the experimental subject whenever there is even the potential for conflict.

Freedom is afforded scientists to pursue problems that interest them because society believes that knowledge is a good in itself or in its application to human problems.

Society recognizes that valid knowledge cannot be obtained without freedom of inquiry. For this reason, we allow freedom in the scientist's selection of problems, methods, and forms of reporting data. Society expects, in return, that the scientists be worthy of the freedom they are privileged to enjoy.

On the strength of this expectation, the scientist is thus allowed a certain latitude or "discretionary space" in the pursuit of knowledge. The dimensions of that space vary with the nature of the subjects and objects under study and with the potential effects of the study on human society. The precise dimensions within which autonomy in trust can be exercised are manifestly difficult to set. Should research on the atomic bomb have been pursued? Is experimentation on the human fetus or embryo permissible? Are studies of the genetic or racial variations in intelligence warranted? Are there limits to the risks a human subject is permitted to undertake - even voluntarily - in the interests of gaining medical knowledge or helping others?

In the specific instance of clinical research, the dimensions of discretionary space must be narrowly defined. Respect for persons and the imperative of beneficence take precedence over scientific curiosity. If investigators choose to be physicians and caregivers, then they must realize at the outset that the needs of the experimental protocol must be subservient to the needs of their own patients. The multiplicity of possibilities for conflict among the values of science, medicine, and self-interest forces us to reconsider whether it is morally licit for one person to be scientist and physician simultaneously.

Arguments can be marshaled on both sides of their question. Those who favor unification of roles of investigator and caregiver place their trust in the binding power of the traditional ethics of medicine, the trustworthiness of the majority of investigators, and the avoidance of interphysician conflict when one physician is clearly in charge. Those who would separate these roles hold that there is a clear advantage when one physician is unequivocally the advocate for the patient's welfare and another for the probity of the experiment. Further, the skills, attitudes, and motivations required for physician-caregiver and physician-investigator roles are different. Different kinds of people are attracted to each role. It is unusual for one person to possess the traits of both.

No general rule can cover all investigational situations, and better surveillance over the possibility of conflicts is needed. In some cases, a separation of roles seems advisable. For example, when investigators receive most of their support from a pharmaceutical firm, own stock in that company, or receive financial emoluments, separation of roles seems the only morally prudent alternative. This is particularly true if the purpose of the experiment is to evaluate an improvement in an already effective treatment. The same is true when the research is clearly nontherapeutic and of no therapeutic benefit to the patient. Protection of the patient's interest should be in the hands of a physician other than the investigator, one whose prime obligation is to the patient and not the experiment.

However, when the intent of the research is to try a new agent in a patient with a serious or fatal disease, and the outcome for the patient-subject is the prime focus of the research, then it seems better for the physician-caregiver and the physician-investigator to be the same person. Here the relationship between scientific knowledge and the good of the patient is so intimate that it is preferable to have one physician who can discuss and weigh both with the patient.

A reassessment of the usually accepted fusion of roles in the physician-investigator is needed. Much depends on the contexts, purposes, and expectations of the research protocol. Autonomy in trust demands a renewed emphasis on care and precision in identifying and resolving the moral dilemmas inherent in different types of clinical investigations.

The safe rule in every case is to favor beneficence over scientific rigor when the two seem to be in conflict or when in doubt. The possible loss of knowledge cannot outweigh the possibility of harm to the subject even if the utilitarian calculus indicated great benefit to many and harm to only a few. This is the case particularly with the mentally retarded, the very young, the terminally ill, and the senile. Whenever valid consent is impossible and the experiment risky, only therapeutic research aimed at benefit to the subject seems morally defensible.

It is especially dangerous to hold, as some ethicists do, that infants and the retarded, for example, owe an obligation to society or to other infants to be subjects of research. No one can presume on the willingness of another to run the risk of experimentation; we cannot presume to attribute activism to those who cannot possibly express their own views on the matter.

Parents and guardians of infants and children below the age of competence do not have absolute rights over their children. Someone must be an advocate for the infant and the child, and this may have to be the physician. The physician may need to protect the child against even well-intended parents who might permit dubious forms of experimentation in hope that it might help others. This is another reason why it is particularly important to distinguish the role of the investigator from that of the caregiver.

Not all experimental procedures in infants and children are ruled out. Therapeutic investigations that could benefit the subject would be licit, provided all other safeguards are scrupulously observed. Nontraumatic studies of a nontherapeutic type - such as examinations of body fluids, excretions, or secretions or noninvasive procedures or observations of various sorts - would be licit if they were done in association with other procedures needed in the care of the subject.

Experimentation on fetuses or embryos, spontaneously or intentionally aborted, is a special subject with its own moral complexities and deserves more than the superficial treatment I can give here. Everything depends upon what we consider to be the ontological status of the fetus and embryo. In my view, they are deserving of the same respect as the infant or child. Their vulnerability is extreme, and the rule of beneficence is particularly stringent upon those who have the unborn in their care.

Even for subjects capable of making their own choices and willing to run risks, there are limits on what should be permissible. A particularly dangerous recent example is so-called "pay-as-you-go" research. This is another manifestation of the growing belief that untrammeled competition will redound to the benefit of patients by providing incentives to investigators to try nonstandard treatment.

In this kind of research a commercial laboratory enters into a contract with a person to try out a new treatment. For example, monoclonal antibodies developed from the patient's own tumor cells that are bonded to an antitumorous agent can be used as treatment. The patient pays all the expenses of the research, plus a profit to the laboratory. In this way, it is argued, bold new treatments will be developed that might flounder in the complex review processes.

The dangers of such research are obvious. All the usual safeguards that surround human experiments are compromised. There is no peer review, no institutional review board or ethics committee, no statistically controlled trial, no monitoring of the results and the dangers. Sharing of information is seriously impeded because investigators are in competition with one another for the market. Finally, there is the serious conflict between the financial interest of the investigator, the interests of good science, and the good of the patient. A more perilous misapplication of the privilege of clinical research can hardly be imagined.

CONCLUSION

I have cited some examples of the ways in which the physician's role as investigator-scientist may be in conflict with the role of caregiver. These examples underscore the need for a more careful scrutiny of the value conflicts possible even in so well-intentioned an enterprise as therapeutic research, but they are not reasons for draconian measures to regulate such research. However, they are reasons for a much greater sensitivity on the part of institutions and investigators to the fact that clinical research places restraints on the autonomy of science and self-interest.

The conflicts between the values of science, medical care, and self-interest have implications for the preparation, selection, and supervision of clinical investigations. Many unfortunate occurrences have resulted from the laxity of senior investigators who are involved in the supervision of too many projects and who are overeager to expand their own publications lists. Some training in ethics should be mandatory for all investigators who are to be involved with human subjects. Some code or explicit set of moral commitments should be developed and subscribed to by all investigators.

Given the present emphasis in Western society on autonomy, the rights of patients, and the wariness about abuses of power by science and technology, clinical investigators must recognize the value conflict inherent in their work. Their best guarantee of freedom in the pursuit of medical knowledge and the good of patients lies in research that is scientifically valid and ethically responsible. To compromise either is, on the one hand, to endanger patients and, on the other, to lose the privilege of freedom without which science cannot thrive.

IV

Health Professionals as Moral Agents

These essays demonstrate Dr. Pellegrino's long-standing commitment to an examination of the collective morality of groups. His perspective will not let us get away with focusing solely on the individual morality and ethics, but requires us to attend to the overall impact of a profession's, a hospital's, an academic health science center's and an Association's behavior as moral agents.

CHAPTER FIFTEEN

THE MEDICAL PROFESSION AS A MORAL COMMUNITY*

Historically and conceptually we have been accustomed to think of medical ethics in terms of the obligations of individual physicians to individual patients. We have largely neglected the obligations of the profession as a moral community, as a group dedicated to a common set of moral precepts. Yet much of the plight and the opportunity of our profession today rests with the way we view the practical implications of being a moral community. Indeed, some of the issues that vex us most are resolvable only through the use of our collective moral power.

This is the thesis that I want to argue this evening. I think this is a particularly appropriate topic at this time, when the Academy, as we have heard this evening, is reshaping its own mission to meet today's challenges. I would suggest that, without some clear commitment to what is required of the profession as a moral community, the full potential of the Academy's new program will not be fully realizable.

THE DILEMMA OF PROFESSIONAL ETHICS

Today, our profession faces an unenviable choice between two opposing moral orders, one based in the primacy of our ethical obligations to the sick, the other in the primacy of self-interest and the marketplace. These two orders are not funda-

* Presented at the Stated Meeting of the New York Academy of Medicine, November 9, 1989

mentally reconcilable and, like it or not, the Academy and the profession will be forced to choose between them. In that choice this Academy can play a central and indispensable role.

Should we, as some prominent medical ethicists urge, reshape our ethical codes to conform to the ethos of the marketplace, which legitimates self-interest over beneficence and makes vices out of most of our traditional virtues?[1] Or should we stand firm in the belief that being a physician imposes certain specific obligations that forbid turning ourselves primarily into entrepreneurs, businessmen, or agents of fiscal, social, or economic policy?[2]

Frankly, I do not know how our profession will respond to this dilemma. Some physicians want to remain faithful to the primacy of the patient's welfare and the idea of a profession. Others see no reason why physicians should be held to a higher standard of ethical conduct than prevails in other professions or society. What is most distressing is the pervasive conviction in both groups that the question has already been answered, and that the ancient citadel of medical ethics has already fallen. Too, many believe that it is no longer possible to be an ethical physician, and that the only choices are capitulation, accommodation, and early retirement with warnings to one's children not to enter the profession. Those who would resist feel powerless and abandoned. Justifiably, they cannot be expected to resist alone. Their burden is too heavy without the support of the whole profession. Only if we have the will to use our collective moral force will the integrity of the profession be preserved.

Medicine is at heart a moral enterprise and those who practice it are de facto members of a moral community. We can accept or repudiate that fact, but we cannot ignore it or absolve ourselves of the moral consequences of our choice. We are not a guild, business, trade union, or a political party. If the care of the sick is increasingly treated as a commodity, an investment opportunity, a bureaucrat's power trip, or a political trading chip, the profession bears part of the responsibility.

Allow me now to set out what I mean by a moral community, why I believe medicine fits that description, and what this means in the practical world of today's sociopolitical climate.

The idea of medicine as a moral community is very old. Yet for the greater part of medicine's history it remained latent or was expressed only in partial or distorted forms. Remnants of these older models remain in the consciousness of the profession even today.

Perhaps the most explicit model is found in both major parts of the Hippocratic Oath - the so-called covenant and the body of the Oath itself. The covenant follows immediately upon the invocation of the gods. It enjoins on the pupil the obligation to treat his teacher as his father, his teacher's sons as his brothers, and to teach the secrets of the art only to his own sons or those of his teacher. There is uncertainty about whether this covenant was added at a later date and about its Pythagorean provenance.[3-5] Whatever its source, its spirit is offensive to democratic sensibilities because it is so frankly sexist, paternalistic, and elitist. But it does impose a set of moral obligations that bind together all who share knowledge of the art, and it does introduce the body of the Oath. The explicit moral precepts shared by the Hippocratic medical community have become the ethical ideals shared by physicians in subsequent ages and in many different cultures.

The Oath and the covenant bind physicians collectively to something other than self-interest, to duties to other physicians and to individual patients. Neither the Oath nor the other books of the Hippocratic Corpus mention social obligations of broader kinds, such as responsibility for the availability, accessibility, and affordability of health care, or collective responsibility for public health, the poor, or public policy.[6] This was largely true of the Stoic physicians as well, despite the cosmopolitanism of the Stoic philosophy.[7]

In the Christian era the Hippocratic Oath remained intact. Significantly, the covenant was omitted, probably because the Church opposed secret societies. Christian belief placed emphasis on community and collective concern for the poor, the outcast, and the sick. Medicine itself became a vocation, a way of salvation, for physicians and patients, a moral community within the larger community of faith.

Non-Christian physicians in the ancient world and middle ages - Egyptian, Hebrew, Moslem, Indian, and Chinese - were also members of moral communities each with its own religious or quasireligious binding force. What is remarkable is the congruence of ethical precepts among physicians who held widely disparate world-views. This suggests something intrinsic to the morality of medicine as a human activity that in some way transcends culture, religion, and historical era.[8] But still, neither the Christian nor non-Christian physicians explicitly developed the idea of a moral community with definitive collective obligations to society of the kind that are of most concern today.

Until very recently, the combination of a religious perspective and a moral perspective internal to medicine united physicians in moral communities. In Anglo-American medical ethics, this tradition was fortified in the *ethics* of Thomas Percival's *Ethics* of 1803, for example, combined the central precepts of the Hippocratic Oath and Corpus, Protestant Christianity, Roman Stoicism, and the 18th Century English Gentleman.[9] Percival's ethical perspective thoroughly permeated the first American Medical Association Code of 1847 and it remains the major influence on Anglo-American medical ethics.

This gentleman doctor was a member of a privileged community to be sure, but to a greater degree perhaps than ever previously, he recognized his profession's responsibility for involvement in such socially important problems as the health of workers, the design of hospitals, care for the poor, and forensic medicine. Benjamin Rush expressed these sentiments this way, "...they entertain very limited views of medicine who suppose its object and duties are confined exclusively to the knowledge and cure of diseases. Our science was intended to render other services to society."

However imperfect they might have been, the earlier models of the profession as a moral community implied, in nascent form at least, the idea of a collective moral identity, commitment, and obligation. In the last 225 years even these incomplete prior conceptions have suffered significant erosion under the impact of several potent social and cultural forces.

Among the most important has been the dominance in our political philosophy for 200 years of the idea of the individual as a free-standing, autonomous social unit, prior to, and indeed standing as the creator, of the community.[10] Granting the importance of individual freedom, this concept does not foster the kind of identification and commitment upon which a moral community must depend. In ethics it has tended to privatism, a focus on negative right, and moral pluralism. The pursuit of private gain and pleasure are also given a primacy and legitimacy inconsistent with a broader social concern.

Within medicine itself many factors tend to divide physicians. Society's moral pluralism separates physicians, especially on the crucial human life issues of abortion and euthanasia. The Hippocratic ethic itself is no longer the moral binding force it used to be. Each of its precepts is being challenged so that it is hard to say what constitutes the ethics of the profession. Moreover, the current interest in medical ethics focuses on moral dilemmas in individual cases and says little about collective responsibility. Finally, the whole edifice of professional ethics is under pressure to legitimate the profit motive and to transform the physician from the patient's advocate into social engineer, entrepreneur, corporate executive, health care manager, or employee. Each new role draws the physician into a community with moral values further and further removed from primary concern for the sick person.

What collective responses we encounter are often far from morally commendable. Physicians have, for example, reacted to onerous policies by defending their prerogatives or remuneration instead of objecting to how such restrictions compromise good patient care. Some physicians take an aggressively retaliative stance, urging physician sponsored corporations, union or strikes. Others retaliate in less overt ways - refusing to see poor, Medicare, Medicaid, or AIDS patients. Clearly, the possibility of collective action is seen in terms of a guild and this is antithetical to a true moral community.

This deterioration of medicine as amoral community has had serious consequences for the profession and society. As a result, no collective voice speaks for the patient, resisting policies and practices that undermine ethics or endanger patient welfare. Physicians are retrenching into a kind of self-protective moral atomism that puts personal survival ahead of moral purpose. No leadership is provided to advocate the care of the sick as a primary concern or to stand for the just distribution of health care or to counter the dominance of the market ethos. When physicians speak there is sometimes little to indicate that they are acting in anything other than their own interests. Those who do resist are often isolated, abandoned, or ridiculed by their colleagues. The enormous moral power latent in the community of medicine is ignored or repudiated. This refusal to act as a moral community is self-defeating. It robs the profession of its most credible and effective means to neutralize the hostile forces besieging it today.

THE IDEA OF MORAL COMMUNITY

A moral community is one whose members are bound to each other by a set of commonly held ethical commitments and whose purpose is something other than mere self-interest. This moral purpose may, as in the case of medicine, arise in the nature of the activity in which the members of the community engage, or, as in the case of churches or philanthropic associations, it may arise from commitments freely chosen by its members. Individual members are bound to support the moral aims of the community to which they belong. Not to do so is to dissociate oneself from that community and to betray the covenant of commitments that gave birth to the community in the first place.

It is important to distinguish between mere commitment to common beliefs and a truly moral community. Groups can be united behind morally erroneous or reprehensible commitments. Simply asserting a set of commitments, therefore, does not make a community morally good. White supremacists are united around a totally indefensible moral belief, as were the Nazi physicians. I have already alluded to some of the self-protective retaliatory attitudes that unite some physicians. These would not constitute the basis of a morally good community. A morally good community is one whose common commitments are grounded in something other than self-interest and meet criteria of moral validity.

Defined in this way, a moral community means several things: First, its members share a covenantal relationship with each other and with society. That covenant is the promise, singly and collectively, to foster certain ethical ideas and standards. Second, the moral community has itself a certain life independent of who its leaders or members might be at a particular time. The ethical ideals of medicine have outlived bad doctors, self-serving medical guilds, and bureaucratic institutions. Third, a community is something more than the simple addition of its individual members: "Whenever men act in concert for a common purpose, they tend to create a body which...differs from the individuals of whom it is constituted."[11] That body has power for good and harm that none of its individual members alone could marshal. A moral community would by definition have to use its power for good. A moral community is therefore one which can be trusted to stand against the values of the society in which it resides if that society's values frustrate the moral purposes to which the moral community is dedicated.

The ethical basis for the idea of a moral community and the ways collective responsibility can or should be exercised are subjects of current philosophical interest. Their theoretical foundations are yet to be firmly established. But I believe medicine affords one of the more concrete and specific examples of those traits that would characterize moral communities.[12,13]

MEDICINE AS A MORAL COMMUNITY

Medicine qualifies as a de facto moral community not simply because its members are dedicated to a common purpose and a common set of ethical ideals but because those ideals are morally grounded. This involves something more fundamental than the arbitrary commitments of physicians. Four aspects of medicine as a special kind of human activity give a moral status to its individual members and to the collectivity that we call the profession: the inequality of the medical relationship, the nature of medical decisions, the nature of medical knowledge, and the ineradicable moral complicity of the physician in whatever happens to his patient.

VULNERABILITY AND INEQUALITY

A central phenomenon of illness is the vulnerability of the sick person and the consequent inequality it introduces into the medical relationship. Even the most self-sufficient person becomes anxious, fearful, and dependent when illness occurs. Patients lose freedom to pursue life's goals, to make their own decisions, and to heal themselves without access to specialized knowledge and skill. Pursuit of relief, cure, and return to health become central preoccupations. In this state the sick person is forced to consult another person who holds the needed knowledge and skill and who therefore has power over the ill person.

These facts impose a condition of inequality on the medical relationship paralleled by few other situations in democratic societies. Taken together they add up to a state of unusual vulnerability. This inescapable vulnerability imposes de facto moral obligations on the physician. In a relationship of such inequality the weight of obligations is on the one with the power. This is very different from the ethos of business where vulnerability is an opportunity to exploit one's adversary. On the contrary, the physician has the obligation to protect the patient's vulnerability against exploitation. He is obliged to be faithful to the trust that is ineradicable in medical relationships. When he offers to help, the physician elicits trust that he will act for the good of the patient, not his own good, the good of society, science, the family, or any other entity.

THE NATURE OF MEDICAL DECISIONS

The second thing that makes the medical relationship a moral enterprise is that the most serious medical decisions combine technical and moral components. The physician must be scientifically correct in his diagnosis and choice of therapy but, at the same time, his recommendation must be for the patient's good. The latter includes more than the patient's medical good.[14] The patient's moral right of self-determination must be respected. The physician must assess the moral status of what he offers to do. He must decide whether his own moral beliefs are consistent with what the patient requests. There are moral issues, of course, in all human relationships, but because of the special vulnerability and exploitability of the sick person they assume overriding importance in medical relationships. The good of the patient is the end and purpose of that relationship. But this is as much a moral as a technical good. To see the relationship of technical and moral aspects of medical decisions and to place them in the right order is itself a moral obligation.

THE CHARACTERISTICS OF MEDICAL KNOWLEDGE

Medical knowledge has certain characteristics that generate obligations in those who possess it. For one thing it is practical knowledge, knowledge intended for a specific purpose - the care of the sick. It is not knowledge to be acquired primarily for its own sake. In addition, medical knowledge is obtained only through the socially sanctioned privilege of a medical education. Society permits the invasions of the privacy of sick persons that medical education demands. Students are allowed to dissect human bodies, see autopsies, engage in experimentation, practice their skills, and gain experience in clinical care. These privileges cannot be bought for a price, like other commodities. No tuition could generate a right to the invasions of privacy required in medical education. Further financial subsidization is provided by society to assure an uninterrupted supply of medical personnel, not primarily to provide students a future livelihood.

We must not forget that physicians are granted a monopoly over medical knowledge. They are allowed freedom to accredit educational programs and to set standards of practice, to admit and to eject from the medical community. This creates in the profession a reciprocal collective responsibility to assure that medical knowledge is available, accessible, and accurate. The physician's knowledge can never be his private property because medical knowledge is entrusted to the profession for the care of the sick. Physicians are its stewards, not its exploiters. As stewards we are obliged to preserve, validate, teach, and extend medical knowledge and to see that it is available and accessible to those for whom it is acquired in the first place.

These three facts about the medical relationship - the vulnerability of patients, the moral nature of medical decisions, and the stewardship of medical knowledge are common to all who profess medicine. It binds them de facto and imposes moral obligations on all who belong to the medical community. Physicians enter an implicit covenant when they accept the privilege of a medical education and the stewardship of medical knowledge that covenant entails. They make that covenant explicit by the Oath physicians take at graduation. This oath is a public promise that those who swear it can be trusted to possess medical knowledge and to use it in the interests of the sick. Significantly, it is the Oath that signals entry into the profession - not the degree or the license to practice. Most medical associations repeat this same promise in some form or another in their official pronouncements.

MORAL COMPLICITY

The physician by virtue of his covenant and the way medicine is practiced is the final common pathway for whatever happens to his patient. No order can be carried out, no policy observed, and no regulation imposed without his assent. He it is who writes the orders that other health professionals carry out. He is inescapably the final safeguard of the patient's well-being. The physician is therefore de facto a moral accomplice in whatever is done that adversely affects his patient. The physician cannot be a double agent - either he serves primarily the patient or primarily the hospital, the economic or fiscal policy, or the law. When they are in conflict, he is the one who acts for or against the patient's well-being. This ultimate responsibility is not transferable to others. Without the cooperation of physicians the Nazi homicides would not have been possible.[15,16] Nor the exploitation of the sick for profit.

THE MORAL COMMUNITY IN PRACTICE

These four facts about the medical relationship make it a moral enterprise in which each physician is a moral agent with specific role-related duties. While each physician is therefore individually accountable, no physician alone can be expected to fulfill the whole spectrum of obligations that belong to the whole moral community. Indeed, without the collective moral support of the entire profession, few individual physicians could fulfill their individual obligations in the practical world. The moral power of the whole medical community is essential.

I do not wish to ignore that in many ways the profession, through its national, state, or local societies and hospital staffs, has manifested sensitivity to the idea of a moral community. We can cite as a few examples affirmation of the moral obligation to treat patients with HIV infection, conscientious fulfillment of peer review responsibilities, updating of ethical codes and guidelines, dissemination of education in preventive medicine, notably with respect to smoking, fatty diets, exercise, use of drugs, alcohol, safe driving, boxing injuries, care for the poor and the homeless, establishing standards of medical education, etc.

These are all commendable evidences of professional responsibility. But they do not address the more sensitive issue of professional self-interest and the advocacy role the professional should play in the conflict between an ethic based on the market ethos and one based in the moral nature of the medical relationship. Without in any way depreciating what is being done by many conscientious individual physicians and their organizations, I suggest that the full spectrum of our obligations as a moral community is yet to be fulfilled. We have yet to use the tremendous moral power we have for good. To do so we must act collectively in certain ways.

We must begin by examining ourselves and admitting that all of the fault for the parlous state of medical care today does not lie outside the profession. To be sure, our *bêtes noires* are not imaginary - the malpractice crisis, inimical public and regulative policies, insurance carrier venality, corporations ducking responsibility for health care, the ethos of the marketplace replete with its advertising, competition, bottom-line-fixated administrators, for-profit hospitals, meaningless paperwork, etc. The list is long and distressing. The tendency to blame our moral desuetude on the "climate" of medical practice is understandable and in part justifiable. But we must also realize that self-righteous complaints are self-serving. They severely compromise our moral integrity. We can restore it only by taking the moral high ground, by acting not on the basis of what external forces do to us, but on what they do to those we serve.

Some of the evils inflicted on the body of the profession are self-generated. Some physicians have refused to see Medicare and Medicaid patients, refused to treat HIV infection, or to go to the emergency room, and even go on strike. Some physicians have defrauded the Medicare/Medicaid system or insurance carriers. Some physicians have charged unconscionable fees, been unavailable, or overly protective of their colleagues in the fact of incompetence or venality. I emphasize some physicians. Most have not done these things but all must recognize that the current climate is not simply the result of a massive conspiracy against the profession. If we are a moral community we are all touched by the virtues and vices of our confreres. We must feel demeaned by them and act to repudiate them.

We must take a stand against the evils inside and outside of medicine on one ground only - the damage and danger they pose for the sick. Every one of the things that disturb the conscientious physician - in his colleagues or in today's social milieu - can be effectively opposed if we are faithful to the central aim of medicine: the care and cure of the sick. Were we to take this position we would have public sentiment with us. We must demonstrate that our first concern is not our own privilege, prerogative, or income but the welfare of those we have a covenant to serve. There is enormous moral power in this position but we have not used it.

But our advocacy will be an empty gesture or interpreted as another public relations gimmick if it is not accompanied by actions. It is not my purpose this evening to write a moral agenda for the whole profession, but there are a variety of efforts organized medicine - or new associations of physicians - can undertake to make the professions' advocacy role authentic and effective.

We should collect the data needed to convince the public and legislators that the free market, commercialization, and monetarization of medicine is unjust and damaging to the welfare of the sick. Anecdotal accounts are not sufficient to make the case, impressive as they may be. If there is clear evidence that a given policy is injurious to patients we must resist and even refuse to carry it out. No policy can make all of America's physicians do what they think is morally wrong. To comply is to be an accomplice in a violation of our covenant with the sick patient.

We should resist the uncritical acceptance of the idea that rationing of health care is necessary in America. Even a superficial comparison of the magnitude of health expenditures with the ways we spend billions of dollars in discretionary income should convince us that needed medical care need not be withheld. Before physicians talk about rationing they can take steps to reduce the waste of resources in unnecessary and duplicated work-ups, procedures, operations, and medications. We can fight to reduce the administrative overhead (perhaps 15-30% in the opinion of some economists) imposed on health care expenditures by "managed health care systems" with their administrative bureaucracies, advertising, and marketing budgets.

The profession can initiate and cooperate in efforts to eliminate excessive fees by adopting a fee schedule and a relative value scale system of compensation. Personal financial investment in health care facilities should be ethically unacceptable. Physicians by virtue of their heavy responsibilities are entitled to just compensation, but they must not regard themselves as entrepreneurs with a monopoly and a franchise to exploit medical knowledge. We should heed the plea of the editor of the *Journal of the American Medical Association* and others for a return to the tradition of pro bono work for the poor as part of the responsibility of every physician.[17]

What America, the sick among us and the health care system, need desperately is moral leadership and medical statesmanship. That leadership cannot be achieved by individual physicians acting alone. But acting as a moral community the profession has enormous power to resist the forces it finds so inimical to the well-being of its patients and its own well-being through that power. We can influence the public, government, and industry to re-evaluate their values, and to appreciate that the fulfillment of each person's potential is impossible without health and medical care for all citizens.

Medicine cannot and should not undertake all of this alone. We must join with other concerned people and legislators. We do not need more reports from Commissions, panels, and committees on how to solve the health care "crisis" by another prescription for tinkering with mechanisms. The answer is clear - America can have health care of quality for all if we order our priorities as a nation, if health professionals dedicate themselves to the care of the sick primarily and not to self-interest, if professional organizations fulfill their moral responsibilities to the public, and if America decides that it wants to be a caring rather than an acquisitive society.

I hope that my arguments for medicine as a moral community with collective responsibilities have some appeal to this Academy at this time, when it initiates its new program. I certainly do not suggest that the Academy follow my agenda. But I hope that it will devise its own way of acting as a moral community - for that is what the Academy cannot escape being. In saying this I am repeating only what one of the Academy's most distinguished presidents, Abraham Jacobi, in his inaugural address in 1885 listed as a major purpose of the Academy: "The advancement of the character and honor of the profession."[18]

CHAPTER SIXTEEN

HOSPITALS AS MORAL AGENTS*

The subject of institutional ethics has significance beyond hospitals. Our country enters its third century in a state of moral disquietude about its own motives. There is widespread confusion about moral values. We suffer from an obsession with means and from a fear of ends and purpose. Institutions are particularly suspect. Most of them - whether we look at business, education, government, or the church - seem to have become disengaged from their human purpose. For economic, political, and fiscal considerations and self-interest are too often their dominant justifying principles. Rarely do our governmental or institutional leaders speak convincingly, as the founders of our country did, of the moral purposes of their enterprise. The inescapable challenge for all our institutions in the next century, the one upon which the revitalization of our national life depends, is to recapture the sense of a moral purpose transcending self-interest and self-preservation.

But it is not my purpose to moralize - this is very different from genuine moral discourse. I merely wish to set the question of the institutional obligations of hospitals against a backdrop of the general deficiency in the assumption of moral obligations that afflicts our nation. Because of the urgent and intensely human milieu within

* Based on a speech entitled "Hospitals as Moral Agents: Some Notes on Institutional Ethics" which was published in Proceedings of the Third Annual Board of Trustees/Medical Staff Executive Committee Conference sponsored by Saint Joseph's Hospital in Saint Paul, Minnesota, on March 26, 1977, pp. 10-27.

which it operates, the hospital must be among the first to attend to its institutional moral obligations. It can, in fact, be the paradigm for others.

In discussing these obligations, I shall reflect on three questions: *First,* What is the actual nature of the human relationship between a patient and a hospital in today's system of health care? *Second,* what obligations are derived from the nature of that relationship? And, *third,* what are some of the practical implications of these obligations?

INSTITUTIONAL ETHICS: WHAT IT IS; WHAT IT IS NOT

Before addressing these three questions, it is essential to clarify two propaedeutic issues - first, what I understand ethics to be, and second, what I *do not* subsume under the rubric of institutional ethical obligation.

While there is a phenomenal resurgence of interest today in biomedical ethics, there is still much confusion and variability in interpretation of the *ethics.* Many still believe ethics is an intuitive domain which consists entirely of personal beliefs that are not arguable and need no rational justification. Others believe that morals cannot be taught or that generally applicable principles cannot be derived. Both views, intuitionist and skeptical, are prominent among health professionals today. Discourse about ethics, they hold, is either impossible or meaningless.

I hold the traditional view of ethics as the systematic search for generalizable and rationally justifiable principles on how we ought to live and act in various relationships with our fellow men. Ethics is, therefore, a branch of practical philosophy. It includes the analysis of ethical statements but is not limited to that analysis. Ethics deals with what "ought" to be rather than with what "is." Institutional ethics, from this view, consists of the general normative principles which define the way institutions "ought" to act with respect to their obligations. It is a branch of social ethics in that it pertains to men when they act as members of a group rather than as individuals. The problems of institutional morality, those which emerge from the actions of organized groups, are more complex than those of individual ethics.

My second propaedeutic centers on what institutional ethics is not. It is not the sum of the ethical beliefs of the people who make up the institution - the individual physicians, nurses, administrators, and board members. Each has his own set of values and beliefs and in a pluralistic society must be permitted to express them as an individual. But institutional ethics consists of a definable set of obligations which transcends these individual beliefs. For example, individual physicians differ in their views on abortion and euthanasia, direct and indirect. What an institution must decide is whether it sanctions absolute or limited pluralism, and whether, on this or that issue, it will take some specific stance to which it feels morally obligated above others. Institutions, as we shall examine further, will be called upon increasingly to make their moral choices more explicit than has been customary.

Nor is institutional ethics to be equated with meeting only the legal requirements for accountability. Many obligations which derive from the nature of the hospital's mission in society are now being transferred to the realm of law. This is a forceful commentary on the tardiness of hospitals in sensing what should be ethical obligations. I refer to the sharpening of the definitions of legal and fiscal accountability of board and administrators for quality of care, protection of the rights of consent, managerial efficiency, equity in provision of services, and assuring rights of due process. Most of these obligations would have, and should have, been derived from a conscious reflection on the moral obligations implicit in what hospitals are all about. Their translation into legislation and patient pleas for a variety of bills of rights are signs of the ethical lassitude of our institutions.

But, if these rights and obligations are now being expressed in law, is this not sufficient? A brief look at the distinction between law and ethics will make the answer clearer. Law and ethics may often coincide, but they are not necessarily and always the same. In fact, as a recent history shows, they may often be antipathetic. Law is in many ways the *coarse* adjustment of society to assure that certain obligations are fulfilled. It has been undeniably a positive force in enhancing human rights and freedom in our country. But as our lagging progress in civil rights and our Vietnam interlude illustrate, there is too often a disjunction between what is legal and what is moral.

Law, for example, can guarantee the validity of consent or minimum standards of quality by requiring hospitals to follow and record certain procedures and by imposing penalties for violations. But law, by its nature, seeks standardized and bureaucratized, often impersonalized solutions. What is transferred to law is by definition taken out of the realm of the voluntary recognition of moral responsibility. Something subtle and exquisite is lost. Law cannot guarantee the quality of human transactions even though it may protect the rights of the parties to the transactions.

Ethics, on the other hand, is the *fine* adjustment of men for the voluntary assumption of obligations because they are demanded by the very nature of certain relationships between humans. Ethics sets a higher ideal than law simply because it is not securable. An ethically sensitive institution takes the full dimension of the medical encounter into account - all those things which flow from the existential condition of humanity in the state of illness.

Law and ethics can reinforce each other, as do the coarse and fine adjustments of the microscope. Law assures that patients' rights will be protected from those who do not act from ethical motives; ethics guarantees that the institutional conscience will transcend law and attend to obligations whether covered by law or not. It also guarantees that law is applied humanely, always in the spirit of serving individual needs rather than justifying itself. Government, therefore, must never be the sanction for ethics but only a re-course when human frailty obfuscates moral sensibilities. Law seems indispensable to human life, but it cannot be totally sufficient for an institution consciously attending to its moral obligations.

Neither should ethics be confused with etiquette, the niceties of conduct between institutions and professionals which protect their mutual self-interests. Even in the so-called ethical treatises of the Hippocratic Corpus, these domains are confused. Intermingled with a few true ethical principles are many more precepts as to the physician's mien, conduct and comportment with patients and families, and courtesies he should afford his fellow physicians. In our times, the proscription against advertising or unseemly publicity and the rules for enlightened self-interest which govern the inevitable but subtle competition between institutions or professionals are in the "etiquette" category. There may be fragments of moral issues here, but they are not mandatory obligations whose violation undermines professional authenticity.

Finally, institutional ethics does not imply that a single rigid set of principles be uniformly practiced by all hospitals. This is manifestly impossible in a society with such a wide range of values as ours. Indeed, our moral pluralism may itself require some declaration by the institution of its values, if the patient's own values are to be fully protected.

Some commonly applicable principles will undoubtedly emerge, so that the final declaration of institutional morality will be an admixture of shared and unshared beliefs. What is important is that the points I have been emphasizing here be adverted to consciously by those in whom corporate responsibility is vested.

Ethics is a legitimate branch of practical philosophy, which systematically examines and rationally justifies claims about how we should live as individuals and members of society. Institutional ethics seeks out these principles as they apply to the moral obligations of institutions to the segment of mankind they profess to serve. There are several things institutional ethics is not: It is not the same as accountability to law, nor the simple addition of the ethical beliefs of those who work in the institution, nor professional etiquette or some unexamined universal set of norms which should be imposed upon all hospitals.

We can now examine briefly three further questions: the nature of the relationships of patients to hospitals that generate ethical obligations, the nature of these obligations, and their implications for everyday hospital practice.

THE HOSPITAL'S PROFESSION AND THE PATIENT'S NEED

We must look first at the genesis of the hospital's moral obligations as an institution to the patient. I find it useful to begin at what I call the hospital's "profession." By this, I mean that a hospital, by the very fact of its existence, makes a declaration - that is, it professes to concentrate and make available those resources which a person can call upon when he is ill. Implicit in that profession is the promise to assist the person in the condition of illness to regain what he has lost - his health - at least to the maximum degree possible.

If it is a community, voluntary, nonprofit hospital, the hospital makes a second declaration, namely, that it is available to all, that it will not profit from the patient's need, and that its self-interests are subservient to the community.

The hospital usually makes its resources available through the medium of the physician. But he too makes a public declaration that he possesses skills he will put at the services of those who are ill. In doing so, He incurs all the moral obligations traditionally delineated in professional codes of ethics: he must be competent, act in the patient's interest, never do deliberate harm, protect confidentiality, and treat the patient honestly, considerately, and personally. These obligations bind the physician within the hospital as they do in his office.

In using the hospital, however, the physician takes advantage of a community resource which he has not personally provided. The community places this resource in the trust of a board of directors, who act as surrogates for the community. The physician's moral obligations to the patient are no longer solely his concern. They now occur within an institutional framework, which modulates the relationship with his patient two ways. First, the physician's decisions directly or indirectly affect others. And, second, he shares his responsibilities with the institution through its board, which must carry out the obligations it incurs by virtue of its own declaration.

As a matter of fact, today an increasing number of patients now enter the same relationship with a hospital which formerly was obtained solely with physicians. The patient with no personal physician, or whose physician is unavailable, or who has an emergency expects the hospital to assume the same obligations for his care a physician would. When the hospital assigns a physician, technician, or nurse, it carries out its moral obligations through them, but it is not absolved of responsibility for how these obligations are fulfilled. When physicians are full-time employees of the hospital, the corporate obligation of the hospital is even more direct.

An even more fundamental and demanding source for the hospital's moral obligations is the special vulnerability of the person who is ill. The fact of illness is an insult to those aspects of existence most integral to being human. The patient is deprived in varying degrees of his humanity: His body is no longer the ready instrument of his will; he lacks the knowledge and skill to repair it or to make free and rational choices; he must place himself in the power of others. In short, illness deprives the patient of his distinctly human freedoms: to act, to make his own decisions, to be independent of the powers of others. The integrity of the patient's self-image as a human is shattered or, at the very least, threatened.

This state of vulnerability and injured humanity of the patient is one of grave inequality. All the power rests with those who have made the declaration that they will assist - the physician and the hospital. Even the most highly educated, powerful, or wealthy patient becomes a petitioner. Healing cannot be humane unless it does everything possible to restore these impaired freedoms, in a sense restoring the patient's humanity along with relieving him of pain, disability, or disease.

It is clear from the foregoing that hospitals as well as physicians incur serious moral obligations by the special nature of the fact of illness and the profession they voluntarily make to heal and assist. The central moral obligation is to make that profession fully authentic by fulfilling the expectations implicit in a relationship of such great inequality as exists between the helper and the one to be helped. A little closer look at the nature of the obligations themselves is now in order.

THE NATURE OF INSTITUTIONAL OBLIGATIONS

We have space to illustrate only a few of the specific obligations which flow from the special relationship between patients and those who profess to heal. Some have been touched upon already.

First, it seems clear that the institutionalization of so many aspects of medicine increasingly demands a moral relationship between the patient and the hospital which can be very similar to the patient/physician relationship. This means a great deal more than simply providing the setting in which medicine can be practiced safely and competently, as well as assuring its managerial efficiency and fiscal integrity, although the latter too are obligations. What is called for is a sharing of the same range of ethical responsibilities which have traditionally been implicit in the relationships between physician and patient. The board of trustees must feel moral as well as legal responsibility for the actions of the professional and nonprofessional workers within the hospital walls. This responsibility, even in presumably professional matters, cannot be delegated. Institutional morality, by necessity, must concern itself with every facet of the corporate life of that institution.

The result should be an overlapping and sharing of moral obligations in which the professional and the institution check and balance each other more intimately than is now customary. On this view, I take some exception to Professor Charles Fried's recent analysis of the partitioning of responsibilities between physicians and hospital authorities.[1,2] He assigns the hospital directors the bureaucratic decisions - those affecting efficiency, equity, and allocation of resources - and excuses them from responsibility for the personal dimensions of care given. These latter he assigns wholly to the physician, excusing him from concern with allocational decisions and suggesting that he must work within the framework of efficiency/equity decisions made by administrators or government.

Fried's division of responsibilities is reasonable so far as primary operational emphases are concerned. But these domains must not be compartmentalized; they must always be in dynamic equilibrium with each other. On the theses I am suggesting here, physicians and hospital directors are morally bound to see that their areas of primary responsibility do, in fact, interact. Each must fulfill the ethical obligation for the whole of what patients have a right to expect.

This mutuality of moral obligation becomes even more impelling in remediation of the injured humanity of the patient which illness entails. Both physician and hospital must reduce the inequalities in the relationship as well as the situation allows. The patient must be provided the knowledge necessary to participate rationally in the decisions which affect him. He must know what is wrong, what can be done, what the chances are for success, the dangers of treatment, the alternative procedures. The physician and the hospital share this obligation to enable the patient to make as free and rational a choice as possible. The obligation goes well beyond the mere legal requirement for valid consent. It demands consent of the highest quality and fullest sense of self-determination by the patient. The right to refuse specific treatment must be protected as well. The physician, the patient, and the hospital share obligations to each other, but because of the patient's vulnerability his needs are foremost.

This particular obligation assumes exquisite significance when a decision involves a moral question - a situation increasingly more pertinent as the capabilities of medicine expand the ways human life can be altered, shortened, or extended by technologic means. The questions in this realm are already matters of widespread public debate: abortion, continuing or discontinuing life-support measures, treatment or nontreatment of terminal or seemingly hopeless patients, participation in experimentation, and the like. The choices involve an intersection of the patient's values and those of the physician and the institution. Respect for the patient and humane treatment demand that these values be respected and that the patient be given the opportunity to act as his own moral agent if he wishes.

There are clear indications that more and more patients will wish to be their own moral agents and not delegate this agency to physicians as in the past. We live in a democratic society in which there is no uniformity of opinion on most medico-moral issues and no recognized authority to settle differences in ethical beliefs. There is also a growing tendency to distrust experts and institutions. The traditional moral authority of the physician has already been substantially eroded. Under these circumstances the moral responsibility of hospitals, like that of the physician, must be to make its values clear so the patient can make his own choice among institutions. We can foresee a time, not too far distant, when hospitals will have to declare their positions on the major medico-moral questions for the patient's guidance. Catholic hospitals have customarily done so on certain specific procedures.

There is room for considerable variation in ethical practices among hospitals. A democratic society should offer each patient the possibility of care in institutions that declare the same moral values he holds. This right can be actualized only if boards of trustees are willing to state clearly, in more specific terms than is now the case, the ethical principles to which they subscribe.

The immediacy of this issue is underscored by the excellent study by Diana Crane of the decisions physicians actually make in the care of the critically ill.[3] She shows considerable disparity between the official medical position, that treatment be continued until the patient is physiologically dead, and actual practice, wherein treatment is discontinued in those patients for whom the possibility of meaningful social interactions is nonexistent. Patients and their families should know of this disparity. Hospitals have an obligation to see that clear guidelines for terminating support measures be developed and monitored. Here again we see the dynamics of interaction on a moral issue between the physician and the institution.

Katz and Capron, in their book, have carefully studied the decision-making process in catastrophic illness. They outline the professional and institutional interactions necessary to assure that decisions are made rationally, equitably, and responsively.[4] Hospitals have the moral responsibility to provide these safeguards before they become matters of law.

What I am suggesting is that most decisions in a hospital are decisions in which technological and value choices are intermingled. Our society has developed a deep concern, not without foundation, that in deferring to the expert in technical matters it has lost control of the values and purposes of that technology. We need ways to control technology democratically, as Arthur Kantrowitz suggested recently.[5] He called for the separation of the technical from the value components in the uses of technology, the delegation of decisions on mixed decisions to judges who are not advocates of science, and finally, wider publication of the deliberations and decisions of judges and advocates.

Some parallel system is needed in hospitals and in society to distinguish between the professional medical advocacy for introduction and use of high technology and the social values of its employment. Institutional morality, if it is to be exercised fully, must grapple with such sensitive and even dangerous issues. Institutions are not immune to irrationality, the abuse of power, or the usurpation of morals.

And analysis of the obligations of professionals and hospitals indicates the need for a new balance between their roles as moral agents. Neither institutional nor individual professional ethics is sufficient for safeguarding the humanity of patients.

Heretofore, professional ethics has been the dominant and even the sole influence. We are now entering a new era in which three-way interaction between the moral agencies of physicians, hospitals, and patients is necessary.

UNANSWERED QUESTIONS WITH PRACTICAL IMPLICATIONS

Many practical questions remain. How does the hospital balance its moral obligations to individuals who work for and with it and its obligations to those it serves, including the community as a whole? How are obligations defined and deployed among professionals, nonprofessionals, and administrators? What mechanisms can be designed to implement the hospital's moral agency? What is the best way to allocate moral responsibility in team care? The team is, after all, a transitory, mini-social system operating within the hospital. It illustrates in microcosm the difficulties of the ethics of group actions. How are conflicts of values and principles among individuals in the institution resolved? To what extent and to what degree of specificity should the institution declare the values it subscribes to? How are the legal and ethical values of everyday decisions reconciled with each other? Law may lag behind ethics in some instances. Can an institution take a stance which society has not yet sanctioned in law?

These and related questions constitute the domain of institutional ethics. They will, I feel sure, be subjected to deeper and more critical analysis in the years ahead. The field of ethics as it applies to humans acting in concert is in need of a sound theoretical base before practical steps can be rationally justified. But the issues are sufficiently urgent to require tentative actions even before a substantial body of theory can be elaborated. Hospital administrators and trustees are already engaging in some of these issues. Some collaboration between ethical theorists and health-care practitioners is essential if the principles developed in this special domain of social ethics are to be practicable as well as theoretically sound.

Even while these fundamental explorations are being conducted, there is immediate need for a more open discussion of the issues of institutional morality among physicians, other health workers, and trustees. These are delicate issues of the kind generally eschewed in our society. The adherents of the intuitionist or skeptical views of ethics will deny the utility of such discussions. Others will shy away from the personal and sometimes emotional tone of ethical discourse. Some authorities even feel that the "tragic decisions" we must make in hospitals should not be the subject of public debate.

In my view, there is no alternative to a more concrete development of the issues in institutional morality at this time in our history. Everywhere there is a rebirth of interest in questions of value and purpose. This is particularly exemplified in medical affairs where the issues of biomedical and professional ethics are receiving unprecedented attention. I have called elsewhere for an expansion of medical ethics beyond its traditional boundaries to incorporate obligations of a new kind.[6] If this scrutiny is happening in professional medical ethics, can we realistically postpone consideration of the new relationships between institutional, professional, and personal ethics?

Moreover, as Professor Renee Fox has pointed out, the new interest in ethical issues in medicine is simply an expression of a deeper concern in America with the values, meaning, and purposes of life and institutions in general.[7] I believe Dr. Fox is right.

The assumption of a more explicit role of moral agency by hospitals is entirely consistent with this trend. I believe further that the hospital is a natural place to raise these questions because of the special sensitivity of its mission in society, one inextricably bound with the most human needs.

Rather than shying away from the undeniable challenges of moral agencies, hospitals can show the way toward a clearer conception of institutional morality. The main tasks of American medicine's third century are not managerial, fiscal, or technological, though such things pressure us daily. They are unequivocally moral and spiritual. The nation must rebuild that sense of moral purpose in the probity of human enterprises without which much of human activity becomes meaningless.

I do not mean to sermonize. But our nation will regain a sense of its worth only if its institutions exhibit the courage to pursue higher ideals than can be accomplished in a lifetime. People are less disappointed with high ideals sincerely enunciated and imperfectly attained than with their abnegation out of cynical or practical motives.

A simple, sincere, voluntary, and expeditious show of concern for moral issues untainted with self-interest must begin in some institutions. Are American hospitals ready for this challenge in their third century?

CHAPTER SEVENTEEN

STATE UNIVERSITY OF NEW YORK AT STONY BROOK HEALTH SCIENCES CENTER

The School of Medicine of the State University of New York at Stony Brook is being developed as an integral part of a comprehensive Health Sciences Center consisting of schools of medicine, nursing, allied health professions, social welfare, dental medicine, and basic health sciences. This fact has conditioned the development of the physical facilities, academic programs, and educational philosophy of the medical school in very significant ways, making it somewhat different from most new medical schools now in development. To delineate the medical school development properly it is essential to devote considerable space to a description of the Health Sciences Center of which it is such an important and essential part.

Details of architectural planning and curricular design have been omitted to save space and to concentrate on the major objectives that they serve. For details the interested reader may refer to published and unpublished documents that describe various facets of the philosophy and planning of the complex Health Sciences Center.

The School of Medicine enrolled its first class of twenty-four students in the late summer of 1971. This is a smaller number than anticipated because of the fiscal crisis in New York State, which has since caused further curtailment of many of the plans described in this essay. Despite the uncertain times and the many alterations of planning objectives caused by fiscal constraints, there are high hopes that the major commitments of the center will be achieved even though postponed.

The center will serve four million, perhaps the largest such population in the United States not now served by a health sciences center. The opportunities and the responsibilities of such an undertaking are correspondingly great. Hopefully the high expectations of faculty, staff, student body, and community will be realized as the physical facilities and academic programs take shape over the next decade.

Presently the center is serving some 500 full-time students in five schools that opened in 1970-1971. Dental medicine will enroll its first class in 1973. For the academic year 1972-1973 enrollments will remain static. A capital construction plan totalling $250 million is now underway with completion set for 1977.

The plan of this presentation will be, first, a brief cogitation of our experiences and lessons learned over the last six years of planning and operation. Particular emphasis will be placed on the impact of delays in decision-making and fiscal curtailments on the attempt to achieve orderly and rational planning for such a complex undertaking.

Some of these observations are based also on the author's prior experiences in "starting from scratch" in two other institutions where, fortunately, the time frame and fiscal determinations were not seriously impaired and it was possible to adhere to a master plan quite closely—Hunterdon Medical Center in Flemington, New Jersey, and the University of Kentucky Medical Center in Lexington.

ORGANIZED PLANS AND REALITY: SOME OBSERVATIONS

It is difficult in any enterprise still in the process of becoming to analyze experiences and to detect errors, wrong turns, and lessons that might be useful to others similarly engaged. The planning and full development of so large and complex an undertaking as the Health Sciences Center at Stony Brook will consume at least a decade from the onset of planning in 1966 to full occupancy of the physical facilities in 1977. At the time of this reporting (December 1971), we are just past the midpoint of this decade. While we are still too close to most of our decisions, some patterns of experience and some problems are already discernible. Out of this emergent matrix we have selected a few for comment—those few that are derived from the testing of our decisions and planning process against actual events, foreseen and unforeseen.

Planning for the health sciences was initiated from "ground zero" in the fall of 1966 with the hiring of the director of the center, E. D. Pellegrino, and an associate, A. G. Knudson. They were presented with a copy of the Muir Commission Report, some 250 acres of trees, and the charge to develop what was the largest and most complex of the new health sciences centers in the making.

The canvas was "clean." Only a few preliminary meetings had been held by the university, itself in process of becoming. Some of the issues in medical education were outlined briefly by outside consultants. The concrete desiderata were few: assurance by the Construction Fund of the State University of New York (SUNY) that some $165 million were available in a bond issue to fund capital construction; the expected date of opening the medical school was set at 1971; opening dates of other schools were still to be determined. A firm of consultants had been engaged to do a preliminary planning analysis and negotiations had begun with the architect who was eventually to be awarded the project contract.

Beyond these few constraints lay the whole panoply of decisions and processes that would eventuate in a comprehensive six-school Health Sciences Center capable of handling more than 3,000 full-time students and presumably geared to a fresh approach to some of the major problems in health care and in professional education.

The planning process began at a time drastically different from the present. Federal support for construction of health educational facilities was available; the university at Stony Brook was at the height of its expectations of becoming a major teaching and research center; the economic stability of the state and the region seemed assured; and the watchword everywhere was innovation, response to challenge, and elaboration of programs of excellence. The contrast in needs between 1966 and the present could not be sharper. Every decision retrospectively analyzed must be cogitated in the light of the changes in the economy of the state and the nation and the disaffection with universities and research that has since occurred.

At the outset, time was afforded for the establishment of an orderly process. Ours may be the last center for some time in which one could proceed from the development of an academic plan to the description of the program requirements essential to implement the plan and then to the design of spaces to enclose the program and facilitate achievement of its objectives. Planning and operation were to be phased into each other; temporary facilities were to be employed to initiate programs that would be moved to permanent facilities as they were completed, so that academic programs could be initiated with a minimum of delay. Careful plans were made to provide lead time for deans, directors of programs, and faculty, so that all preparations for initiating a given program could be made well in advance.

The result of this overall approach was a highly articulated, closely integrated academic and facilities program, carefully interdigitated with operating budgets and enrollment dates. If these plans had been followed and decisions made on the pre-agreed time frame, all programs would have been in operation by 1972 and all facilities occupied by 1975. The impact of delays in decision-making outside the Health Sciences Center, defaults in funding, and the changed economic situation in the state demanded innumerable alterations in the process. The cumulative effect of the resultant compromises now determines the nature of the program as much as the original conceptions of what the center would and could be.

By the end of the first year, 1967, the following had been accomplished: An academic plan was completed that defined in detail the objectives of all programs in the center as a whole and in each of the component schools. Detailed programs describing the functional uses, equipment, and sizes of all rooms were complete, as was a master architectural plan. The architect had initiated preliminary designs and was prepared to go rapidly to more detailed drawings. The original plan called for development of the facilities in a series of closely integrated but separate buildings; as each building was completed programs would be moved from temporary or surge spaces.

The first serious damage to this plan was sustained when the SUNY Construction Fund rejected the idea of multiple successive buildings in favor of a megastructure to be constructed as one massive unit. Another complication occurred when the approval for temporary quarters was delayed from the time of first request in 1966 to late 1969. The most serious disruption of plans, however, followed upon the unexpected announcement that funds originally allocated for the project had been spent for other purposes and that funding would have to be reauthorized by the legislature. As a consequence the megastructure itself had to be constructed in stages. Meanwhile escalation in construction costs had increased precipitously—by about 40 percent.

The impact of these events was to disrupt the entire academic plan and enrollment schedules. The university hospital has yet to be authorized and plans for temporary buildings have yet to be fully implemented. All academic programs have been delayed by at least two to three years.

Concomitant with the disruptions in architectural plans came deficiencies in operating budgets. These undermined the concept of "lead time" for planning and orderly acquisition of personnel, equipment, and facilities. In no budget period have facilities, equipment, faculty, staff, and operating funds been made available in a congruent fashion. Characteristically, one element or the other was authorized and the others withheld. The orderly procedure from academic plan to implementation was unsuitably compromised and in place of a carefully designed plan we were forced by events to numerous changes in design, program objectives, and target dates. With the growing disorder of state finances these incongruities of necessity became even more serious.

Despite these problems the Health Sciences Center has opened five of its schools on schedule and there is little doubt that the total plan will eventually be carried out, although with considerable delay. The confrontations of a well-designed and highly articulated plan with unforeseen fiscal realities in the setting of complex decision-making machinery outside the center itself is unique to our system. Recognizing the uniqueness of our program and the special problems of planning in a very large university system, as well as the peculiar nature of the times, some of our observations may yet have value for others.

1. There are problems inherent in a highly integrated, closely articulated planning process. Given the conditions that existed in 1966, development of a large-scale, carefully laid-out plan which synchronized development of temporary and permanent facilities with development of staff and initiation of program seemed justifiable. Such a plan has great cogency and if it is possible to carry it out it is the most effective way to achieve stated objectives.

What was not foreseen was the impact of delays in making decisions by central university authorities, the Construction Fund, and the Division of the Budget. These delays coincided with unexpected dissolution of funds for buildings and operating budgets. Under such circumstances a closely integrated, rationally developed plan suffers in ways a less ambitious and more fragmented plan would not. The time delay in the availability of building produced very serious effects on morale and faculty recruitment. The decision to build an integrated megastructure was a good one in terms of the objectives to be achieved but it suffered much in the time frame imposed upon it by reality. A plan built upon stepwise development, with a short time frame for each step and completion of each unit at the end of each period, would have been preferable under the circumstances. We have been forced to face clearly the fact that the time frame must match the design and that every attempt should be made to ascertain the time frame well in advance of the initiation of any design.

2. In the development of temporary spaces the matching of time frame with program and design is just as important as in permanent facilities. Indeed with the delays one can expect in program facilities any viable plan should be so devised that whole and complete programs can take place in temporary spaces and for indefinite periods of time. The availability, utility, and efficiency of temporary structures today make this a realistic approach and one might contemplate periods of five or ten years in such temporary spaces to allow for the proper development of a permanent physical facility. The expenditures, while considerable, would be worthwhile as programs can start with a minimum of delay and be developed to a high degree in the absence of permanent physical facilities.

While the impact of reality on a highly articulated program of physical facilities may be severe, the impact on academic planning and the process of establishing an institution with common goals and objectives may be even greater. Some comments on this aspect of our planning process might be useful.

3. We were afforded the opportunity in the early days of the center to adhere to some of our most important requirements for academic planning. One of these was the early recruitment of the deans of the six schools and the directors of all the major supporting programs. This was essential in development of the concept of a unified Health Sciences Center with a clearly defined mission and a cooperative approach to problems of education, research, and patient service. There is no question that this has been a most significant element in our program commitment to the concept of the Health Sciences Center as a unified and integrated entity. Deans and directors were permitted to become acquainted with one another, to define goals and objectives, to learn about each other's programs, and to assist one another in recruitment and in facilities design and planning.

As each dean began to recruit faculty members, however, the process was disrupted by great reductions in operating budget requests and delays in the approval of appointments of faculty and supporting staff. Thus after enjoying about one-and-one-half years of an orderly process of recruitment the plan was thrown into disarray. Each dean had to scramble for faculty, bring them in with short time periods of preparation, and introduce them to teaching with little opportunity to become acquainted with the institution, its goals, and its objectives.

Everyone acknowledges the very great opportunity provided in developing a new institution from its inception, for one need not deal with established precedents. We must not forget, however, that individuals do bring their own precedents and experiences with them. There must be a suitable period during which the faculty and staff members are allowed to unpack their "cultural baggage," so to speak—that is, to display the techniques and modes that provided success in their previous institutions—and to modify their preconceptions in the light of the objectives and goals of the new institution. Because of the disruption of the time frame we had envisioned and planned for, this opportunity for "acculturation" to the ideas and objectives of the new center was not available to enough people.

This is a very serious deterrent to attempting to strike out in new directions and to develop the unity of perspective we deemed so important to the development of the entire program. This is not a defect in the planning process but in its implementation. One may avoid it with a less ambitious plan or by developing smaller and more complete units before integrating them into the whole. Thus the academic program probably is better developed in these uncertain times in a stepwise fashion and with less ambitious attempts to integrate the whole at the outset.

Whether or not one can ultimately put these small packages together into a large unit which really has a definable unity of purpose is difficult to ascertain. Probably the end result would not be the same as what we have envisioned. Hence while our planning was rational it was simply out of phase with the unexpected events that seriously impaired the full evolution of the plan we had elaborated.

4. Very clearly the half-life of human enthusiasm is relatively short. One of the very serious problems caused by the delays in obtaining facilities, equipment, staff, and personnel was the notable dissolution of the initial zeal of faculty members. Human beings need to see the results of their efforts and most of us need to see them within a reasonable time span. As a consequence of the author's previous experiences in establishing new institutions he is thoroughly convinced that if innovation is to occur this period of enthusiasm must be captured and put to work in the first four or five years. After that there occurs a rapid attenuation of eagerness for change, even in those who came originally with high purposes and determination to strike out in new directions. When crises impinge upon an institution, the tendency to revert to type and seek the safe solutions of the past is overwhelming.

The alternative again involves establishment of a less ambitious plan that would concentrate on a few new innovations rather than an across-the-board attack on a wide range of problems. This is a serious decision to make. Many feel that truly fundamental changes cannot be made in education and service without change in the total pattern of function and organization of a new center. In a new institution such broad changes in concept, organization, and philosophy are possible. But global approaches must also take the time frame into account and perhaps the more cautious piecemeal approach is preferable, even in a new school.

5. One of the most serious problems at Stony Brook has been the delay in authorization of funds for the university hospital. This problem will be with us for at least another four or five years since building has not yet begun. The original decision in 1966 to build the hospital as part of the total structure was the rational one, given the considerations then existing. But in retrospect in would have been better to hold out for hospital construction first and delay the building of permanent academic and laboratory spaces, using temporary facilities instead. The opening of the new general medical and surgical Veterans Administration Hospital at Northport, twenty-five minutes away, has also been delayed by two years. We are therefore totally dependent upon cooperative but distant institutions for our clinical teaching.

Absence of a hospital has seriously impaired the rate at which clinical faculty can be recruited. Prospective clinical chairman are willing to defer clinical activity for one or two years but understandably not for four or five. When one must travel up to one hour to reach a hospital the difficulties of integrating clinical teaching into first- and second-year curricula are manifest.

Another consequence of the unavailability of a clinical facility for full-time faculty is a lack of a means of supplementing clinical faculty salaries. The budget division of the state of New York has reluctantly accepted the fact that full salaries comparable to those at other SUNY medical centers must be paid, but the lack of clinical funds to offset these expenditures is a source of constant difficulty and delays in making appointments.

Over and above all of this is the tremendous effect of a hospital and the presence of patients in impressing students and faculty with the ultimate justifications of all their activities—human beings in need of assistance. The intellectual center of gravity of an institution becomes displaced whenever it lacks the daily reminder of patient needs to modulate every decision and orient every educational effort. This loss of the presence of patients cannot be estimated in dollars but it is so serious that we would advise any new school first to secure its clinical facilities and to do so in the closest possible proximity.

None of these comments should be construed as indicating lack of commitment to the idea of a consortium of clinical campuses. These campuses are essential in expanding the capacities of the center to handle students, to provide a wider range of clinical experiences, and serve as nodal points in a total system of education for a region. The university hospital is, however, an essential core requisite of the consortium idea without which the concept itself suffers from lack of academic directions.

6. Many facets of the Stony Brook plan are unique or at least new in conception, but our major contribution will probably be less in the originality of individual programs and more in the synthesis of a series of interlocking synergistic programs in one center with a unity of perspective and mission. It is too early to make useful observations about our major academic commitments as outlined in the subsequent pages of this report. Whether the consortium plan, the commitment to multitrack curricula, the efforts toward interdisciplinary education, or any of our other programs is successful will take more time to evaluate.

It does appear clear that change can be built into a new institution only on the basis of a clarity of objectives and the fortunate confluence of funds, facilities, and people in a time frame that does not exceed that half-life of human enthusiasm. Our highly articulated and integrated program plan depends upon many things and events happening on a time schedule and in a social atmosphere that we cannot control. The value of this center to the world of education and service in the health professions may well be more in the breadth of its hopes, aspirations, and conceptualizations than in the actual realization of each and every program as described herein.

It has always appeared preferable to the author to aim for the ideal, realizing that it can be approached in the world only asymptotically, than to plan for the merely feasible. When we fall from the ideal we are still on a more elevated plateau than when we fall from the merely possible. Hopefully the asymptote we reach will approximate the ideals we have set for ourselves. After all, the very magnitude of our problems may be the most valid indication of the worth of the goals we have set for ourselves.

THE MUIR REPORT

In December 1961 Governor Rockefeller appointed a special New York State Committee on Medical Education and directed it to project the needs of New York

State for the next two decades and to recommend the number of health professionals that would be required, appropriate ways of producing these additional personnel, and a satisfactory timetable for the expansion of existing schools and the establishment of any new schools that might be considered necessary. Under the chairmanship of Mr. Malcolm Muir and the directorship of Dr. Lester Evans, the committee submitted this report in June 1963.

Medicine

The Muir Committee stated that in order to maintain the existing ratio of physicians to population in New York State it would be necessary to increase the number of practicing physicians from 30,700 to 39,900 by 1980. The committee recommended the creation of 325 additional first-year places in medical schools by 1970 and 425 first-year places by 1980 and stressed that these were minimum requirements that might well need to be increased if other factors did not remain favorable.

Dental Medicine

The Muir Report estimated that in order to merely maintain the current ratio of dentists to population it would be necessary to provide seventy-five additional first-year dental school places in New York State by 1970 and 100 first-year places by 1980. These figures presuppose continuance of the same high migration rate of dentists trained in schools outside of New York.

Nursing

The report concluded in discussion of nursing needs for New York State with the following strong recommendation for the development of new baccalaureate programs: "The development of such school is essential if the nursing profession is to be supplied adequately with practitioners of the broad background in the social, behavioral, and physical sciences that is eminently desirable in the bedside nurse, and vital to the supervising and teaching nurse. They are the schools most heavily depended upon to supply leadership in the profession."

Allied Health Professions

The fact that "many health services that began as vocations on the periphery of medicine have evolved into professions of increasingly central importance to the provision of comprehensive medical care" was recognized by the Muir Committee in its report. No university-level institution currently exists on Long Island with a strong commitment to the allied health professions. Three community college-level institutions have made beginnings in the limited number of vocational-level health programs, but these schools have until now had no center of higher education to which to turn for faculty, consultation, and other expertise.

General Comments

As a component of the SUNY, the Health Sciences Center at Stony Brook has a clear responsibility to work toward the resolution of problems of health manpower in

New York State. To the extent that graduates of the various programs of the center choose to reside within the state they will be filling that need. In addition, it is likely that a significant number of health professionals educated at this center will choose to locate elsewhere in the country and in so doing will be helping to close the health services gap on the national level.

THE ACADEMIC PLAN

It is difficult to elaborate an imaginative academic plan even in a fully developed university. The attempt to do so for the new Health Sciences Center at Stony Brook while it is in its earliest stages of development is fraught with obvious uncertainties.

Detailed planning for the center began in September 1966 with a staff of two physicians. While many of the questions requisite for the development of an academic plan were faced then, all projections have since been subjected to critical and expert review by deans and staff as they were recruited. These plans will remain flexible until the senior faculty is recruited in all units of the Health Sciences Center.

The unique chance to create something new in each of the health professions will be the single most attractive factor in recruiting a high quality faculty to Stony Brook. To predetermine any program too rigidly would not only be imprudent but would seriously impair our ability to attract creative academic leaders to our campus.

Every facet of education in the health sciences is currently the subject of widespread critical re-examination. In the rapidly changing health field today's projections and hopes may be outmoded by the time the center is in operation. Flexibility is an essential ingredient in planning for so large a complex, and this implies freedom to change objectives as new dimensions and challenges make themselves apparent.

Academic goals and philosophy must in consequence be treated broadly and in principle. Nonetheless the major commitments outlined in our academic plan should be valid for at least the next decade. This plan will undoubtedly undergo maturation, emendation, and refinements as the faculties grow, and it should be regarded as a definition of the philosophical compass points that will guide the development of the programs in the health sciences at Stony Brook.

Implicit in the charge to plan and develop any new educational institution is the responsibility for a critical and imaginative interpretation of its mission in terms of current and future scientific and social forces. This responsibility is all the more compelling in the genesis of a comprehensive health sciences center, for in few situations is the intermingling of the traditional and the innovative so urgently demanded. The half-life of human enthusiasm for innovation is rapidly shortened as planning imperceptibly yields to the exigencies of operation. To effect the synergism of new ideas with the traditional it is mandatory that the short fertile period of the early days of planning be utilized maximally.

The new Health Sciences Center will develop within the favorable environment of a growing comprehensive university dedicated to a fresh approach to teaching, research, and service. The opportunity is unexcelled for a vigorous confrontation with some of the major problems of service and education in the health sciences. The primary responsibility of the planning staff is to create a center that is scientifically based, sensitive to the needs of the community it serves, and courageous enough to initiate experimentation. It must explore ways to generate new knowledge simultaneously with improving ways to deliver what is already known in a socially responsible and effective manner.

THE HEALTH SCIENCES CENTER

Academic Mission and Commitment

Academic programs will range from molecular biology through the usual clinical disciplines to community medicine and service. The majority of the programs are to be at the baccalaureate, master's, and doctoral levels, geared to the future and present health needs of our region and the nation. We hope to confront some of the major issues in providing optimal health care in a socially relevant way. Such an undertaking demands a heavy commitment to early planning for physical facilities, but concern for building must not obscure the ideas which alone will distinguish this new center and justify expectations and expenditures.

Certain academic commitments will characterize the Health Sciences Center at Stony Brook. These commitments are the basis of this academic plan; they define the mission of the center and will guide planning for the next decade. They are particularly relevant to the academic programs in medicine and dental medicine.

First, the Health Sciences Center is committed to the cultivation of all the health professions as university disciplines. "The task of the university," in the words of the philosopher, A. N. Whitehead, "is the creation of the future." In the thirty years since this utterance, society has even more explicitly charged the universities to confront the relevant issues of the day and to use their resources for the direct betterment of the human condition. For a new university such as Stony Brook, Whitehead's words have particular acuteness. With the center as an integral part, the university can extend the range of its concerns to some of man's oldest problems: disability, disease, and the maintenance of health.

The Health Sciences Center could not fully "create the future" in health care without the most intimate relationship with the biological sciences, humanities, social sciences, and other professional schools in the university. While most medical schools in this country are under university aegis, the association is best characterized as uneasy. Mutual advantages have nowhere been fully developed. How to make the potential of a health sciences center available on a wider basis to all disciplines is one of the major academic issues of today. Stony Brook has the advantages of physical cohesiveness, of concurrent growth and cooperative planning, and of conscious efforts to interrelate the Health Sciences Center and the University. Stony Brook has an opportunity shared by only a few new institutions: to develop a health sciences center simultaneously with a new university.

A *second* major commitment is to develop a viable conception of the Health Sciences Center from the outset—there are many "medical centers" but few which have developed all the health sciences and professions in a genuinely unified and cooperative way.

One of the major deterrents to the delivery of optimal medical care today is a failure of communication and of a precise definition of functions among the steadily increasing numbers of health professions. Too often the health professions have approached patient care in isolation from one another; it is essential that medicine, dentistry, nursing, and the other health professions develop their programs of education, research, and patient care in close collaboration with one another from the outset. The health sciences center is the major instrument whereby the health professions can jointly examine the health needs of patients and society and determine what roles must be developed to meet these needs in new and more effective ways. Public interest in health is too strong to permit dalliance or blind defenses of professional prerogatives to interfere with the cooperative efforts so urgently called for if we are to provide optimal care for all our citizens.

A *third* major commitment is to the fullest development of the interface with the communities of Nassau and Suffolk counties. Medical centers are belatedly awakening to their responsibilities to make their resources available to the communities they serve. A few of the new schools have pioneered in this direction but most established medical centers are still effectively isolated from their communities.

The planning staff at Stony Brook has already begun to make contact with voluntary health agencies, hospitals, public agencies, professional societies, and the lay public. Under the provision of the legislation on heart disease, cancer, and stroke, Stony Brook has already played an important role in the establishment of the Nassau-Suffolk Regional Medical Programs. Its staff and faculty members are working in Comprehensive Health Planning, community councils, and the Hospital and Health Planning Council. Effective liaison has been established with the departments of health in both counties and with community groups interested in health care for the disadvantaged and for migrant workers. A two-way relationship is contemplated involving continuing education, hospital affiliations, and the sharing of facilities and specialized personnel and equipment. Our center will be a resource available to all segments of the Long Island community.

In addition, a community-based experience of some kind is considered essential for students and faculty in all the health professions. It is planned to make the Department of Community Medicine one of the broadest and strongest and to give it centerwide responsibilities. It will cultivate all aspects of the community's health needs and provide medicine *of* and medicine *in* the community. Affiliations with community hospitals and health departments, public education programs, assistance to community planning groups, development of models of health care delivery—these are among the plans for community *interaction.*

A *fourth* commitment is to experimentation in how best to deliver to every patient in every community the knowledge and technology needed in contemporary health care. Here, too, medical centers have lagged. Recent federal legislation, such as Regional Medical Programs and Comprehensive Health Planning, reflects public awareness of the need for new patterns of medical care that is running ahead of professional perceptions.

Health sciences centers must wrestle more directly with this question by designing and operating experimental models of patient care. In the living laboratory of actual medical care we can study such things as the best alignment of roles and functions between health professional, optimal organizational patterns, and the optimal use of computers and other technological equipment. With such models, students in all the health professions can be taught to work together cooperatively and to examine their own effectiveness in objective ways in relation to the contributions of others.

We are planning experimental models of patient care delivery in several contexts: the university hospital itself, selected community hospitals, low income areas, and migrant labor camps. In each, students at all levels of sophistication and in all the schools of the center can familiarize themselves with possible future patterns of care and learn something of the problems of delivery of optimal care.

A *fifth* major commitment is innovation in the educational process and in the curricula of our schools. The details of each curriculum are developed by deans and faculties now being appointed.

There is a veritable revolution in the sphere today. Every new medical school is impelled to design a new curriculum defined in terms of what will be demanded of its health professionals tomorrow. The outlines of the curricula in medicine will be described in more detail later in the document. Certain general features will, however, characterize the curricula in all the component colleges of the Health Sciences Center.

In place of the present standard curricular programs we can expect variable programs adjusted to student needs and interests and more in keeping with the principles of graduate education. Thus in place of complete coverage of all subjects, emphasis is placed upon learning a smaller number of widely applicable concepts. "Core curricula" have been designed to teach two "languages," one in the basic sciences and the other in the clinical. Students will share these core curricula but then take alternate and multiple tracks to their degrees. Some who have not made a definite career decision will follow standard courses; others will pursue one of several tracks—basic sciences and research, clinical specialties, general and family medicine, etc. Each track is designed to teach different skills and prepare graduates for specific roles in the health care system. Admission to advanced standing, earlier or more varied entry points into professional curricula, and transfer from one curriculum to another are contemplated. Earlier contact with patients is planned as this is essential for today's students who need to see the "relevance" of the work they are pursuing. We plan work-study programs of various types. All curricula obviously must be flexible enough to permit these excursions into the health care arena.

We also expect greater emphasis to be placed on the students' learning processes as well as on the techniques of teaching. Technologic aids such as the computer, television, films, and automated carrels will often replace lectures and long laboratory sessions. Seminar and tutorial teaching will assume a more prominent place as the curriculum becomes more flexible. A system of advising is essential to many of these concepts.

We plan to combine preprofessional and professional education into assimilable packages in which the student can more readily see the goals before him. Collaborative efforts are being developed in order to relate existing university undergraduate courses more closely to the later needs of the health professions.

With the effective application of some of these measures the total time spent in acquiring a professional education can be shortened appreciably. The details of implementation of these general ideas will be found in a later section of this paper.

A *sixth* commitment is to continuing education that will equip each physician to combat the invariable obsolescence of knowledge that follows so rapidly upon graduation.

Present methods of continuing education are admittedly inadequate to meet the needs of today's practicing professionals. Use will be made of audiovisual techniques, closed circuit television, and computer assisted educational programs, but these must be supplemented by the more lasting effects of education of physicians, nurses, dentists, and others in their own hospitals and in the course of their daily work. The Health Sciences Center will assist every community hospital to become an educational institution. Provision of faculty, consultation in educational methods, and training of an indigenous faculty are responsibilities the center will undertake. A plan for involvement of all hospitals that wish to participate has already been developed.

A *seventh* major commitment of the health professions must be to maintain the human and compassionate aspects of health care in the tightly organized and highly technical systems of care now emerging. Special attention in education must be given to underscoring the humanistic, ethical, social, historical, and economic dimensions of health. This implies a much closer interchange with the university disciplines and their actual involvement in clinical teaching. Opportunities for continuation of a student's general education while in the professional schools must be developed.

Finally we are of course committed to building all of the above on a firm basis of scientific medicine—on the physical, biological, and social sciences that nourish it. In a university such as ours, and in the modern world, to do less would be to damage the wellsprings of knowledge that have transformed medical care in the past 100 years from a conjectural art to a reasonably rational process.

The real challenge is how to do all the things which must be done to update education in the health professions without sacrificing the scientific fundamentals of each profession. We are committed to the idea that all our programs must be both scientifically based and socially responsible. The great intellectual task before us is to make these goals mutually reinforcing rather than competing elements in the life of our center.

Challenge and Opportunity

To create a health sciences center today is among the most exciting and complex tasks imaginable. It is pregnant with possibilities that no one institution can fully encompass, even one as large as Stony Brook will be. There is danger of succumbing, on the one hand, to tried and true safe formulae that insure success and, on the other, to the evanescent triumphs of trivial innovation.

The critical problem is to select the most significant intellectual and practical challenges in a world continuously transformed by science, technology, and social change. The foregoing brief listing of commitments is a configuration of the challenges now being faced at Stony Brook; they will inevitably define its ultimate character and delineate its special mission.

The major commitments that have been described are applicable to each of the component colleges, modified to meet the needs and future developments of each of the health professions. Dedication of each of the colleges to a series of common commitments, albeit somewhat differently expressed, is an important way to unite the health professions in a common endeavor. The ultimate aim is the betterment of the health care delivered to the American public. The opportunity to develop the health professions in close collaboration with each other in the planning and operational phases of the new Health Sciences Center is unique and may constitute one of the major opportunities open to Stony Brook.

TABLE 1. DEGREES TO BE CONFERRED AT FULL DEVELOPMENT
PHASE 1—1967-77

	Degree	No. of Students	No. of Faculty
School of Medicine	M.D.	600	200
School of Nursing	B.S., M.S.	700	50
School of Dental Medicine	D.D.M.	150	86
School of Allied Health Professions	B.S., M.S.	600	60
School of Social Welfare	B.S., M.S.W., D.S.W.	550	75
School of Basic Health Sciences	M.S., Ph.D.	500	150
		3,100	621

Organizational Structure

In achieving the objectives of cooperative teaching, research, and service, the Health Sciences Center is organized so that each health profession has an opportunity to participate equally in policy making and implementation. Accordingly the administrative deans of each unit—basic health sciences, medicine, nursing, dental medicine, social welfare, and allied health professions—report directly to the vice president for the health sciences on all matters of budget, academic programs, and policy. Also reporting to him are the directors of laboratory animal resources, university hospital, health sciences communications, and health sciences library.

The vice president for the health sciences is the executive officer responsible for all matters relating to the health professions. He in turn reports directly to the president of the university on matters of budget, programs, service, and administrative policy. He processes all academic matters, such as appointments, curricula, and new academic programs, for the president through the academic vice president, in keeping with general university policy.

The design and implementation of the curriculum and courses in each of the component colleges is the responsibility of the deans of the component schools and their faculties. Recruitment, processing of new appointments, promotions, and advancement to tenure are initiated by departmental chairmen and transmitted through the appropriate dean to the vice president for the health sciences.

The vice president's cabinet is composed of the deans of the six schools, the associate directors of the center for academic affairs and patient and administrative services, and the directors of laboratory animal resources, health sciences library, health sciences communications, and the university hospital.

Relationship to University Administration

The size, complexity, and specific nature of the programs in the Health Sciences Center are such that considerable decentralization of administrative functions will prove necessary. Further, the special problems of patient care, university hospital business affairs, and relationships with community professional and lay groups require specific coordination in the center. The vice president for the health sciences needs a staff of coordinating administrative assistants for such functions as business and fiscal affairs, personnel, community relations, purchases and supplies, plant and maintenance, grants and research administration, planning and development, student affairs, and instructional resources. Each of these assistants will maintain liaison with his counterpart on the general campus. Administrative procedures and policies are those established for the general campus unless by specific arrangement some facet of patient care or clinical activity requires modification.

Cooperative efforts are as essential in the administrative sphere as they are in the academic. Decentralization should be regarded as a tool for efficiency of operation geared to meet the somewhat specific needs imposed by the size of the Health Sciences Center and the complexities of its operation. In addition very special dimensions are introduced by the need to respond quickly and effectively whenever the needs of patients are concerned.

Relationship to University Academic Organization

1. *Relationship to Undergraduate Departments*: All departments of the university, including those in the Health Sciences Center, are universitywide departments, that is, they are not duplicated and each is expected to meet the teaching responsibilities at the undergraduate and graduate levels and in continuing education

The component schools of the Health Sciences Center depend upon university departments to provide the nonprofessional instruction requisite to their programs. In the cases of nursing and allied health professions, at least half of the requirements for the baccalaureate degree consist of general education in the social sciences, humanities, and physical sciences. Manifestly the deans in the Health Sciences Center are dependent upon provosts in the university disciplines and their department chairmen to arrange suitable and relevant course work in general education for their students.

Conversely, suitable nonclinical courses offered by schools in the center—physiology, microbiology, anatomical sciences, social welfare, community organization, and epidemiology, for example—are available to students in the divisions of the general university. Much of the commitment of the center to integrating with the university is expressed in this cross-participation in courses and interchanges of students and faculty.

2. *Graduate Programs:* Doctoral programs in the sciences basic to medicine are planned, as well as master's and doctoral programs in nursing, social welfare, dental medicine, and the allied health professions. The same policies that apply to graduate programs in the university apply to all nonprofessional doctoral and master's degree programs in the center. Students are expected to meet the criteria for admission to the graduate school and are registered therein. All academic programs are submitted by the faculties and deans of the schools in the Health Sciences Center to the Graduate

Council for review and approval. Interdisciplinary graduate programs are encouraged involving members of the health sciences faculties and those in university disciplines, but these will not preclude doctoral programs of departmental origin.

THE SCHOOL OF BASIC HEALTH SCIENCES

The sciences basic to health are organized in the School of Basic Health Sciences headed by a dean who is under the administrative direction of the vice president for the health sciences for purposes of budget, academic programs, appointments, research, and service functions. Departments in the School of Basic Health Sciences will include anatomy, physiology, microbiology, pharmacology, and pathology. Biochemistry is physically located in the Department of Biological Sciences. These departments are university departments in the fullest sense of the word and have responsibility for undergraduate as well as graduate, professional, and continuing education. In conjunction with appropriate components in the biological sciences these departments have the principal responsibility for what is traditionally thought of as the basic health sciences for students in all schools of the Health Sciences Center.

Organization of these departments into a School of Basic Health Sciences rather than under the exclusive jurisdiction of the medical school represents a departure from the traditional pattern. This is consistent with the breadth of educational responsibility being assumed by the center and the need to assure the access of all professional schools to basic science resources. The School of Basic Health Sciences will be organized in a fashion similar to that of the other schools in the center. For administrative purposes this school will also include departments of medical social sciences and humanities and bio-mathematics.

Because of its size and the specificity of its mission a health sciences complex places certain strains on the organizational patterns of any university. These are particularly noticeable in the relationships between the Department of Biological Sciences and departments traditionally considered basic to education in medicine and the other health professions. On few campuses have these relationships been defined optimally.

In establishing a Health Sciences Center on a new campus such as Stony Brook there is a responsibility to re-examine a critical question: How can the Health Sciences Center best be made an integral part of the university? And how can the university disciplines have their impact on education and research in the health professions? The arrangement described here is considered most feasible at this time. It must be re-examined periodically to see whether or not it achieves the purposes for which it is designed.

The specific assignment of a division or department to either the Department of Biological Sciences or the Health Sciences Center was determined after consideration of a number of factors: the degree of involvement with undergraduate teaching in biology, the direction of research and service interests, and the need for both the center and the department to administer certain disciplines with a deep commitment to their own academic programs and curricular development. Using these criteria, cell biology, genetics, developmental biology, marine biology, ethology, and ecology are placed in the Department of Biological Sciences. Pharmacology, pathology, anatomical sciences, physiology, and microbiology are most suitably placed in the School of Basic Health Sciences.

Biochemistry poses a somewhat more complex problem. It has strong traditional ties to medicine, on the one hand, while on the other it is increasingly essential to undergraduate and graduate teaching in biology. The need for a strong commitment of biochemistry to undergraduate teaching and its relevance for all divisions of the biological sciences determined its assignment to the Department of Biological Sciences.

It is essential that the deans of the schools of medicine, dental medicine, nursing, and allied health professions have a voice in the selection of faculty for the basic sciences departments as well as those assigned to the Department of Biological Sciences. In addition, chairmen of the departments in the School of Basic Health Sciences and the divisions of the Department of Biological Sciences participate in the curricular planning of all schools requiring basic science instruction.

Some specific mechanisms at Stony Brook are useful in the integration of the Health Sciences Center and the biological sciences department and help to remove barriers to communication and cooperation that plague health centers and their component universities. Physical placement of the center on the university campus is a clear advantage. Sharing the use of the Health Sciences Library can bring basic scientists, biologists, and clinicians into contact with one another. The provost for the biological sciences and/or his designee sits as a member of the Health Sciences Council. The vice president for the health sciences and/or his designee participates in the Biological Sciences Council. Interdisciplinary cross-departmental and intercollege cooperation is fostered by the development of graduate programs, research projects, and conjoint courses. A system of joint appointments also enhances cooperation.

The dean for basic health sciences in the Health Sciences Center has a specific responsibility for assuring cooperation between the basic sciences departments in biology and in the School of Basic Health Sciences. The multitrack system being considered for all curricula will permit students to spend substantial parts of their predoctoral careers in many of the divisions of the Department of Biological Sciences. Also the provision of liberal elective time should further encourage participation by medical and dental students in biological sciences courses.

The School of Basic Health Sciences will include the departments listed in Table 2. Biochemistry will be physically located in the Department of Biological Sciences.

TABLE 2. SCHOOL OF BASIC HEALTH SCIENCES—FUNCTIONAL STAFF

Anatomy	20
Biochemistry	20
Biomathematics	7
Medical social sciences	12
Microbiology	20
Pathology	30
Pharmacology	19
Physiology and biophysics	22
Total	150

SOCIAL SCIENCES AND HUMANITIES

The necessity for a close working relationship between the physical and biological sciences and the health sciences is relatively easily accepted. The equal dependence of the health sciences on the university departments in the social sciences is still largely unrecognized in most institutions. Yet major developments in the health sciences and the social sciences are not possible without viable cooperative efforts between them.

Because of the special needs of the health sciences for closer contact with the social sciences and humanities at Stony Brook, we are establishing a group of social scientists with primary appointments and commitments to the health sciences. For appointment they must first be well grounded in their own disciplines and acceptable to those disciplines for appointment and participation in graduate programs.

This group consists of sociologists, social psychologists, social and cultural anthropologists, political scientists, and social historians; theologians are to be added. They participate in planning the medical curriculum and also develop courses and seminars designed to introduce all students in the health sciences to the principles of social science. A unique opportunity is thus provided to influence the development of the philosophy of patient care and clinical teaching in our emergent institution.

This group has a close identification with all programs in the Health Sciences Center but not with any particular college. Its members use the patient care facilities of the center laboratories for their own studies and encourage interrelationships between medicine and the university social science departments. Graduate training programs for physicians and social scientists should provide a cadre of skilled professionals for the future who can work cooperatively on some of society's most urgent problems.

The interfaces of medicine with the *humanities* must be as well developed as those with the physical and biological sciences and the social sciences. This interfacing might well be the most important of all for the future of medicine and the health professions. Future medicine will certainly be practiced within the framework of a highly organized, highly institutionalized, complex system of institutions and persons. Such an organization is essential if the maximum benefits of scientific medicine are to be available to the largest number of people. It will of necessity emphasize specialization, the fragmentation and analysis of the patient's problem, and the application of highly specific diagnostic and therapeutic techniques.

To balance these trends there must be a concomitant development of a high regard for personal and human values on the part of all future health professions and institutions. Simple exposure to courses in the humanities is not in itself a sufficient condition for producing "compassionate" or socially responsive physicians or students. Nonetheless the possibilities of achieving these ends through inculcation of the attitudes of mind fostered by certain of the humanities is much in need of exploration. Such attitudes are most effective if interwoven with clinical education at the bedside and in the clinic—those points at which the student sees the concrete problem and is himself involved in its resolution.

The members of the humanities group, like those in the social sciences, should carry appointments in their own university disciplines. They would, however, be paid from the Health Sciences Center budget and constitute a division within the health sciences, working with all of its component colleges and faculties. This group includes philosophers, theologians, ethicians, historians of medicine and science, and lawyers.

The social sciences and humanities groups have several clear responsibilities arising out of their commitment to students and to problems in the health sciences. They use the specific clinical experiences of students in the health sciences and professions as a basis for consideration of larger questions of ethics, philosophy, and history. In this way health science students can be exposed to a liberal attitude of mind toward their own work and enlarge their appreciation of the wider implication of their own work and enlarge their appreciation of the wider implication of their professional acts. They participate with the faculty of the health sciences in developing policies on such broad issues as human experimentation, the social responsibilities of the health professions, the moral problems of medical practice, definition of value systems, and the relations of cultural and medical history. They serve as a point of contact with the social sciences and humanities faculties in the university to allow a freer interchange of students and faculty than is ordinarily encouraged in a health sciences center. They stimulate graduate studies and programs in which philosophical, ethical, theological, social, and other questions can be investigated in the context of the existential laboratory of a Health Sciences Center.

Experiences in attempting to draw upon the presumed liberal education of medical students indicate that a premedical liberal education has too few lasting effects. It must be reinforced in the context of the specific problems of daily life in hospital and clinic. When this is done, a liberal education can be more securely founded, will prove more "relevant," and will more surely affect the physician's behavior and style of life. We look to our social sciences and humanities groups, as well as to the main university departments, to assist in this liberal education, which can in part be given concurrently with professional education.

FACILITIES

Permanent Facilities

Some comments on architectural planning were included in the early sections of this report. Only the barest outline of the scope of the project is presented here.

A preliminary planning analysis was prepared in 1967 by the consulting firm of Lester Gorsline Associates in collaboration with the director of the center and his associate. This was followed by the appointment of Bertrand Goldberg Associates, Incorporated, as architects of the master plan and the design of the entire project. A site of some 250 acres was available on sloping terrain.

The academic plan had been elaborated before building design was initiated. As a consequence the buildings were designed as a three-dimensional expression of some of the major functional requirements of the academic plan. Some of the factors that influenced the building configuration were:

1. It was important to develop an integrated set of programs involving six schools. This required the sharing of all services such as classrooms, computer center, library, animal facilities, student-faculty center, and teaching laboratories.

2. The building should encourage fortuitous as well as planned contacts between faculties and students of the six schools. Dining areas and other facilities were designed with this end in view.
3. Maximal flexibility of spaces was needed so that additions or alterations could be easily achieved as the needs of the health professions changed in response to the needs of society.
4. Physical connections and easy accessibility of clinical sciences to the hospital and to the basic sciences, with floor-to-floor connections, were desired.
5. The identity of each school must be preserved, while making each school part of a larger entity—the Health Sciences Center.
6. Accommodation of the building to the sloping terrain and preservation of trees, green areas, and recreation areas out-of-doors was stipulated.

The design finally decided upon was a single massive building following the megastructure principle. A network building built into the hillside contains all the common, shared supporting services and administrative and ambulant facilities. Three towers—clinical sciences, basic sciences, and the hospital—rise from this network. A carefully distributed vertical and horizontal transport system facilitates communication between all parts of the megastructure.

Construction of permanent structures for the Health Sciences Center began in April 1970 and will proceed in three stages. When the building program is completed in 1977 it will comprise a single multistoried complex building occupying approximately 1.3 million net square feet of space. Listed in Table 3 are the functional areas of the center that will be erected in each stage of construction.

The scheme for construction of the center in stages was devised in keeping with several important factors. No spaces completed in one stage will require alteration in a later stage. Functional entities will either be constructed entirely in a single stage, or arranged so that upon the completion of several stages no inconvenience to the users will result. While observing these requirements it has been possible to organize the staging in a way that will not require a change in the anticipated timetable of student enrollment.

Temporary Facilities

While awaiting completion of permanent construction, all programs have been accommodated in temporary space. Some 12,000 net square feet are rented in a former supermarket for the Health Sciences library, already holding some 60,000 volumes and receiving some 2,500 serials. A laboratory-office building containing some 62,500 net square feet is being used for basic science instruction and research. An additional 90,000 net square feet, in semipermanent steel prefabricated buildings, house administration, animals, communications center, classrooms, and research laboratories. The acquisition of an additional 100,000 net square feet is contemplated to house expansion of all programs, including the School of Dental Medicine, until permanent facilities are completed.

TABLE 3. CONSTRUCTION DESIGN OF THE HEALTH SCIENCES CENTER

	Function		Area (Net Sq. Ft.)	
Stage I				
	Administration		15,470	
	Basic science instruction		60,900	
	Faculty offices and laboratories		198,930	
	School of Allied Health Professions		22,320	
	School of Nursing		24,370	
	School of Social Welfare		16,510	
	Library		49,720	
	Lecture Halls		19,380	
	Health sciences communications and computer services		30,450	
	Student faculty center		20,600	
	Animal facilities		36,035	
	Research support shops		11,720	
	Physical plant services		43,340	
		Total	549,745	
Stage II				
	Administration		10,000	
	Physical plant services		20,600	
	University hospital		456,322	
		Total	486,922	
Stage III				
	Faculty offices and laboratories		123,230	
	Auditorium		11,140	
	Student-faculty center		19,200	
	Community medicine		4,320	
	Continuing Education Center		7,000	
	Administration		12,320	
	School of Dental Medicine		123,710	
		Total	300,920	
		Total, All Stages		1,337,587

SOME ISSUES IN MEDICAL EDUCATION: THE BASIS FOR CURRICULAR DESIGN

Although physicians will become increasingly dependent upon the cooperation and assistance of members of the other health professions, medicine for the next decade will remain the central discipline in the delivery of health care to the American public. Indeed many of the problems it now faces prefigure those soon to be encountered by the other professions.

Medicine and medical education are at the most critical point in their long histories. In 1910 the Flexner Report pointed up the great problems we faced in our country in achieving quality in medical education commensurate with the improved state of scientific knowledge. The last fifty years have been devoted to making medicine a university discipline, ridding it of proprietary and inadequate schools, and firmly basing it in the physical and biological sciences. As a consequence we are today enjoying the most fruitful period ever in medical care. Medicine now has the capability to alter man's life and environment in unprecedented ways.

The present crisis is of a very different sort than that of fifty years ago. In the midst of a wealth of new discoveries we face what are essentially problems of human organization. How can we most efficiently deliver scientific medicine to the entire population in each community? Can we devise a system of medical care that will reach every citizen and at the same time be humane and as considerate of the individual as it is scientific? How do we meet the challenge of primary medical care?

The task of medical educators is admittedly complex. We must continue to secure and advance the scientific bases of medicine and educate physicians to function as technicians and scientists. Simultaneously we must anticipate future patterns of medical care that will be vastly different from our own. We need urgently to discern the changes in the physician's role that will occur in the net quarter-century and the numbers and kinds of physicians needed. Based on our answers to these questions we must prepare students to fill new, changing, and still undefined roles. Their intellectual equipment must help them adapt to a world transformed by computers, increasing technology, and an ever more complex social organization.

To approach even workable approximation on how best to satisfy future needs, the medical school at Stony Brook must epitomize the commitments already outlined for the center as a whole and take forceful leadership in their attainment.

The instrument that both the faculty and students will use to prepare themselves to meet the urgent problems of today and tomorrow is the curriculum. Certain general and specific remarks should therefore be made about the contemplated curricular configuration we can expect at Stony Brook.

The medical curriculum is an instrument for ordering the intellectual attitudes and the behavior of students in such a way as to make them serviceable to society as physicians. So considered it is in large measure defined by its "*terminus ad quem*": the conception we entertain of what the physician is, will be, or should be. As a consequence, the curriculum is really an epitomization of a faculty's conception of the social uses of medicine, a veritable physiognomy of their collective beliefs, prejudices, hopes, and fears.

Today's revolution in the medical curriculum has been incubating since the close of World War II. It is now far more than a recurrent exercise in academic prestidigitation or a saving diversion from the exacting labors of laboratory and bedside. The conviction is well-nigh universal among medical faculties that, present success notwithstanding, a linear extrapolation of current methods cannot be anything but inadequate in a world governed by exponential charges. A fundamental reworking of all our educational instruments is the only way to meet the changing character and motivations of today's student, the processes by which he learns, and the altered roles he will play in the twenty-first century.

A striking feature of the current curricular inquiry is the emergence of a common lattice of ideas about which future curricula will inevitably crystallize. Definition of the objectives of a medical curriculum is dependent upon what we think the physician's role will be, the types of students who will seek to prepare for those roles, and the learning processes they will follow. We shall look briefly at each of the factors that are responsible for stimulating much of the present unrest with existing curricula.

Future Medicine—The Matrix and the Physician

The end to which a medical education is directed is the severest constraint and the final test of any curriculum. It is just at this vital point that our hopes for a rational attack on curricular design falter badly. We simply do not know precisely what society's needs will be or what will be expected of the physician; there is no alternative to a series of semi-intuitive estimates; this is the serious business of medical educators who in years hence will be distinguished by the accuracy of their estimates.

The medicine of the future seems certain to be a highly systematized operation extending over the entire nation in such a way that the civic rights of each individual to optimal medical care be actualized. This means regionalization of facilities, techniques, and personnel, and a further extension of specialization to encompass and organize the vast mass of information the laboratories will continue to bring forth. The system of medical care will resemble a vast and complex organism integrated by a nervous system of computerized communication and information processing. In such a system many of the physician's manipulative functions will be assumed by others to protect his time for the more demanding judgmental tasks. The physician will have to keep the system effective, handle the unexpected events outside the preset program, and coordinate the entire process. He will function increasingly as a member and coordinator of a group of experts and almost never as an isolated individual.

Such a system requires more, not fewer, specialists of all kinds and also the conscious development of a generalist who is essentially a specialist in social engineering—capable of assessing a patient's needs, designing a plan for meeting them, with a host of people and facilities available, and coordinating all in a sensible and understandable way. The physician as a helper of humans may well find that this is his most important contribution in the years ahead. A system so far-reaching and so complexly organized will by its nature be dehumanizing, and every attention must be given to minimizing this effect while retaining the utility of a systematized approach.

The demands of such a system of care will call for an ever wider spectrum of specialists as medicine extends its concerns from the molecular to the social, the international, and the ecological levels. The decision for specialization will have to be made sooner if the physician is not to be obsolescent by the time he graduates. Every ten years at least half of what a physician learns will become outdated, so that any attempt to turn out a finished product is scarcely imaginable.

The emphasis of present curricula on a rigidified program for all students, and insistence on exposure to all specialties in the vain hope of providing a liberal education in medicine, can hardly cope with such transformations as have already occurred in medical practice patterns, to say nothing of unforeseen changes certain to occur.

To meet the demands of the system we describe, a curriculum must allow for the development of a wide variety of socially relevant roles as soon as possible. Emphasis is best placed on the use of knowledge and its sources rather than on its mere acquisition. Continuing education becomes a mandatory requirement. Sufficient educational flexibility must be allowed to permit later entry into specialties as they are born in increasing numbers and unforeseen variety.

The Student Profile

Certainly, much of the stimulus for curricular changes derives from the metamorphosis in the ways a medical education will be useful to society. Equally profound stimuli arise from changes in the preparation, interest, and motivation of the student seeking entry into medical college, even in the years immediately before us. Today's medical students are intellectually better prepared than their predecessors and are more likely to have already taken advanced courses in the physical and biological sciences. More of them are coming from advanced placement, honors, or innovative programs, and they are still too homogeneous in their socioeconomic profiles and in their bias toward the practical and scientific. However, greater dishomogeneity is certain to result as soon as financial aid for medical students becomes a reality, as it must. Also, the wider scope of medicine as an applied social and behavioral science, as well as its community and institutional functions, will demand a larger intake of students with interests in the social sciences and the humanities. Indeed we shall have a plan deliberately to admit such students if the broader responsibilities of medicine to society are to be adequately fulfilled.

Perhaps more significant than the changing intellectual qualities and interests of medical students is the discontinuity between their goals and those of medical faculties. This discontinuity is already an established fact in other branches of the university. Today's student is interested in the relevance of his educational experiences and its immediacy for the life of mankind. He looks upon education, even professional education, as a means of knowing and finding himself—as the more extreme put it, finding their "thing." Students with these goals regard as irrelevant the postponement of acceptance and involvement characteristic of medical curricula. The abstract notion is simply not acceptable to them.

To make effective contact with today's and tomorrow's students any new curriculum must be broad enough to meet their varied interests. It must emphasize practical experiences early and must permit more flexible arrangements of time, fewer formal courses, and more chances for self-exploration and development. Rather than being deleterious these tendencies open up medicine to a whole group of young people who might ordinarily not consider it; these are the students most likely to develop interests and later careers in the socially relevant areas of better delivery of health care, new patterns of usage of health personnel, and better community medicine. If medicine is to respond to public pressures for active involvement in the real problems of health care in the community, medical schools will need more students interested in relevance. From this group will come the future practitioners and teachers so badly needed in social and community medicine.

The Learning Process

The third great stimulus to curricular revision insistently demanding our attention is the parallel revolution in the process of learning. There is no doubt that audiovisual, television, and other types of nonlinear learning will become familiar to coming generations of students. Nor can we deny the potential utility of computer-assisted methods for teaching at least the core of a subject that formerly was taught by drill methods. The use of mechanized methods of instruction must increase in medical education—basic as well as clinical. A curriculum that does not deal with these modalities is unrealistic and missing a major point of engagement with today's students.

Some Features and Objectives of the Medical Curriculum

This brief delineation of the major stimuli to revolution in the medical curriculum provides a base for a more specific consideration of the objectives of the Stony Brook curriculum in medicine.

It might be well to point out what a curriculum *cannot* be. An adequate curriculum today cannot hope to transform a student into a totally competent physician ready to practice all branches of medicine; it cannot hope to inculcate all the knowledge of the basic sciences or the clinical fields; it cannot even pretend adequately to introduce the students to all the branches of medicine; it cannot provide for the same student an education that has meaning simultaneously in medical sciences, clinical medicine, social and preventive medicine, medical history, and behavioral science. Nor is it possible to achieve that much talked of objective of the postwar years—the undifferentiated physician. The serious decision to choose a more limited and more socially useful role should be made as expeditiously as possible. To delay is hardly justifiable in the face of the obvious need for more and more varied types of physicians.

What are some of the definable features of a medical curriculum that tried to adapt itself to the stimuli for change outlined above? Patently, a medical education must provide the intellectual tools and attitudes essential to the later pursuit in depth of a large number of specialties that will be entered upon much sooner than is now the case. We must realize that each of the basic sciences and the clinical specialties has a varying utility for any student, dependent upon his later role in medicine.

Manifestly, two essential tools are fundamental for any field of medical specialization: the "language" of the basic sciences and the "language" of the clinical sciences. But they must be taught as just that—languages to comprehend a given field in medicine. The sciences basic to medicine are now taught too globally. What seems indicated instead is emphasis on understanding in depth a few widely applicable concepts rather than a total coverage of each of them as is now the case. These concepts are best taught in an integrated, interdisciplinary fashion. Full use of programmed and computer-assisted methods to permit self-testing will enable the student to assess his comprehension as often as necessary whenever a major concept reappears.

Such a framework of ideas in molecular biology, structure, and function at the cellular and systems levels becomes the framework for later specific application at the bedside. It can be modified when some essential advance is made. Laboratory exercises can be reduced in number and designed to explicate these common concepts.

The objectives should be to teach ways of knowing, the rules of evidence, and the critical assessment of data.

The first two years in such a system can be considered as a unit extending from cellular concepts to tissue and system levels or organization, proceeding from normal to abnormal, and thence to clinical manifestations. They would merge into the introduction to the *clinical language*—how to collect data from the patient by interview, physical examination, and laboratory, and how to analyze such data, order it into probabilities by diagnostic process, and arrive by value judgments at prudent decisions as to action. These latter skills and attitudes could also be learned in a single general clerkship rather than in the usual round-robin of the clinical specialties, each competing for a clerkship, some as short as ten days.

This introduction to the two essential languages need not consume more than two years on the average. The student should then be ready to make a selection of one of a number of alternate pathways to the M.D. degree. With the help of a Faculty Advisory Committee he can select a "major" field adapted to his interests, abilities, and personality. The design of the remaining years would then be highly individualized. Few students would have the same curricular program. Some definable pathways could be those of the clinical specialties, the medical scientist, generalist and family medicine, community medicine, a university discipline such as sociology, anthropology, or any other field related to human health and disease. An "undifferentiated pathway" or track would be reserved for those who wished to postpone choice of a field for a time. Or, after the introductory language, the student might decide that he preferred to pursue a Ph.D. in a basic science and not take further clinical education.

After the two-language introduction the student going on to a clinical specialty could, under university aegis, devote the next four years to becoming a specialist, taking six years to accomplish what now takes an average of eight years. If this could be preceded by two instead of four years of premedical work, as I think it could, the total span of education could be nine instead of twelve years.

After a student chose one of these specific pathways he would return to a fuller and more detailed contact with the basic sciences, but only those relevant to his clinical concerns. In the case of the surgeon, for example, his initial introduction to anatomy would take place with the other students as a general introduction to the structure and language of anatomy with little dissection and much use of prosected material. If he majored in surgery, however, he would undertake a much more detailed dissection. Likewise the other clinical specialties can reintroduce the basic sciences most pertinent to their disciplines. For a clinician the most effective stimulus to learning the basic sciences is the usually belated realization of their significance for his functioning as a specialist.

Certainly one of the constant features of new curricula is the need for earlier introduction to the patient, not only in the first year but perhaps even in the later premedical years. Students have for years sampled some of the dimensions of clinical medicine, by taking summer jobs, for example, and today many students want to see the "relevance" of the field they choose. Opportunities must be allowed for medical students to drop out and to engage in community, hospital, or welfare work during the medical course.

Last, an experience in the social, ecological, and epidemiological dimensions of health and illness has become essential for anyone in medical school who thinks seriously about the social responsibilities of the physician.

Another necessary feature of a new curriculum is to allow for the entry of students with more varied backgrounds than is now the case. This can be accomplished by a system that permits entry at several points in the curriculum, admits to advanced standing, and allows for make-up of science background for those who wish to enter with majors in the social sciences or humanities. I envision, for example, a make-up year in which those with nonscience backgrounds might acquire the necessary chemistry, physics, and mathematics. Students would therefore proceed at differing rates and take differing times to finish the medical curriculum. If we abandon the notion of a "class" going through each of its courses all at the same time, the mechanical problem of a free entry system should not be unmanageable.

There are some clear implications for premedical education in these curricular trends. First, there is a tendency to shorten the premedical portion to three or even two years. Second, the curricula we expect in medical school would allow of advanced placement; such courses as biochemistry, molecular biology, biophysics, and genetics would be useful for those students who are willing to spend longer periods in college. Third, there will be more opportunities for nonscience majors to enter medical medicine and they should receive help and encouragement. Such students are often dissuaded from a career in medicine by premedical advisors who are being "realistic" in terms of today's medical curricula but not tomorrow's. Fourth, shorter periods of premedical education will probably be far more acceptable than they are today, while entry to advanced standing will be possible for those who have delayed their decision to enter medicine. Finally, if such features as flexibility and advanced standing are to become realities, it is very clear that a much closer integration of undergraduate and graduate curricula with medical school curricula is mandatory.

The School of Medicine at Stony Brook has an unusual opportunity to develop a true continuum extending from high school through premedical, medical, and postgraduate education. Discussions have already begun with the Department of Biology and will later include chemistry and physics. New courses are needed that will recognize the new trends in medical education and that will prepare students to enter professional education earlier and at different points. For example, those with science majors could be admitted to advanced standing in the medical school; those with nonscience majors could enter after a specially designed make-up year to familiarize them with the language of the sciences; transfers from other medical school could enter at the beginning of the clinical years and go directly into a specially selected pathway.

The clinical block of four years will carry the student through his clinical education to the point at which he will be able to function as a specialist in a selected field. This innovation enables the university to retain supervision over postgraduate as well as undergraduate education, a trend not yet fully developed in this country.

PATHWAYS OF ENTRY AND PROGRESS

The School of Medicine is responsible for the organization and teaching of the clinical sciences in the undergraduate, postgraduate, and continuing education setting.

Traditionally a school of medicine includes a basic science faculty but, as discussed earlier, in the Stony Brook Health Sciences Center for cogent reasons this custom has been altered. The dichotomous arrangement allows the clinically oriented school more latitude in curricular development and educational goals, while still retaining strong ties to the basic sciences necessary for support.

Although clinical arts and skills are taught immediately after entry into the medical school the early focus must be on teaching the student the language of the basic sciences. Subsequent to this core of information, pathological physiology, the matrix of clinical science, is taught within the framework of coordinated teaching arranged within organ systems. Clinical encounters are designed for this system to give special relevance to each system. After demonstrating competence in the clinical language the student will move to a general clerkship in medicine or pediatrics where opportunities are presented. This continuum from entry through clerkship will take two years and will be followed by a multitrack elective clinical experience.

The core curriculum was primarily developed to provide earlier career decision-making for an ultimate professional lifestyle and to shorten the period of time necessary for the student to establish competence in a chosen track. Clinical specialty, community medicine, family medicine, biomedical engineering, and academic medicine are among the present well-defined tracks. Obviously many more will develop with time, and even today within the clinical specialties there are innumerable options.

The two-year core curriculum is primarily given at the Health Sciences Center although many of the clinical encounters are given at various community clinical facilities integrated into the Health Sciences Center under a variety of arrangements. In each clinical facility the instructional goals will be supervised by a full-time faculty presided over by a dean appointed by the Health Sciences Center. Additional instructional support will be provided by the clinical faculty of the School of Medicine.

A student may deviate from the standard curriculum by demonstrating proficiency in any course of study to the satisfaction of the department concerned. The use of this released time will be determined by appropriate discussion with the student's faculty adviser. Each student will be initially assigned a faculty adviser who will be responsible for assisting him or her through the years of the curriculum. This arrangement should be mutually beneficial; if not, it may be altered by either partner and restructured with different partners.

Following the two-year core curriculum the student will be assigned to a *clinical campus* for the implementation of his chosen track. (See section on consortium, p. 259.) The Long Island Jewish-Queens Hospital Center has qualified for this designation as have the Veterans Administration Hospital at Northport, the Brookhaven National Laboratory, and the Nassau County Medical Center.

Another feature of the curriculum is the establishment of field experiences in the health delivery system; these are planned at several points depending upon the year of instruction. The exercises afford an opportunity to introduce the medical student to the health delivery system while he is playing a variety of roles in mental health clinics, migrant camps, visiting nurse associations, doctors' offices, emergency rooms, welfare departments, etc. These exercises, as well as the environment created by the concept of the Health

Sciences Center, should allow for the interaction of the neophyte physician with other students within the health delivery system, such as nurses, allied health professionals, and social welfare workers. It is through such interaction that the physician will develop an understanding of and respect for his colleagues in the other health professions.

At the end of the first year a student-directed field study, using student teams from the center, will identify, research, and address problems that exist within the health delivery system. Support from the faculty of the center will be available as needed.

Toward the end of the second year of the core curriculum there are two mandatory clerkships: the general clerkship described previously and one in community medicine. Because the clinical encounters encompass a wide variety of experiences—coronary care units, dialysis units, chest services, emergency rooms, etc.—none of which last for less than a week, the student can be prepared for an informed decision in choosing the track for the rest of his clinical experience.

The third year may be the first year of this track or the student may choose a rotating clerkship. Whatever the choice, it is freely elected and on its completion he will be awarded the degree of doctor of medicine. The opportunity to obtain the degree in three years does not preclude other students from opting for a four-year sequence if there are substantial reasons for not completing the three-year curriculum.

THE MULTITRACK CLINICAL CURRICULUM

The multiple track curriculum has the following objectives:

1. To take the student from his basic science and clinical introduction through a graded series of responsibilities to the point at which he can function as a specialist in the track or field he has chosen.
2. To provide clinical skills in depth in a limited and specified field of medicine.
3. To enable the student to pursue clinical education in a highly integrated manner providing the basic sciences relevant to each field simultaneously with clinical experiences.
4. To provide university and medical school supervision of post-graduate as well as undergraduate clinical education, emphasizing the continuum and making the residency years a formal educational experience.
5. To provide flexibility and mission orientation in clinical education while reducing the amount of time required to educate physicians for socially important roles in the health care system.
6. To provide university certification of specialty training much in the same fashion as it does in graduate education in the university disciplines.

The multitrack curriculum comprises an educational module, beginning with what is now the third year and terminating at the point when the student is ready to function within his chosen field. What is ordinarily a period of six years (junior and senior years of medicine plus four years of internship-residency) can be reduced to four years by earlier concentration and telescoping of undergraduate and graduate medical education into one "package." The number of years for each module will vary somewhat depending on the requirements of each specific field.

Selection of a track is a difficult and delicate matter. However, more students in college and medical school are seeking to begin work on a specific field as soon as possible. They can be more highly motivated to learn both clinical and basic sciences if these are related closely to what they wish ultimately to do in medicine and life. We wish to capture that motivation and also to prepare the student for a useful role in the health care system as soon as possible. The multitrack system can and should be exploited for these ends.

Several general principles will apply in each track:

1. Choice of a track will be made with advice; a track can also be changed with advice. The student need not be "locked into" any field.
2. The track is a major field of study, the details of which will be designed in advance by each department and section. The curricular details for each track must be approved by the clinical curriculum committee. Flexibility will be encouraged, but vagueness disallowed.
3. Tracks will be of variable length, depending upon the requirements for competence in a given field. They will all provide:
    a) Graded increasing clinical, investigative, or administrative responsibility under supervision.
    b) A basic science component will be included in a variety of ways, such as courses in the basic science departments, correlation seminars, or independent research. It is by this route that the student will achieve depth in the relevant basic science and supplement the introductory and general basic sciences of the first two years.
    c) Experiences in related clinical sciences will be arranged as "minors" relevant to the major field.
    d) A thesis in investigative tracks or equivalent demonstration of clinical competence in the chosen field will be required to obtain university certification in a field.

Some tentative details of preparation in sample tracks include:

1. *Investigative Medicine:* This track is designed for those who wish to pursue careers in medical investigation. Students can select either a problem or a discipline of interest to them. Essentially the graduate school approach will be followed. The first year or two will be devoted to basic science course work and seminars with simultaneous work in the laboratory with a senior investigator. The last two years will be devoted to intensive research on a specific problem and preparation of a thesis. Where the problem involves clinical disorders the student will be provided with clinical experiences of an appropriate nature.

This pathway will be pursued either at the university campus at Stony Brook or at the Brookhaven National Laboratory. The latter is uniquely equipped for such training, having a forty-eight-bed clinical research center available for this purpose. Students may also work with investigators in the university Department of Biology or in the interdisciplinary graduate programs in molecular biology or development biology. The award of a Ph.D. degree at the conclusion of this curriculum is under consideration.

2. *Clinical Specialty:* This pathway would be divided into a series of subpathways: medicine, cardiology, nephrology, general surgery, otolaryngology, ophthalmology, psychiatry, etc. The number of years required would vary depending upon the field chosen. The student would start as a clinical clerk and proceed to responsibilities of an inter-resident and resident or fellow. The aim of this path is to prepare the student for clinical specialty practice. The major portion of his time would be spent at either the university hospital or one of the designated clinical campuses (Nassau County Medical Center, Long Island Jewish-Queens Hospital Center, Northport Veterans Administration Hospital, Brookhaven National Laboratory).

Each specialty will arrange for the basic science correlations necessary to that field, for example, anatomy of musculoskeletal system for orthopedics; physiology and biochemistry for endocrinology; or psychology and psychopharmacology for psychiatry.

A student may, on mutual agreement of both departments, change his major from one clinical department to another.

At the termination of the prescribed work in any of the clinical specialty tracks the student is expected to demonstrate competence sufficient to enable him to function as a practitioner in that field. The university will certify to this fact in addition to conferring the M.D. degree.

3. *Family and General Medicine:* This track will take a total of four years: two of undergraduate and two of graduate education. The family medicine major will be under the aegis of the Department of Family Medicine, which will establish the requirements for competency and examine for them.

The experiences in the first year will be similar to those described above for the junior year of interim clerkship. The fourth year will have a more prolonged experience in community medicine, ambulatory medicine, and psychiatry. The last two years will be divided among a variety of experiences. One year will be spent in several models of practice under the supervision of faculty members who are general practitioners. The last year will be devoted to elective experiences related to family medical problems, behavioral sciences, additional clinical specialty experiences, and research in environmental, community, or family medicine, medical sociology, medical economics, industrial and occupational medicine, school health, and health education. These are some examples of the experiences that can be provided.

At the termination of the prescribed period of study the student will be examined for competence in his ability to manage family and general medical problems in a variety of community settings. We regard the family medicine track as one of the most important and one in which much experimentation can be conducted. The plan may change considerably when the Department of Family Medicine is formed.

4. *Social and Community Medicine:* This track will prepare students for a variety of socially important functions as future health officers, health planners, workers in international medicine, health care administrators, etc. The emphasis will be on general familiarity with clinical problems, but major emphasis will be placed on subjects such as sociology, economics, anthropology, ecology, epidemiology, systems and operations, and industrial engineering. The first year could be like that described above for the interim clinical curriculum and the last three years divided between field experiences,

course work in the relevant basic sciences, and research project in some aspect of community medicine.

5. *Biomedical Engineering:* This track is under joint development with the College of Engineering and a precise set of requirements is being defined. It is planned that students may enter this pathway either from the medical or the engineering curricula. Those from engineering would receive clinical and medical orientation; those from medicine would be provided with the requisite engineering "language." Both groups would work on basic and applied research in biomedical engineering problems, for example, instrumentation, materials, computer technology, and industrial and systems engineering. The schools of medicine and engineering would jointly certify to competence according to predetermined standards.

6. *University-Medical Pathway:* This pathway is designed for those who wish to occupy a middle position between medicine and the university disciplines, particularly in the social sciences and humanities. Students would be prepared specifically for such roles as medical sociologists, anthropologists, economists, philosophers, and law-medicine and law-religion experts.

A major portion of the time would be spent in a research project involving some aspect of health sciences and relevant university discipline. Part of the time would be devoted to course work and seminars in the university disciplines. The last year might be devoted to research, field work, and thesis preparation. Graduates of this program would probably become teachers and consultants in either the health sciences or university departments.

These pathways or tracks are examples of some of the major options open to students who have completed the common core portion of the curriculum. Other tracks will undoubtedly develop as the needs of our health care system expand and new disciplines appear. The precise delineation of the content and requirement of each track will be continually refurbished in the light of advances in medicine and related disciplines.

FACULTY

Faculty Projections, Size, and Composition

Instruction in the clinical and basic sciences will be carried out predominantly by full-time faculty supported by "hard money" from state funds. The number of basic and clinical science faculty projected is based on the needs for teaching 150 medical students per class. With the multitrack curriculum we have proposed, and the use of clinical campuses, it is very likely that larger numbers of students could be handled without increasing the faculty size. In addition 200 Ph.D. candidates, 200 postdoctoral fellows, and some 300 fellows and house staff are to be served by the same faculty.

One hundred and fifty full-time basic scientists are being recruited and their distribution has already been outlined. In addition, 100 biological scientists in the Department of Biology will be available for medical school teaching in such fields as genetics, molecular and cellular biology, developmental biology, ecology, and marine sciences.

The distribution of full-time clinical faculty is given by department in Table 4. In addition, part-time and voluntary faculty members drawn from the practicing community will participate in the teaching program. To date more than 1,000 practicing physicians have indicated an interest in clinical teaching. To this must be added the participation of the full-time staffs at the Nassau County Medical Center, the Long Island Jewish-Queens Hospital Center, the Northport Veterans Administration Hospital, and the hospital of the Brookhaven National Laboratory. The combined total of these full-time clinicians will be in excess of 200.

TABLE 4. SCHOOL OF MEDICINE FULL-TIME CLINICAL FACULTY—FULL ACTIVATIONS, 1977

Department	No. of Faculty
Medicine	48
Psychiatry	24
Surgery	24
Pediatrics	21
Radiology	16
Community medicine	12
Obstetrics and gynecology	12
Neurology	10
Anesthesiology	8
Dermatology	5
Orthopedics	5
Ophthalmology	5
Otolaryngology	5
Physical Medicine	5
Total	200

Departments or Not?

Every new school goes through the difficult process of deciding whether or not to perpetuate the departmental system, the many disadvantages and advantages of which are well known to medical educators. At Stony Brook we have attempted to optimize the advantages and minimize the disadvantages in the following way:

We will preserve the departmental organization to provide a homebase and identification for the major disciplines. The department is thus responsible for assessing faculty standards in appointment and research and providing space and facilities.

The department *does not*, however, control curriculum time, either in the basic or clinical sciences. Teaching in the basic sciences is coordinated by the dean for the basic sciences; teaching in the clinical departments becomes departmental only after a student has chosen a path he wishes to follow. Each department must therefore provide a worthwhile experience or it will not attract students either to its electives or to its major program.

Moreover, greater flexibility is provided by the interdisciplinary nature of the systems teaching in the core curriculum. Graduate programs are also interdisciplinary in nature, for example, molecular biology. Hence departmental members may participate fully in graduate and research programs that interest them and that cross departmental boundaries.

Each faculty member can thus be considered to belong to a "department" on one coordinate and to a "program" of teaching or research on another. His place on the grid will depend on his discipline, his interests, and his abilities.

UNIVERSITY HOSPITAL AND OTHER CLINICAL FACILITIES

A 600-bed university hospital is planned as the central teaching facility for all of the educational programs of the Health Sciences Center. In addition a variety of affiliations is planned with hospitals throughout the area, not only to provide additional educational facilities of the Health Sciences Center but to fulfill the social purposes of the university hospital as a major health resource for Long Island.

Purposes of the University Hospital

The prime function of the university hospital is educational; it will serve as the major teaching facility for students in medicine, dentistry, nursing, social work, and the various allied health professions. It will also serve as a teaching facility for interns, residents, postdoctoral fellows, and postgraduate students in all of the health professions. In addition, the hospital will be a major resource for the continuing education programs of the Health Sciences Center.

Although the prime mission of the university hospital is an educational one, it is our deeply rooted conviction that such a facility cannot educate members of the health professions unless it provides services of the highest quality. This does not mean provision of patient care more or less as "a necessary evil" in order to provide a pool of "teaching material." It means the creation of an institution that recognizes its role as a primary health care resource for its entire region and accepts the challenge to function as a social instrument serving the needs of a "community" that embraces the entire Long Island region.

Patient Care

The hospital of the Health Sciences Center will be the only university-based hospital in the entire Nassau-Suffolk region, which comprises almost all of Long Island. The nearest medical school is the SUNY Downstate Medical Center in Brooklyn, which is concerned primarily with the Borough of Brooklyn and with some parts of the adjacent Borough of Queens. The university hospital will therefore be a key resource for referral of patients by physicians, hospitals, and other health facilities from all parts of the Nassau-Suffolk region.

The hospital will have a major ambulatory facility capable of handling well over 100,000 patient visits annually. Outpatient services will be organized along group practice lines, with family medicine as a major component.

A special objective of the Health Sciences Center will be to develop new patterns in the delivery of patient care and to provide a variety of models of patient care within which students may learn by direct experience and develop the concept of the health care team. Both the inpatient and outpatient programs of the university hospital will be designed so as to further these objectives. Patients from all socioeconomic levels will be accepted for both outpatient and inpatient care. All patients will be involved in the teaching program and every aspect of the quality and quantity of services provided to every patient will be the responsibility of the faculty and administration of the center.

Professional Staff Organization

The administration organization of the Health Sciences Center has been structured so that the university hospital will be responsible directly to the vice president for the health sciences. The underlying philosophy is that the hospital should serve the educational needs of *all* of the schools and that it can accomplish this objective most effectively if it is independent of any individual school and is under leadership committed to the concept of rendering high quality patient care within a broad community-oriented context.

The directors of all divisions of the medical and dental staffs will be the chairmen of the corresponding departments in the schools of medicine and dental medicine. All other members of the medical and dental staffs will hold faculty appointments and will be members of the staff of the university hospital.

A somewhat unusual feature of the professional organization of the hospital is the fusion of education and service responsibilities in all services. The deans of nursing, social welfare, dental medicine, and allied health professions will also be responsible for the clinical services in the hospital, and directors of these services will hold associate deanships in the respective schools. In this way we hope to avoid some of the service/education dichotomies that vex university hospitals and interfere with both education and patient care. The advantages to the student, who can see education and practice so closely integrated, are obvious.

Architectural Design of the Hospital

The university hospital is being planned as an integral part of the Health Sciences Center. In the interest of efficiency and economy of operation, certain facilities that might otherwise have to be duplicated in the hospital and in other components of the center will be combined into integrated support units: functions such as food preparation and distribution; receiving, storage, and distribution of supplies and equipment; plant maintenance; personnel; and various other administrative activities. Most of these services will be contained in the large base or "network" building and will not be readily identifiable as space allocated exclusively to the hospital or to any other component of the center. Allocation of costs will be made to identify and distinguish among expenses attributable to the hospital that will be situated within the network building include laboratories, surgical suites, delivery suites, diagnostic suites, diagnostic radiology, radiotherapy, emergency facilities, and ambulatory outpatient facilities. In particular, the emergency room, diagnostic radiology, and surgical suites will be located in close proximity to each other, with traffic pathways designed to facilitate ready movement of patients from one to another of these areas.

The inpatient services of the hospital will be located within a "bed tower." This tower will rise from the network building and will be adjacent to and connected with the "clinical science tower" housing the offices and laboratories of the clinical faculty.

The distribution of clinical services within the hospital and the location of clinical faculty within the clinical sciences tower will be such that the specialty occupying any given floor in one tower will correspond generally to the specialty located on the same floor of the other. For example, pediatric patients will be housed in the bed tower on the same level as the offices and laboratories of the pediatric faculty in the clinical sciences tower. This of course is intended to facilitate faculty traffic between the patient areas and their laboratory-office areas and thereby assure intimate involvement of the faculty in patient care functions. Ample conference space for teaching purposes will be provided close to the patient area on every floor.

Relationship of the Hospital to the Community

It has been noted above that the university hospital's geographic area of concern will be the two largest Long Island counties-Nassau and Suffolk. It is fortunate that this area coincides exactly with the boundaries of the local Regional Medical Program, the local Comprehensive Health Planning agency, and the local Health and Hospital Planning Council. Efforts are currently underway to assure that these three agencies complement one another and work cooperatively rather than competitively. Senior staff of the Health Sciences Center have been working closely with all three, and it is hoped that a cohesive—indeed a truly "comprehensive"—plan will gradually be evolved for all health services in the region.

The hospital will seek to maintain close relationships with hospitals and other health-related agencies throughout the area. In addition to our sense of responsibility to serve as a central resource for all of these agencies, there are several specific reasons, directly related to the educational objectives of the Health Sciences Center, for our interest in maintaining such relationships:

1. The sheer number of students who will be in the process of education at any one time is such that the center will need additional educational facilities over and above those of the university hospital. This will be particularly true during the first four years of the center's existence, as the hospital will not have yet been completed, but it will continue to be true even after completion of these facilities.
2. It will be important for students to be exposed to the community hospital environment so that they do not complete their education having seen patient care rendered only in the Health Sciences Center and the university hospital.
3. Affiliations with a number of different hospitals will facilitate the development of a variety of different models of patient care that will be of importance both for the educational exposure of students and for research in the field of delivery of health services.

Altogether in Nassau and Suffolk counties there are forty-two hospitals of which eighteen are voluntary nonprofit, eighteen are proprietary, and six are governmental; twenty-eight are general hospitals, most of which have under 200 beds; only one has over 400 beds.

During the initial planning period, the vice president for the health sciences visited most of these hospitals. The visits generally consisted of a review of physical plant and meetings with the professional staffs and boards of trustees of the hospitals to ascertain their attitudes in possible affiliation with the Health Sciences Center. Each hospital was assessed from the point of view of its potential as an auxiliary teaching facility.

THE LONG ISLAND-STONY BROOK HEALTH SCIENCES CONSORTIUM

The community-oriented philosophy of the Health Sciences Center and its university hospital has been interrelated with the need to expand educational opportunities and capacities of the center in a "health sciences consortium" that will be described briefly at this point.

There is universal acceptance of the need for a drastic increase in the number of health professionals in all categories. This need has been amply and repeatedly documented in local, state, and national studies. The crucial issue is how fast can both the numbers and kinds of health professionals be increased at a reasonable cost and without detriment to the development of other socially necessary services. The usual methods are to expand the facilities of existing medical centers or to develop new centers; both methods are being employed and both have serious limitations. New schools are expensive and require a delay period and thus far they have not resulted in the drastic upturn of the production curve so urgently needed. The physical facilities of a new medical school cost about $1 million per entering student and a time delay of almost a decade from the decision to establish a school to the graduation of its first physician. In an existing school some expansion can occur with its present facilities and faculty. Beyond a certain threshold number, however, new facilities and faculty are requisite.

The major deterrents to a drastic expansion in the ranks of health professionals are the limitations imposed by classic curriculum structures and insistence on providing the major experiences for all students within the medical centers themselves. Only in a few instances—Illinois and Indiana in particular—is attention being given to expanding the state capacity to train physicians by more imaginative use of large community hospitals and medical centers. By a judicious combination of curriculum revision and the conversion of a number of community hospitals into major clinical teaching units, it can become realistic to think in terms of significantly larger entering classes in all the health professions. The program proposed here outlines a new and unique consortium of this type.

Clinical Campus

We plan at Stony Brook to establish a new kind of health sciences consortium, one in which the state-supported Health Sciences Center would become the functional center of a network of institutions providing basic science and clinical education under a unified academic plan and equivalent academic standards. All units in the consortium would derive their degree-granting authority and academic supervision from the state university center. Cooperative efforts are being developed with institutions under a variety of auspices—federal, state, county, and private. The ultimate plan envisions a student entering for his basic science training at any one of several clinical campuses for completion of his curriculum and granting of the appropriate degree.

A "clinical campus" is a community hospital of a sufficient size to provide a wide variety of patients, sufficient spectrum of clinical specialties, and a wide range of inpatient, outpatient, and community services. It serves as a major base for the clinical portion of the education of medical students and students in the other health professions. In medicine the clinical campus would carry a student from the end of basic sciences through his residency period. Such a clinical campus is to be academically administered by a clinical dean jointly appointed and working full-time at the clinical campus; all the chiefs and most members of the major clinical departments will be full-time physicians and appointed to the faculty of the medical school.

All patients in these institutions are to be teaching patients in the fullest sense of the word. Close correlation in research and teaching programs between these hospitals and the medical school will be essential. Rotation of staff members between the university and the clinical campus and participation in the teaching at the university by clinical campus faculty would facilitate the integration of teaching and research progress. A cadre of clinical teachers thus would be established at these clinical campuses and their counterparts at the center would constitute a council for each discipline. This council would have the responsibility for determining the M.D. educational requirements in that discipline at the pre-M.D. and post-M.D. levels.

Students may transfer to the clinical campuses after completion of a "core" of basic sciences and an introduction to clinical medicine, a period totaling one-and-one-half to two years. At the clinical campus the student is to be taken to the point at which he can function as a specialist in any one of the major clinical fields as well as in family and community medicine treated as specialized tracks. The period at the clinical campus will vary depending on the area of major study chosen. Under this concept the four years ordinarily devoted to residency and the last two years of medical school are telescoped into each other and accomplished in four years.

In addition exchange of students and rotation between clinical campuses will be encouraged to enrich and broaden a student's clinical education. Each clinical campus is expected to develop a character and a mission of its own, achieving depth and emphasis in certain clinical fields but not others. Duplication of expensive facilities, personnel, and equipment can be minimized if this expectation is fulfilled even partially.

Each clinical campus will be under the academic direction of a clinical dean. This person will be responsible for coordinating the academic programs in all disciplines and for effecting liaison with the state university center. The academic program at each institution will be determined cooperatively under final supervision of the appropriate academic department at the university center. Equivalency of academic programs is a basic objective so that a student will be able to transfer credits from one campus to another without difficulty and in response to changes in his interest and career development.

Besides the full clinical campus arrangements, there are five additional ways in which the smaller community hospitals can be integrated into the educational programs. In essence the plan is to be geared to the needs and capacities of every local hospital which, to the extent its size and facilities permit, will contribute to one or several levels of education in the consortium.

In addition to hospitals, plans can be developed for association with other health agencies, neighborhood clinics, Regional Medical Programs, and Comprehensive Health Planning, that will further solidify the concept of an integrated educational and research approach to the entire community under the academic aegis of the consortium.

Basic Sciences Campuses

A plan similar to that developed for the clinical campuses could be developed for the basic sciences. Selected four-year colleges and universities would be encouraged to expand their biological and physical sciences departments so they could provide the preliminary basic science education for students in all the health professions. This expansion would be carried out under the academic supervision of the appropriate departments in the state university center. As in the clinical campuses the aim would be to achieve unified basic sciences curricula at the several campuses. The chairmen of the departments at the basic sciences campuses would constitute councils for their disciplines in parallel fashion to the councils on the clinical campuses. Deans for basic health sciences programs would be appointed at each associated campus to coordinate programs and effect liaison with the appropriate dean at the state university center. Transfer and rotation of students and credits among the basic sciences campuses would become the common practice. After completion of the common core basic sciences curriculum the student would transfer to the university center for upper division studies in the schools of medicine, nursing, allied health, or dentistry, or to one of the clinical campuses for completion of his clinical education.

This combination of clinical and basic science campus offers the student multiple entry points to an education in the health sciences, multiple opportunities for pursuit of areas of special interest, and a completely flexible curriculum that could be pursued over a period of years and not locked into the usual four-year sequence.

Community and Private Colleges

Community colleges are already actively engaged in education for the health professions at the associate degree level. Plans comparable to those for the clinical and basic sciences campuses are being developed so that students with the ability and motivation who wish to transfer to upper division work at the state university center after completion of the associate degree would be enabled to do so as expeditiously as possible. Many cooperative academic arrangements are envisioned as well as joint planning for curricula, equivalency, and transfer of credits. Similar arrangements can be made with two-year and four-year programs in private institutions so that an integrated set of education opportunities can be offered for the region.

Clearly there are many complex questions to be answered in any program such as this, with interlocking arrangements between public and private institutions. Yet such arrangements offer the most promising solution to our current needs to expand manpower resources quickly and at a cost that society can tolerate without compromising essential programs of social welfare, general education, housing, and other needs.

Through such arrangements and consortia we estimate that the number of entering places in medicine alone could be doubled or tripled without expanding the physical facilities or faculty of the Health Sciences Center at Stony Brook. Similar expansions of enrollment would be possible in the other health professional schools.

Of equal importance is the fact that such a consortium for educational purposes would also facilitate the development of an integrated and coordinated, regionalized, and functionalized care system in each of the institutions involved. This is, from the public point of view, an essential element in any large-scale solution to our local and national health crisis.

The four clinical campuses under contract now have a total of almost 3,000 beds available for programs in the schools of the Health Sciences Center. Each of the campuses has a clinical dean who serves as a chief academic officer for all programs and as a liaison officer with appropriate offices and departments at Stony Brook. A brief summary of the resources of these hospitals is as follows:

1. *Nassau County Medical Center:* This is a 613-bed general hospital owned and operated by Nassau County as a county institution with a large full-time medical staff. The hospital is presently undergoing a major rebuilding program that will increase its size to about 800 beds and add conference, laboratory, and office facilities. It maintains approved rotating and straight internships and approved residency programs in anesthesiology, internal medicine, obstetrics and gynecology, orthopedic surgery, pathology, pediatrics, plastic surgery, psychiatry, radiology, general surgery, and urology. The hospital has about 15,000 admissions per annum, with an average stay of eleven days, and 85,000 outpatient visits.

2. *Long Island Jewish-Queens Hospital Center:* This is a 268-bed, acute, general, voluntary, nonprofit hospital. The hospital is now completing an expansion program that will increase its capacity to 450 beds and add conference, laboratory, and office facilities. The hospital has full-time chiefs of service and supporting staff. It has approved rotating and straight internships and approved residency programs in anesthesiology, internal medicine, obstetrics and gynecology, pathology, pediatrics, pediatric cardiology, radiology, and surgery. The hospital has about 11,600 admissions per annum, with an average stay of eight days, 35,000 outpatient visits, and 23,000 emergency room visits.

The Queens Hospital Center, part of the metropolitan New York hospital system, is a general hospital of some 1,200 beds.

3. *Hospital of Brookhaven National Laboratory:* This is a forty-bed hospital devoted to clinical research. An affiliation with this hospital will of necessity be more specialized in nature and students will be selected to receive clinical experience there primarily on the basis of demonstrated interest in clinical research.

4. *Northport Veterans Administration Hospital:* At the present time the VA maintains this as a 2,200-bed psychiatric hospital. Plans call for a considerable reduction in the number of psychiatric beds and for the construction of a 480-bed general medical and surgical facility that is already underway and is scheduled for completion in the summer of 1972. This institution has already been designated as a dean's committee hospital and all of its professional staff will be nominated by the Health Sciences Center and will be closely associated with it.

In addition to the comprehensive affiliations with the clinical campus hospitals, affiliations of somewhat less comprehensive nature are in existence with six other hospitals in the Nassau-Suffolk area. These affiliations serve a variety of purposes in providing clinical experiences for all of the schools in the center.

CHAPTER EIGHTEEN

ACADEMIC HEALTH CENTERS AND THE MEDICAL MARKETPLACE: A Faustian Compact Examined

"This is apparently the law of human progress, that upon attaining a certain point in its course a movement only escapes detrimental exaggeration by recoiling in the opposite direction."
Desiderius Erasmus, On the Education of Boys

INTRODUCTION

I should feel a little guilty appearing before you today. For the first time in thirty-four years, I am not responsible for the administration of an institution or a significant part of one. I reside now in the nirvana of a professorship which permits me to refer all real-world decisions to someone else and to devote myself to such recondite - and safe - pursuits as today's assignment - expatiating on values and value conflicts. My memory of the decision-making arena is recent enough not to have been entirely obliterated, however. I hope the mixture of closeness and distance with that arena that I now enjoy will grant me a certain empathetic and possibly helpful objectivity with which to examine the issues you face individually as executives of academic health centers and collectively as an Association.

Let me recall the difference between a surgeon's and an internist's beside prayer: The surgeon prays, "My God, what have I done?" The internist prays, "My God, what should I do?" Monty Duval has played the surgical role well. Now it is up to me to say what we *should* do. Monty wisely gave no prescription; I will foolishly try one. Monty also said he would "set the stage," for me. What he did not tell you is the name of the play or the role I am to play. I think he expected me to play Hamlet, the surgeon's paradigm, of the internist, the paragon of velleity and indecision.

I don't think Hamlet's dilatory and irresolute tactics will help very much in facing the choices we are forced to make. So I'll forgo the role of vacillation and venture at

Edmund Pellegrino. Academic Health Centers and the Medical Marketplace: A Faustian Compact Examined. Speech presented at: Annual Meeting of the Association of Academic Health Centers; September 29-October 2, 1982; Kiawah Island, Charleston, South Carolina.

least a strategy for resolving the conflicts of values that run through Monty's predictions. While avoiding Hamlet's indecisiveness, I must also circumvent Laertes' importunateness and Polonius' circumlocution.

I will hold that the ethos and values of the marketplace are incompatible with the social and academic mission of academic health centers. Accommodation or compromise with the values of a competitive marketplace must ultimately corrupt the academic enterprise. Only a genuine reappraisal of what is intrinsic to the academic mission will suffice. Such a reappraisal must raise painful questions about the present viability of the Flexnerian belief system. The challenge is either to sharpen the academic mission of academic health centers or enter a Faustian compact with the marketplace which must ultimately prove self-destructive.

VALUES, VIRTUES & VICES

Anyone who speaks about values today ought to give an operating definition first. There are many such definitions, I prefer to consider values as the criteria on which human choices are made, the justifications we use for our actions, the things that give us satisfaction, fulfillment, meaning, and worth.[1,2] Values are the things we are willing to work for, suffer for, pay for, and sometimes die for. They orient our choices and thus impel us to select certain alternatives over others. They link thought and action by framing our perceptions of what is good and worth doing. Not all values are moral or ethical. They are social, cultural, academic, economic, political - indeed, values exist in every dimension of human action. Only those values that relate to the goodness and evil of human actions or are used as moral justifications are ethical.

Every human decision involves an assessment of fact (what is the case), and evaluation (is it worthwhile doing), and ethical judgment (is it right or wrong). The value or evaluative decision thus links knowledge with action through choice.

Without values or with the wrong values institutions become their own moral arbiters with obvious dangers to society. Man is the only valuing animal and value choices are critical to all his endeavors. The values we choose reveal the kinds of people, institutions, or societies we really are, or want to be.

Value desiderata, therefore, are a central concern for the chief executive in any organization: It is the executive's task to spell them out in a mission statement, to articulate them within the institution and externally, and to make value choices when policy decisions are in dispute.

There is an inverse law of values in decision-making: The higher one's authority, the less one decides matters of fact and the more matters of value. Managers make largely technical decisions. Their value choices are over a narrow range only. Their choices do not decide the mission, shape, or direction of an institution. Executives depend on subordinates for facts; they must obviously know how to be critical about facts. But their special task is to choose among values in opposition. They must make the "tragic choices." The quality of an executive and of the institution he directs is often best defined by the way he resolves value conflicts.

Values are not synonymous with virtues nor are they good simply because someone sincerely believes in them. A virtue, to use Alasdair MacIntyre's definition, is "an acquired human quality the possession and exercise of which tends to enable us to achieve those goods internal to practices and the lack of which effectively prevents us from achieving any such goods" ... "External goods are therefore characteristically objects of competition in which there must be losers as well as winners. Internal goods are indeed the outcome of competition to excel, but it is characteristic of them that their achievement is good for the whole community who participate in the practice."[3] On this view, medicine, physics, or painting are practices. Courage, honesty, and justice are virtues internal to every human practice; riches, honors, or pleasures are values but not virtues in this sense.

A value which when translated into an action enables us to attain the end for which the act is ordained is a good value - or a virtue. A value that frustrates that end or is peripheral or external to it is, or may become, a vice. Virtues may be values, but all values are not virtues. When value and virtue coincide - as they do all too infrequently - we have a good society.

For academic health centers, we must discern which values are "virtues" in the sense of being internal to the practices of education, research, and patient care and without which those practices cannot be accomplished. Values "external" to those practices - competition, profit, price - are not virtues in the strict sense, and may even become vices. The rest of this essay tries to clarify the distinction between what is internal and what external to the mission of academic health centers.

VALUE DESIDERATA FACING ACADEMIC HEALTH CENTERS

We can now turn to our second subject - the value desiderata underlying the decisions we must make about medical and health care in today's socio-political and economic climate. Monty Duval's enumeration of the major socio-political forces now acting upon academic health centers is accurate: 1.) The ethos of competition and the marketplace - both spawned by the need to control costs. Competition is here, deregulation is the order of the day and price is the "name of the game." 2.) The FTC ruling which challenges the idea of medicine as a profession and unequivocally classifies it as a commercial enterprise, thus reinforcing the power of the marketplace. 3.) Virtual abandonment of the idea of a right to health care and willingness to accept the idea that there must be "winners and losers" in society and in health care.

These three features of our current national attitude about health and medical care clearly focus on the central question: To what degree are the values of the marketplace compatible with the responsibilities and functions of academic health professions? Few would argue against the desirability of cost containment or against conscious decisions about the allocation of our national resources between health and the other requirements of a civilized life. The choices, therefore, are not between good and evil, but between good things in conflict. These are the so-called "tragic" choices when good things conflict with each other, when both cannot be achieved simultaneously, and the dilemma cannot be circumvented. 4.) The values of the marketplace, however desirable they may be for other purposes, do conflict with the values underlying the care of the sick, the advancement of medical knowledge, and the education of health professionals. Let's look at some of these conflicts more closely.

A remarkably sharp shift in values has occurred in the nation and correspondingly in academic health centers in the last few years. A decade ago, most academic health centers were agreed that they had a central role in meeting the nation's health care needs. As a group, they subscribed to most of the following: 1.) health care as a right of all Americans; 2) equity in access, distribution, availability and quality of services; 3.) elimination of financial barriers to health care; 4.) government as a supporter, partner, and provider in achieving these ends; 5.) regionalization and outreach of academic health center resources into the community; 6.) matching the number and kind and health personnel trained to the health care needs of the nation; 7.) basic research and education in service of national needs; 8.) closing the gap between basic research and application as rapidly as possible.

These commitments found their practical expression in the central role academic health centers played in programs like Regional Medical Programs, Comprehensive Health Planning, primary care, family practice, team care, "physician extenders," Area Health Education Centers, PSRO, and minority student recruitment, to mention just the commonest examples. As a result, there was a remarkable agreement between the socio-political values of the nation and those espoused by most academic health centers.

This agreement was not without its tensions, of course. Academicians worried about the dilution of their traditional functions of education and research; politicians argued that the centers were not "responsive" enough to national health care needs considering the fiscal support they were receiving. Consumer expectations sometimes exceeded anything academic centers could provide. But on the whole, the centers responded to the stimuli of federal funds well enough to achieve a large number of new and socially relevant goals.

That they did so was not really the result of any deep-seated idealism about meeting the nation's health needs, except indirectly. Rather, it resulted from a practical tradeoff: Academic health centers accepted certain functions in exchange for support for their central enterprises. With federal funds, the physical facilities, faculties, academic and research capabilities of almost every center expanded phenomenally. The usual tensions between service, teaching, and research were submerged because there was enough money to go around. The choice was rarely "either-or," but rather "who" should get the lion's share of government largesse.

The temptation then was to initiate programs because funds were available rather than because of their relevance to the academic mission of an institution. As a result, many programs were shaped, and perhaps somewhat subverted, by medical centers to meet their own needs rather than those for which they may have been intended by Congress. The dissolution of so many federally funded "experiments" and programs following the withdrawal of government funds speaks eloquently to their peripheral position in academic health centers.

No one really knows what academic health centers would look like today if government money had not been available in a quantity sufficient to serve both the Congressional intent and academic interests. We do know, however, what the central values of the academic enterprise have always been, and remained even in the face of their involvement in publicly sponsored programs. Then, as now, they were: 1.) the preparation of scientifically competent physicians - specialists, clinical investigators, and entists; 2.) bio-medical research, both basic and clinical; 3.) teaching medicine as a scientific endeavor by full-time teacher/investigators who are not primarily practitioners; 4.) teaching in a university-controlled hospital in a tertiary care setting.

These are the essential values of the Flexnerian doxology - the educational credo of medical schools for more than half a century. These values were not threatened by the expansion in the functions of academic health centers in the '60s and '70s. But today, they are threatened directly and seriously by economic constraints and the current shift to an ethos of competition and the marketplace. Now the university hospital and the clinical faculty are forced to compete with other providers who do not carry the additional costs and responsibilities of education and research. As a result fiscal survival threatens to become the overriding value, replacing and compromising the socially vital functions only academic centers can perform.

When fiscal survival becomes a dominant value, an institution turns to alternative sources of revenue or improving the revenue from its usual operations.[5] Academic health centers are doing both. Tuition has been increased to unprecedented levels. The volume, income, and fee structures of faculty-provided patient care are geared for greater profits. Contracts involving privileged access to faculty research capacity are being concluded between medical schools and universities and the chemical and pharmaceutical industries.[6]

The clinical faculty becomes a revenue-producing resource; the basic scientist a revenue consumer, teaching is a "loss item," research contracts, targeted research, and development become new market opportunities for faculty talent. Some may even "invest" in nursing homes, patenting techniques or equipment.[7]

Each of these devices for survival poses a potential danger to the central academic enterprise. Each resembles a Faustian compact that must eventually be paid off. Medical institutions, however, cannot hope for Faust's last-minute redemption and so it is essential that the longer-term consequences be examined before these compacts are made.

The pressures on academic health centers today are not for a broadened, but a constructed, role in society. We hear no more talk of health care as a right; equity of availability and accessibility are no longer explicit goals; health care is now a private matter in which the consumer purchases what he wants or needs. Competition has become the new redemptive theme. Under its aegis the consumer will purchase only so much health care as he wants after shopping among providers eager for his business and therefore impelled to cut prices and maintain quality. Or so the untested assumptions glowingly suggest.[8]

On this view the university teaching hospital is another provider and is expected to compete for its share of the market. Instead of advancing new technologies, the university hospital must cultivate referrals not for their teaching and research value but for economic survival. It becomes not a "back-up" but a competitor to the community hospitals. The university's competitors are the many suburban hospitals which can often provide equivalent technical expertise, because the university's own graduates staff them in impressive numbers. Even more formidable is the growing competition of the hospital corporation, the proprietary hospital and the multi-hospital systems with their built-in referral networks. These hospitals can be fully dedicated to profit-making, since they are unencumbered by costly and time-consuming teaching and research.

In a competitive environment, cutbacks in public support for indigent or less than full-pay patients will force university hospitals and their faculties to turn away from their traditional service to those at the economic margins of society. Many of today's value questions derive from demands for fiscal survival and the commercial spirit an unregulated marketplace engenders. Profits, revenue production, and good bond rating, market penetration, product diversification, cornering the market on profitable techniques, management efficiency, cost-cutting innovations - these are the new values that will measure administrative success. None of these things is bad in itself. But they can easily corrode, erode, and subvert the fiduciary nature of the healing professions and the institutions dedicated to their education. There is an unavoidable conflict between the canons of business and the canons of medical morality.[9]

To compete successfully, faculty members must be encouraged, and sometimes coerced, to engage increasingly in private practice. Faculty practice plans are already indispensable to assure current levels of faculty income. These incomes, especially in the narrower and technique-oriented societies, are at unprecedented levels. Serious questions already can be raised about the motivation, commitment, and moral propriety of some supposedly academic clinicians. The distinction between being primarily a teacher and primarily a practitioner is becoming blurred in the rush to compete.

The justifications for increasing revenues from faculty practice are reasonable enough—the rising costs of quality education, the need to take up the slack in government support for research, patient care, and replacement of physical facilities and equipment. But their effects on the value system of academic health centers and all who function within them must be more carefully weighed.

What happens to a faculty forced to engage in patient care, to compete for as much of the "market" as they can corner. To be driven by incentive programs that make financial gain the prime target rather than teaching or research? What does a climate of such values, and the model of patient care they foster, do to the values of medical students and house-staff trained by such a faculty? What happens to the traditional ideals of service? How much teaching and how much supervision can reasonably be provided by faculty members who must pursue their own private practice goals? One need not advocate an unrealistic return to a romantic past of starvation salaries to question the propriety of today's levels of compensation and their impact on the motivation of academic clinicians. What will the already compromised physician-patient relationship look like after its full commercialization is realized? When ethics and economics conflict, it is not the usual experience that ethics prevails.

The FTC may end up being right, after all, in labeling medicine as a commercial enterprise and therefore subject to its jurisdiction. The issue of advertising is really trivial against the ethical and sociological implication of the FTC ruling. What is at issue is a direct challenge to the idea of a profession, of a human activity that makes the good of those it serves an overriding consideration. Can individual physicians and their institutions transcend self-interest in a society whose mores and law make profit the incentive for treating the sick and the troubled? Are healing and helping primarily a commercial transaction or is the fee they produce secondary to something more critical to society than profit? Is medical care, as some seriously suggest, a commodity transaction no different from buying beer, refrigerators or taking a disabled auto to a mechanic?[9,10]

The implications of the FTC ruling are clear. It says that no group can be trusted to police itself, that professional ethics is self-serving, that no more can be expected of a physician than of a used car salesman, a funeral director, or an auto mechanic at worst, or a competent plumber at best. This is no caricature - one has only to read the optimism with which some very creditable scholars foresee the salvation of medicine and the health care system through the combined efforts of the FTC, procompetition legislation, and more rigorous application of the Sherman Anti-Trust Act. Hospital appointments, accreditation, certification, licensure, cooperative planning for health care delivery provided dominated prepayment plans, negotiations with third-party payers over reimbursement, constraints on how service is provided - all are on the anti-trust agenda.[11,12,13]

I do not wish this to be a diatribe against sincere efforts to gain control of costs and overutilization and to improve the efficiency of our patterns of provision of health care. My purpose is to question the moral costs of health care. My purpose is to question the moral costs of substituting the ethics of the marketplace for the traditional ideals of medical practice. Where do the ideals of service, of trust, compassion, and equity fit in a commercial transaction? Do we not have responsibilities as advocates for the sick that transcend economic theories?

We must not compromise the one thing that really distinguishes us as a profession - our promise to the patient to be competent and to use that competence in the patient's interest.[13] That promise is made to someone who is ill and therefore vulnerable, anxious, dependent, and literally at the mercy of the professed healer. Business and money do not mix well with morals and covenants as even the most casual observation of the marketplace will attest. What is so significant about the FTC ruling is not that organized medicine must be regulated and restrained from anti-trust activity. The FTC in fact has some basis for its claim as a detailed review of its arguments will reveal.[14] The real question the FTC raises is whether the very idea of a profession is compatible with a competitive ethos and a profit-making economic philosophy. Without changing the American free-enterprise system, are there not some human activities - medicine, ministry, teaching, and the law—that, by virtue of the needs of those they serve, incur obligations that demand more than the minimal moral demands of a competitive marketplace? The "helping" professions must invite trust in order to help the person who needs help. The necessity for trust, and the implied assurance that it will be respected, is of a different order than we expect from tradesmen.

The academic health center is caught in a painful dilemma. Without other sources of fiscal support, the pressure to conform and compete in the medical marketplace can be overwhelming. Yet even if a procompetition ethos were acceptable for other hospitals (and this is highly debatable), it cannot be for the academic hospital. The academic health center shapes the values of the health professionals it trains. How it conducts the care of its patients becomes the model for what is acceptable as future practice. How authentic or convincing can its teaching of ethics, the meaning of a profession, or the obligations owed the patient be when the academic center adopts the values of commerce in place of the values of covenant and commitment?

When fiscal survival, profit, and cost containment become ends, rather than means, traditional professional ideals are not likely to survive for very long. Whatever their shortcomings, academic health centers have at least generated some sanctions for idealism in the pursuit of knowledge, and the care of patients. If these sanctions are weakened, few sources of legitimatization will remain for the young physician who still cherishes altruistic ideas about his profession. Indeed, the altruistic student may find medicine a repelling rather than an attractive occupation. Already, some very sincere young people are turning away from medicine because of its deteriorating moral image.

The dangers of the new environment in which patient care and teaching must take place do not, by any means, exhaust the agenda of choices that must be faced. The academic health center has always been caught in a maelstrom of contradictory and powerful value systems and expectations which threaten its special functions. We need only recall the conflicting demands and interests of legislators, administrators, patients, basic scientists, clinicians, students, consumer groups, third-party payers, hospital corporations, "investors" in the "health industry," and practitioners. Each group expects its own ends to be served by the powerful array of resources an academic health center represents. Each group espouses a different set of criteria for choices and actions that have in the past, and certainly can in the future, pull the center off course.

My strong emphasis on the marketplace as a new and powerful source of values is not to deny the continuing complex interaction of all these old forces. If the functions proper to an academic center are further compromised by the values of the marketplace, however, the task of adjustment will be more vastly complicated than it has ever been.

Three Strategies and a "Scenario"

Monty Duval showed wisdom in diagnosing but not prescribing how the challenges of the new marketplace environment should be met. I will be less prudent. I cannot offer specific resolutions for each of the value conflicts I have outlined. I do think we need a strategy that will enable academic health centers to retain some semblance of leadership and control over what they will become in the years ahead.

Academic health centers could continue to allow themselves to be shaped passively as they have in the past, molding their characters to fit the exigencies of national fiscal policy more or less without resistance. By adapting they will make survival their prime ordering principle, hoping for better days when the national economy has turned around. This is the easiest strategy, and one which many will no doubt adopt.

It is not a responsible strategy. Today's challenges are too directly aimed at the central mission of academic health centers to allow for such passivity. Academic centers cannot in good conscience be allowed by default to become proprietary hospitals or proprietary medical schools. Some centers at least will have to take a more active role, seeking a more creative adaptation or society will surely be the loser.

A second strategy has been proposed by James T. Howell and his associates.[15] They propose that medicine become a competitive "fifth force," by organizing as "doctor corporations." These corporations could serve as instruments to preserve the autonomy and integrity of the profession in the face of their erosion by the other four "forces"- government, hospitals and hospital corporations, business, and the health insurance industry. Howell's proposal is that a management core be established within corporate structures composed of physicians to provide the mechanisms for providing quality care, preserving the values of the profession, and developing its own competitive strategies. The essence of this philosophy is "beating them at their own game" - always a powerful strategy.

This strategy has the advantage of keeping academic health centers an active force in shaping the future of health care and assuring them a "share" of the marketplace. The emphasis on improved management and planning is commendable as is the challenge to shape the marketplace to fit more closely the more traditional values of the profession. Whether such corporations would be considered in violation of anti-trust law is problematic.

Howell's strategy, however, accepts a significant part of the ethos of the marketplace. Ultimately, I believe that ethos will compromise the values of the academic enterprise. Price, profit, and marketplace tactics are incompatible with the socially indispensable functions of research and teaching only academic health centers can perform. The virtues of the marketplace notwithstanding, to embrace them in the name of fiscal survival is to conclude a Faustian compact. Some functions essential to society are simply too important to be left to the fortunes of a competitive marketplace. Nonetheless, Howell's strategy is worthy of careful consideration. It is certainly preferable to passive adaptation to market forces. It has a contact with reality that is very appealing.

The third strategy - and the one I would favor - is unequivocally and responsibly to re-focus our enterprise on the two things academic centers do that is their unique function in a progressive society - to advance basic and applied medical knowledge and to assure an uninterrupted supply of competent practitioners, teachers, and investigators in the health sciences. These two purposes must be reestablished as the organizing principles, the architectonics that will guide the choices we must make and the future shapes our academic health centers must assume.

To be successful, this strategy must be unequivocal and responsible, and not a virtuous and defensive recitation of everything we now do. A pious and self-righteous incantation of the Flexnerian doxology simply will not suffice. This calls for the practice of an unaccustomed "economy of pretensions," a critical re-examination and re-selection of what is truly essential to carry out the unique social responsibility of academic health centers. Such a redefinition of purpose demands a willingness to give up those things others can do as well or even better.

The questions to be addressed are painful, unattractive, and threatening to cherished beliefs about medical education. Their difficulties, however, do not absolve us from addressing them.

Which of the large array of things academic health centers now do, and feel they must do, are essential to their singular social mission? Is a large university hospital, run or controlled by the medical school, a necessity as we have believed since Flexner? How many of the vast array of specialties and subspecialties, each with a faculty appointment, is necessary for undergraduate medical teaching or research? How large does a medical faculty need to be in both the clinical and basic sciences to fulfill its teaching responsibilities? Must undergraduate and graduate medical education be an administrative continuum to qualify as an intellectual continuum? Should the idea of a full-time clinical faculty engaging in intensive practice be re-examined? Is the notion of large clinical departments embracing practice, clinical investigation, and teaching academically viable? How dedicated to undergraduate teaching, or even the supervision of residents, is the academic clinician who needs large financial incentives to remain in academia? Is not the rewarding of financial success inimical to the academic goals of a medical school? Is not the escalation of academic salaries more related to the need to bring in patients and enable the university to compete than the result of any academic requirement? Should not the costs and sources of funding of undergraduate, residency, continuing education, and research be sharply differentiated? Would clinical research suffer if more of it were done outside the medical school? Can a university hospital and a clinical faculty that try to "compete" in the medical marketplace really remain part of a university?

To raise such questions is to invite charges of unspeakable heresy. What is being questioned are the very things medial educators have argued as essential to quality education and have struggled hard to introduce and preserve. The triple threat clinician will not respond kindly to partitioning his functions. Before labeling these questions as insolent or in disregard of what medical education is all about, we ought to examine them a little more carefully. It is not outside the realm of possibility that some of the things we deem so essential were added to medical education simply because funds were available and not because of any intrinsic connection with quality education or research. Even if we end up retaining most of what is now extant, a "dusting off" of our objectives is in order. If the marketplace forces a rigorous rethinking of what we are all about, it will have served a useful social purpose.

To address these questions, academic health centers may be forced to disarticulate some things they labored hard to forge together: undergraduate education, residency training, the training of biomedical scientists, the conduct of research, and the operation of tertiary care hospitals. For each function we need to re-examine how many teachers we need, how each should be funded, and whether our assumptions about teaching methods are correct. When we have engaged in such exercises in the past - as individual institutions or as a corporate educational establishment- we have ended up too often by reasserting the importance of almost everything we are doing.

That kind of outcome is no longer acceptable. The forces Monty Duval outlined are potent enough to re-shape academic health centers in their own image. The only alternative may be a revised model of the academic health center defined and defended on the basis of its social indispensability and not its survival in its present state.

I have not the time to examine these questions in detail. Yet I cannot raise them and expect to escape without pointing at least in the direction some of the answers might go. Were we to examine the questions critically and emotionally in the light of the powerful forces not acting on academic health centers, I believe that a trimmed down, but no less effective and socially indispensable, model of the academic health center might emerge.

In such a "scenario," the medical school would concentrate on undergraduate medical education - preparing practitioners, and investigators, in the clinical and basic sciences. Its faculty could then be much smaller. They would be primary full-time teachers and investigators. They would not be required to carry major responsibilities for large clinical services or engage in extensive clinical practice. The prime task of the academic clinician would be to provide the basic clinical skills, and a foundation in the major clinical disciplines. The subspecialties, especially those with a highly technical orientation, would be reserved for house-staff training in the hospital.

Academic clinicians could be hired on "true" full-time salaries, independent of income from practice. Those salaries would by necessity be less than is currently the case. They would be paid for teaching and research and their salaries funded through tuition, endowment, and grants. They would be responsible for operating a clinical research service within the hospital but not for the operation of the major clinical services. The clinical research center would be the locus for their own clinical investigations, as well as the training place for clinical investigators.

Full-time academicians could go on "service" in the university hospital to maintain clinical skills but not out of necessity to enhance income or support their salaries. There are still enough faculty members who would hold a truly academic career to assure that the ranks of this kind of a medical faculty will be filled.

Academic clinicians would thus be true full-time academics, more comparable to their university colleagues. They would not be expected to do all the clinical teaching for students or house-staff. The university hospital would have the major responsibility of the education of house-staff, clinical clerkships for undergraduate medical students and continuing education. Its orientation would be to tertiary level patient care, and the training of residents in clinical specialties. Its research would be clinically oriented.

The hospital staff would consist of clinical faculty members not on a tenure track, paid out of patient care income and not medical school or university funds. Their salaries could then be competitive with those of their peers in community hospitals of like stature. The hospital could then "compete" with other tertiary care institutions and its staff could concentrate primarily on patient care. House-staff salaries would come from hospital and professional income for patient care. The major teaching hospital would continue to be part of the medical or health science center but not owned by the university or the medical school. It should have a separate board of trustees concerned with patient care, and closely affiliated, but not identical with the university or medical center board.

On this plan, the academic departments would be smaller and fewer in number, being limited to the disciplines basic to undergraduate medical education. The clinical subspecialties would be organized in hospital departments rather than medical school departments. Most medical schools encompass a large number of departments because they are needed for tertiary care, rather than medical education per se.

Some of these arrangements have been existent for many years in those medical centers that do not own their own hospitals but include a major teaching hospital in the medical center organization. The difference is that the organization of the academic departments would no longer be synonymous with the organization of the hospital services. The chairman of the department of medicine, for example, would be an academic chairman and not necessarily the chief of the medical service in the hospital. Nor would he be the director of the residency training program. His "residents" would be those preparing for careers in research and getting the bulk of their training on the clinical research service.

The basic science faculty would also be reduced somewhat in size. Instead of teaching snippets of a course - those few hours related to their research expertise - they would teach a whole course as their university colleagues do. Their prime mission would be to educate medical students in the basic sciences, prepare graduate students for advanced degrees, and pursue research in biomedical science. The basic sciences could be seriously affected by the forces now reshaping medical centers, if some measures are not taken to buffer them from the marketplace.

I have said little of the other health professional schools. A like re-examination of dentistry, nursing, and allied health education is necessary in the light of dipping enrollments. This is a subject worthy of its own considerations. Suffice it to say that to remain as true academic "health centers" requires involvement with education of more than medical students and residents. Indeed, the opportunity to educate all health professionals in one place is a strength of academic health centers still to be fully realized. The forces of competition and the marketplace will probably have a lesser impact on education in professions other than medicine since they have not become dependent upon professional practice for their academic sustenance. In dentistry this immunity is sure to be challenged. Faculty dental practices promise to become a necessity with the same impact on the academic enterprise that I have outlined for medicine.

Academic health centers will, in the light of the new forces acting upon them, be forced consciously to choose some variation of the three strategies I have discussed here. The "scenario" I have developed is not to be taken as an optional model of what should occur in every center. My purpose was merely to indicate what kinds of questions must be asked and what kinds of answers might emerge from a strategy of conscious re-examination of what is deemed essential to the prime social functions of an academic health center as contrasted with a tertiary health care institution. That the university hospital and the medical school must remain as integral parts of an academic health center seems indisputable. That their administration, funding, and personnel need to be intermingled as they have been in the recent past is problematic and I believe untenable given the present socio-economic and political climate.

The only way, in my opinion, to retain what is essential about academic health centers - their academic responsibilities - is to make the case for their support on the basis of a cogent analysis of what they require to fulfill their socially indispensable role. Some privileges, power, prestige, and personal income may be lost. But the advantages are not insignificant - a clarity of purpose, a streamlining of functions and mission, and very likely an increase in the quality of pedagogy, graduate training, and research. These are solid grounds for a statesman-like appeal for public support of our endeavor, more likely to succeed than our past practice of defending everything we do.

In that effort I believe, too, that we must recover some of the moral credibility we have lost in recent years by arguing from what appears to be self-interest rather than social obligation. There is an urgent need for statesman-like leadership that will counter the values of the marketplace with a reconstruction of medical morality. We need to reassert the values of service to others, of the primacy of trust and obligation to the sick; we need to exercise restraint in financial gain from the illness of others and to combat the commercialism already in medical care and sure to be legitimized by the mores of pro-competition.

The present quarrel of the profession with the FTC is before the Congress. However, the issues it raises are less legal than moral. They may be settled by taking jurisdiction from the FTC but that would be a pyrrhic victory indeed if we did not reassemble, reaffirm, and reinstate our commitment to the moral center of our enterprise.[16] If academic health centers do not fulfill their obligation to teach and practice a morally sound model of patient-physician relationships, who will do so?

Recapitulation

I remain convinced that the academic health center is an important and irreplaceable social asset. It concentrates resources - people, facilities, techniques; it links education with research, patient care with social and public policy; it brings together the education of all health professionals; it is a tertiary care referral center par excellence; it links the university with the community and the practical world. Its potentialities for shaping health and medical care are still, in my view, a long way from being fully realized. These potentialities must not be lost by a passive adaptation to the current cycle of political and economic strategies.

Like Toynbee's civilizations, social institutions pass through cycles of development and decline. They grow in response to environmental challenges.[17] When their responsiveness in the face of those challenges is lost they go into decline and disappear. A few can recapture their vitality before this happens. The majority decay and recede from power and influence, to be replaced by new civilizations or institutions.

Academic health centers have run through a telescoped Toynbean cycle of sorts in less than two decades of existence. First conceived as administrative devices whereby universities might contain their burgeoning medical schools, they grew to unexpected proportions on the aspirations and funding of the Great Society. Today with the Great Society a deflated dream they face decline in an environment of economic and social minimalism.

It is problematic whether academic health centers can redefine their roles in the face of the powerful forces Monty Duval has so neatly dissected for us - the economy, science and technology, health care corporations, the ethos of competition. Each of you, as the chief executive of an academic health center, must determine where in these cycles you would place your institution and whether it can recover its vitality. Each of you must make the choices among values that will determine whether your institution is a passive instrument or an active creator of its own future. The CEO of an academic health center, like a head of state, must determine whether his institution is in a beginning state of decay and losing its vitality and creativity in responding to external challenge, or whether it is still at that point when a recovery of vitality is possible.

Academic health centers - through this organization, the AAHC - have a corporate and collective responsibility for the kind of assessment I have urged upon you. This is a unique obligation of the AAHC - since it represents all the health professionals, their educational and service components, and their social mission.

I believe as strongly as ever in the potentiality for social good inherent in academic health centers and the AAHC. For those potentialities to be realized, the academic health centers have something more than a role of passive acquiescence and adaptation to external forces. They must be not only servants of social and economic policies but critics as well. This is impossible without being sure of who they are, what they deem important, what values they espouse, and how those values advance the good of the society they purport to serve. In that self-examination, you, the CEOs and this association, have a major and indispensable moral responsibility.

did not mention health care specifically, I believe it fits his criteria for that set of human needs that must be accessible to all citizens by some mechanism other than the marketplace.[4]

Moreover, health care is not, and cannot be, a commodity like any other. Hence its distribution cannot be left to a mechanism suitable for commodities. But what makes medical and health care a moral claim that imposes an obligation on society to make it accessible to all?

Health care has three characteristics that distinguish it as an individual and social good and puts its distribution primarily in the moral not the economic category.

1. Health and medical care are essential if other human goals such as life, liberty, and the pursuit of happiness are to be possible.
2. Health care is not a property that belongs solely to the health professional or providing organization.
3. Commodification, rather than a professional ethic with serious consequences for patients, legitimates a business.

Medical and Health Care: As Human Good

Health and medical care, like education, justice, liberty, and public safety, are universal needs necessary for human flourishing. It is true that many people, despite serious or chronic illness, can be happy and productive. But, for many more, illness impedes realization of their full potential and undermines their capacities to cope with other less remediable misfortunes. Serious illness disrupts life even for the relatively well-off, and is disastrous for those on the margins of society.

Health care and relief of suffering are also good for society. Human beings are social animals, dependent upon association with other humans for fulfillment. A healthy society—as a social organism—depends on the health of its members. We acknowledge this in the extremity of an epidemic when all is set aside to stem the spread of disease. But we do not recognize the silent epidemic of treatable, preventable disease and disability and the burden of suffering for their negative impact on the healthy functioning of society.

Daniels[5] has argued that health is necessary to assure equality of opportunity for each person to realize his or her potential. On this fact of human life, Daniels et al.[6] ground a moral claim for access to a just health care system and go further to define the sociological criteria for its fulfillment. I would agree but can see additional reasons for a moral claim to health care. Health care, especially the knowledge upon which it is based, is a common possession. Health professionals have no exclusive rights to such knowledge. It is not a product they "own" and can offer for sale as a commodity.

Medical and Health Care Are Not "Owned"

Where does the medical knowledge come from that health professionals offer to those who need it? As medical students, we were allowed a set of privileges closed to others not in medical school. We were allowed to dissect human bodies, to participate in the care of sick persons, and to enter the private realms of their bodies, psyches, and even, at times, their souls. We were permitted to learn and "practice" technical procedures that, in our novice hands, were more time-consuming, clumsier, and more painful or uncomfortable to the patient than in the hands of an experienced clinician. We were given increasing responsibility for independent decisions regarding care. We were allowed to gain further experience during the years of residency as we progressed from the incompetence of the neophyte to the "safe" practice of a qualified physician.

We did all of this through a societal mandate or a presumed societal contract. We were granted privileges that, taken outside of medical education, would be legally actionable. These privileges were not granted for our own benefit or ceded to us as private property. We were given sanction to "learn" medicine for one reason, namely, that society would be assured of a continuing flow of qualified practitioners that could meet the universal human needs of the sick.

Certainly, we paid a tuition, worked hard, and denied ourselves. But none of this could pay for the privilege of invading the privacy of body, mind, and psyche of patients whose objective in seeking medicine was relief of pain or suffering, not becoming instruments of our education. To be sure also, some of us have added to medical knowledge, developed our skills to exceptional degrees, or provided pro bono care. Most of us, even as students, also provided sympathetic care for our "patients." But the equation is still unbalanced in our favor. Maturing in medicine is not like making a product where raw material is purchased, processed, and marketed. A product is proprietary; our medical knowledge is not comparable.

Along the way, we have had free access to all the "raw" materials. The world's medical literature past and present is ours for the asking, and we use freely the new information garnered from clinical investigations involving willing human subjects. These studies are supported by public funds or philanthropies to which we all contribute through taxes, contributions, or volunteer work.

Thus, health professionals are stewards of the knowledge required to heal. They are entitled to a just compensation for their effort in using that knowledge for the benefit of others. But they are not the sole proprietors of the information that they dispense and from which they earn a living.

Business versus Professional Ethics

Commodification legitimates leaving issues of access to the vagaries of competition. If access is profitable, "providers" will compete for it; if it is not, they will decline to compete. There is no moral obligation in business ethics to compel a provider to meet a social need no matter how fundamental the need. In fact, there is evidence that managed competition, which focuses on price competition, leads to higher costs and lesser care for those who cannot pay the price, and, thus, to inequalities of access and availability.[7,8]

Business ethics is not to be belittled. It is an important constraint on unfair business practices and serves to restrain the grosser injustices of the profit and market ethos. But it differs from professional ethics in medicine, which begins with a commitment to something other than self-interest, namely, the welfare and good of the sick person.

Professional ethics requires some degree of effacement of self-interest, whereas business ethics does not.[9] Business ethics is contract-oriented, but physician-patient relationships cannot be reduced to legal contracts. Clinical relationships are fiduciary and, implicitly, covenantal relationships. Contracts are written between persons who do not trust each other. Clinical relationships center on trust.

When there is time, patients can and should find out about their physicians' reputations, credentials, results, and other qualifications. In any case, contracts are negotiated between persons with roughly equal power to accept or reject terms. A sick person is dependent on the physician's knowledge and usually cannot access whether the physician is competent or trustworthy in advance. Thus, in the end, some physician must be trusted with one's well-being. This kind of trust cannot be spelled out in terms of legal obligation except in the broadest and roughest way, making a contract in the usual sense a practical impossibility.

Thus, access to health care and health care reform cannot be primarily determined by an economic paradigm, as is currently the case in the United States. Health care is a human good and a universal need that all humans sooner or later must experience. It is a good to which all citizens of a good society have a moral claim. It is not simply a right (as it is in many countries); a legal right can be granted and taken away by societal choice. Health care as a moral claim is grounded in the very fact that we are humans and live in human societies; it cannot be taken away without violating our humanity itself.

If individuals are to thrive, they need a healthy society (physically and morally); society also needs healthy individuals (physically and morally) to thrive. Individual and social good cannot be disengaged. Ethics and politics are, therefore, reciprocally related. To argue for access as a moral obligation is not to deny economics but to put it into the right order with respect to ethics. Ethics is suited to defining good ends and purposes (i.e., the kind of society we want). Economics is a science of means. It provides the knowledge for attaining those ends and purposes when the resources are scarce or limited. It is ethics, however, that defines whether the ends we have chosen are morally defensible or not.

To make access a moral obligation of a good society does not eliminate the possible need for rationing, for priority setting, or for reform. What it does mean is that health care reform should be driven by ethics and not by economics, commerce, or business. It means that both projected and existing policies must be measured by their impact on the patient and not by the money they save or the profit they return to investors.

Seeing access to health care as a moral obligation does not mean providing everything to everybody or putting health care ahead of every other social good. It does mean placing health care high among our societal priorities. It also means that we bear a mutual accountability for the suffering, hardship, and missed opportunities that ill health engenders, especially when illness is remediable.

Over and above all of these considerations is the way our attitude to people without health care access reveals the kind of society we want to be and the kind of society that we, in fact, are. Compassion for the sick and rescue of the sick among us from suffering is a measure of our sensitivity to solidarity with our fellow humans. A society that blandly accepts remediable suffering without helping, even at some sacrifice, is hardly a moral society. But sacrifice is a difficult appeal to make in a society oriented to self-gratification.

IMPLICATIONS FOR ACADEMIC HEALTH CENTERS

A shift in paradigms from the economic to the ethical carries definite implications for the essential role of academic health centers in our society. First, an ethical imperative does not in any way curtail the efforts now being directed to improve access to the services each academic health center provides in its own clinical components. Indeed, such programs now take on moral urgency. Those centers that have not moved in the direction of improved access are being impelled to do so to the extent possible.

Each center, within the limits of its financial, creative, and organizational capacities, should feel responsible for some program of improved access. However, academic health centers by themselves cannot expand access on a national scale, which is what true reform of health care requires. The efforts of academic health centers should go toward conceiving, operating, studying, and evaluating models of expanded access. The centers can provide empirical data about the relative merits of plans, thereby giving to those policy makers and legislators disposed to improving access the information they can use to mobilize public opinion.

Academic health centers will also be more effective if they cooperate with each other in establishing regional experimental delivery systems. I am realistic about the difficulties of intercenter collaboration, especially now when each center may be under a different economic management organization. But the difficulty does not remove the obligation.

Conclusions

Perhaps the most powerful means for improving health care access is mobilization by academic centers to use their unused power for moral suasion. Such advocacy is an untapped resource. However, if they are to convince the public and legislators, academic health centers will need to avoid conflicts of interest in the plans they advocate or propose. Too-close associations with and dependence on health maintenance organizations will make this a difficult task, especially if our centers profit from those associations that limit access to care.

It is my experience that legislators at state and federal levels see academic health centers as simply another lobbying group seeking special privileges. We must also convince a suspicious public that we are motivated by a moral objective: the improvement of access to satisfy a human need and also for our own benefit. Toward this end, we will do best by maintaining our stance as academic institutions educating future health professionals to view access as a major health concern and have the attitude, motive, and know-how needed to expand access.

In this respect, there is the counter caveat that overinvolvement in the pursuit of access, either in one's own institution or as a national advocate, can dilute the academic purposes of academic health centers. Their irreplaceable role in society is educating health professions, fostering basic and applied research, and providing models of optimal patient care. If forced to choose, academic health centers must put more effort into their academic mission than in improving access. When it comes to pursuing access, they can be replaced by nonacademic institutions. Ultimately, however, it is the academic nucleus that defines the role in society of academic health centers; they cannot be replaced.

Unfortunately, the academic enterprise is eroding and, as a result, America's world leadership in medicine is at risk. Some of our institutions have struck compromises with managed care thus raising the suspicion that our lament is more a matter of self-interest than of genuine concern for what society loses. If academic health centers simply become larger-scale corporate providers competing with other academic and nonacademic institutions, their unique mission is destroyed.

Eighteen years ago, I expressed my ideas about the erosion of the academic soul of the academic health center, which Lewis and Sheps[10] called "the sick citadel," and some of the things that needed to be done to recapture that soul.[11] Today, I perceive the tasks and burdens to be heavier and more complex than they were in my time.

The tone, spirit, and character of institutions, however, still depend on the chief executive. If our academic health centers are to exert advocacy for universal access, this visible symbol of what the organization strives to be will need to articulate the institution's position. Furthermore, the advocacy must go beyond pious pronouncements. Every policy and action at the institution must also demonstrate that the leitmotiv is to advance the interest of the sick and that this standard perforce includes, as a first step, access to what is available and making available what is needed.

The leaders of academic health centers may be among the very few who can marshal the enormous moral power of cooperative advocacy for access and justice in health care. Imagine the impact if a united effort with nurses, allied health workers, dentists, physicians, pharmacists, pastoral counselors, and social workers together advocating ethically driven health care reform. Provided they do not do so for self-interested reasons, health professionals speaking out on behalf of their patients would be hard to ignore by the public or their elected legislators.

The difficulties notwithstanding, the challenge is steeped with possibility for good. The public and policy makers look for this kind of leadership. It is what is required if the "sick citadel" is to regain its health.

REFERENCES

FOREWORD

1. Pellegrino, E.D. *Humanism and the Physician.* Knoxville, TN: The University of Tennessee Press, 1979; and Pellegrino, E.D. "Toward a Reconstruction of Medical Morality: The Primacy of the Act of Profession and the Fact of Illness." *Journal of Medicine and Philosophy* 4 (March 1979): 32-56, 54-65, 79, 95-116, 123, 141-152, 157-163, 168-169, 187-202, 229, 265.
2. Pellegrino, E.D., and D.C. Thomasma. *A Philosophical Basis of Medical Practice: Toward a Philosophy and Ethic of the Healing Professions.* New York: Oxford University Press, 1981: 47, 50, 80, 125, 148, 149, 159-160, 192-220, 224-225.
3. Thomasma, D.C. "Antifoundationalism and the Possibility of a Moral Philosophy of Medicine." In: *The Influence of Edmund D. Pellegrino's Philosophy of Medicine,* D.C. Thomasma, ed. Dordrecht: Kluwer, 1997: 127-143.
4. Pellegrino, E.D. "The Metamorphosis of Medical Ethics: A 30-Year Retrospective." *Journal of the American Medical Association* 269 (1993): 1158-1162.
5. Beauchamp, T.L., and J.F. Childress. *The Principles of Moral Ethics,* 4th ed. New York: Oxford University Press, 1994.
6. Veatch, R.M. *A Theory of Medical Ethics.* New York: Basic Books, 1981.
7. Jonsen, A.R., and S. Toulmin. *The Abuse of Casuistry.* Berkeley: University of California Press, 1988.
8. Jonsen, A.R. "Casuistry as Methodology in Clinical Ethics." *Theoretical Medicine* 12 (1991): 295-307.
9. Brock, D.W. *Life and Death: Philosophical Essays in Biomedical Ethics.* New York: Cambridge University Press, 1993.
10. Carse, A.L. "The Voice of Care: Implications for Bioethical Education." *Journal of Medicine and Philosophy* 16 (1991): 5-28.
11. Sharpe, V.A. "Justice and Care: The Implications of the Kohlberg-Gilligan Debate for Medical Ethics." *Theoretical Medicine* 13 (1992): 295-318.
12. Sherwin, S. *No Longer Patient: Feminist Ethics and Health Care.* Philadelphia: Temple University Press, 1992.
13. Purdy, L.M. *Reproducing Persons: Issues in Feminist Bioethics.* Ithaca, NY: Cornell University Press, 1996.
14. Chambers, T. *The Fiction of Bioethics: Cases as Literary Texts.* New York: Routledge, 1999.
15. Fins, J.J., M.D. Bacchetta, and F.G. Miller. "Clinical Pragmatism: A Method of Moral Problem Solving." *Kennedy Institute of Ethics Journal* 7 (1997): 129-145.

16. Singer, P. *Rethinking Life and Death: The Collapse of Our Traditional Ethics.* New York: St. Martin's Press, 1994.
17. Gert, B., C.M. Culver, and K.D. Clouser. *Bioethics: A Return to Fundamentals.* New York: Oxford University Press, 1997.
18. Engelhardt, H.T. *The Foundations of Bioethics,* 2nd ed. New York: Oxford University Press, 1996.
19. Fletcher, J.F. *Situation Ethics: The New Morality.* Philadelphia: Westminster, 1966.
20. Pellegrino, E.D., and D.C. Thomasma. *For the Patient's Good: The Restoration of Beneficence in Health Care.* New York: Oxford University Press, 1988: 51-58, 76-83, 106-110, 116, 120.
21. MacIntyre, A. *After Virtue: A Study in Moral Theory,* 2nd ed. South Bend, IN: University of Notre Dame Press, 1984.
22. Pellegrino, E.D., and D.C. Thomasma. *The Virtues in Medical Practice.* New York: Oxford University Press, 1993: xii, 18-30, 31-50.
23. Hippocrates. "Aphorisms." I.i. In: *Hippocrates,* vol. IV, W.H.S. Jones, trans. Cambridge, MA: Loeb Classics, Harvard University Press, 1992.
24. Veatch, R.M. "Against Virtue: A Deontological Critique of Virtue Theory in Medical Ethics." In: *Virtue and Medicine: Explorations in the Character of Medicine,* E.E. Shelp, ed. Boston: D. Reidel, 1985: 329-345.
25. Jansen, L.A. "The Virtues in Their Place: Virtue Ethics in Medicine." *Theoretical Medicine* 21 (2000): 261-275.
26. Davis, D. "Phronesis, Clinical Reasoning, and Pellegrino's Philosophy of Medicine." In: *The Influence of Edmund D. Pellegrino's Philosophy of Medicine,* D.C. Thomasma, ed. Dordrecht: Kluwer, 1997: 173-195.
27. Van Leeuwen, E., and G.K. Kisma. "Philosophy of Medical Practice: A Discursive Approach." In: *The Influence of Edmund D. Pellegrino's Philosophy of Medicine,* D.C. Thomasma, ed. Dordrecht: Kluwer, 1997: 99-112.
28. Veatch, R.M. "Is Trust of Professionals a Coherent Concept?" In: *Ethics, Trust, and the Professions: Philosophical and Cultural Aspects,* E.D. Pellegrino, R.M. Veatch, and J.P. Langan, eds. Washington: Georgetown University Press, 1991: 159-173.

CHAPTER ONE

1. Hippocrates. "The Art." *Hippocrates II,* W.H.W. Jones, trans. Loeb Classical Library 148. Cambridge, MA: Harvard University Press, 1981: 193.
2. Collingwood, G.R. *An Essay on Philosophical Method.* Oxford: Clarendon Press, 1933: 2.
3. Pellegrino, E.D., and D.C. Thomasma. *A Philosophical Basis of Medical Practice: Toward a Philosophy and Ethic of the Healing Professions.* New York: Oxford University Press, 1981.
4. Pellegrino, E.D., and D.C. Thomasma. *For the Patient's Good: The Restoration of Beneficence in Health Care.* New York: Oxford University Press, 1987
5. Pellegrino, E.D., and D.C. Thomasma. *The Virtues in Medical Practice.* New York: Oxford University Press, 1993.
6. Caplan, A.L. "Does the Philosophy of Medicine Exist?" *Theoretical Medicine* 13 (1992): 67-77.
7. Pellegrino, E.D. "Philosophy of Medicine: Problematic and Potential." *Journal of Medicine and Philosophy* 1-1 (1976): 5-31.
8. Engelhardt, H.T., Jr., and E. Erde. "Philosophy of Medicine." In: *A Guide to the Culture of Science, Technology, and Medicine,* P.T. Durbin, ed. New York: Free Press, 1984: 364-461 and 675-677.
9. Szumowski, W. "La Philosophie de la Médicine: Son Histoire, Son Essence, Sa Dénomination, et Sa Définition." *Archives Internationale d'Histoire des Sciences.* 2-9 (October 1949): 1097-1139.

10. Temkin, O. "On the Inter-Relationship of the History and Philosophy of Medicine." *Bulletin of the History of Medicine* 30 (1956): 241-251.
11. See also articles by Doroszewski, J., Lamb, D., et al, Qui, R., Walton, D.N., in Metamedicine, vol. 3 (1982) for philosophy of medicine in Poland, United Kingdom, China, and Canada. For philosophy of medicine in Austria, Germany, Scandinavia, The Netherlands, and the U.S.A., see articles by Kenne, T., Kottow, M., Lindahl, B.B., Ten, H., Have, et al., and Thomasma, D.C., in Theoretical Medicine, vol. 6 (1985).
12. Engelhardt, H.T., and K.Wm. Wildes. "Philosophy of Medicine." *Encyclopedia of Bioethics*, 2nd ed., W.T. Reich, ed. New York: Macmillan Publishing Company, 1995: Vol. 3: 1680-1684.
13. Pellegrino, E.D. "Medicine and Philosophy: Some Notes on the Flirtations of Minerva and Aesculapius." *Annual Oration of the Society for Health and Human Values*, Nov. 1973. Philadelphia: Society for Health and Human Values, 1974.
14. Engelhardt, Erde. "Philosophy of Medicine," 364.
15. Caplan.
16. Engelhardt, Erde. "Philosophy of Medicine."
17. Engelhardt, H.T., Jr., and K.F. Schaffner. "Philosophy of Medicine." In: *Encyclopedia of Philosophy*. London: Routledge and Kegan Paul, 1996.
18. Engelhardt and Wildes. "Philosophy of Medicine."
19. Pellegrino, Thomasma. *A Philosophical Basis of Medical Practice.*
20. Pellegrino, Thomasma. *For the Patient's Good.*
21. Pellegrino, Thomasma. *The Virtues in Medical Practice.*
22. Tauber, A.I. "From the Self to the Other: Building a Philosophy of Medicine." In: *Meta Medical Ethics: The Philosophical Foundations of Bioethics*, M.A. Grodin, ed. Dordrecht and Boston: Kluwer Academic Publishers, 1995: 158-195.
23. Caplan.
24. Ibid: 69.
25. Engelhardt, H.T., Jr. and Spicker, S.F., eds. Round table discussion, *Evaluation and Explanation in the Biomedical Sciences, Philosophy and Medicine I.* Dordrecht: D. Reidel Publishers, 1975: 215-219.
26. Sadegh-Zadeh, K. "Toward Metamedicine" (Editorial). Metamedicine, (1980): 3-10.
27. Lindahl, B., and B. Gemar. Editorial. *Theoretical Medicine* 11 (1990): 1-3.
28. Engelhardt, Schaffner. "Philosophy of Medicine."
29. Audi, R., ed. *The Cambridge Dictionary of Philosophy.* Boston: Cambridge University Press, 1995.
30. Edwards, P., ed. *Encyclopedia of Philosophy.* New York: Macmillan Publishing Company, 1967.
31. Van der Steen, W.J., and P.J. Thung. *Faces of Medicine: A Philosophical Study.* Dordrecht: Kluwer Academic Publishers, 1988.
32. Sinha, A.K. *Philosophy of Health and Medical Sciences.* India: Associated Publishers, 1983.
33. Department of Philosophy of Medicine and Science, Institute of History of Medicine. *Philosophy of Medicine and Science: Problems and Perspectives.* New Delhi: Institute of History of Medicine and Medical Research, 1972.
34. Hippocrates. The Art. *Hippocrates I*, W.H.W. Jones, trans. Loeb Classical Library 148. Cambridge, MA: Harvard University Press, 1972: 185-218.
35. Hippocrates. "Ancient Medicine." *Hippocrates I*, W.H.W. Jones, trans. Loeb Classical Library 148. Cambridge, MA: Harvard University Press, 1972: 1-64.
36. Jaeger, W. *Paideia: The Ideals of Greek Culture*, vol. III, G. Highet, trans. New York: Oxford University Press, 1944: 3-45.
37. Rosen, S. *Plato's Symposium.* New Haven: Yale University Press, 1968: 119.

38. Plato. "Laches." In: *The Collected Dialogues of Plato.* Bolligen Series LXXI, E. Hamilton and H. Cairns, eds. New Jersey: Princeton University Press, 1978.
39. Moon, R.O. *The Relation of Medicine to Philosophy.* New York: Longmans, Green, and Co., 1909.
40. Temkin, O. *Hippocrates in a World of Pagans and Christians.* Baltimore: Johns Hopkins University Press, 1991.
41. Pellegrino. "Medicine and Philosophy."
42. King, L. *The Philosophy of Medicine: The Early Eighteenth Century.* Cambridge, MA: Harvard University Press, 1978.
43. Sydenham, T. "Medical Observations Concerning the History and Cure of Acute Diseases." (3rd ed., 1676). In: *The Works of Thomas Sydenham,* vol. I, R.G. Latham, trans. London: The Sydenham Society, 1848: 11-21, reprinted in King, L., ed., *A History of Medicine.* New York: Penguin, 1971: 118.
44. Peek, H.T., ed. *Harper's Dictionary of Classical Antiquity.* New York: Cooper Square Publishing Company, 1965: 9552.
45. Riche, P. *Education and Culture in the Barbarian West, from the Sixth to the Eighth Century,* J.J. Contreni, trans. Columbia, SC: University of South Carolina Press, 1978: 46, n. 206.
46. Wilson, C. *The Invisible World, Early Modern Philosophy and the Invention of the Microscope.* New Jersey: Princeton University Press, 1995.
47. Engelhardt, Schaffner. "Philosophy of Medicine."
48. Pellegrino, E.D. "The Metamorphosis of Medical Ethics: A 30-Year Retrospective." *The American Medical Association* 269(9) (March 3, 1993): 1158-1163.
49. Sundström, P. *Icons of Disease.* Linköping, Sweden: Linköping University, 1987.
50. Van der Steen, W.J., and P.J. Thung. *Faces of Medicine: A Philosophical Study.* Dordrecht: Kluwer Academic Publishers, 1988.
51. Wulff, H.R., S.A. Pedersen, and R. Rosenberg, eds. *Philosophy of Medicine: An Introduction.* Boston: Blackwell Scientific Publications, 1986.
52. Grodin, M.A. *Meta Medical Ethics: The Philosophical Foundations of Bioethics.* Boston Studies in the Philosophy of Science, vol. 171. Dordrecht: Kluwer Academic Publishers, 1995.
53. Gillon, R. Philosophical Medical Ethics. New York: John Wiley and Sons, 1986.
54. Ibid.
55. Culver, M.C., and B. Gert. *Philosophy in Medicine: Conceptual and Ethical Issues in Medicine and Psychiatry.* New York: Oxford University Press, 1982.
56. Baldini, M. *Epistemologia Contemporanea e Clinica Medica.*
57. Reznek, L. *The Nature of Disease.* New York: Routledge & Kegan Paul, 1987.
58. King, L. *Medical Thinking, A Historical Preface.* New Jersey: Princeton University Press, 1982.
59. Wulff, Pedersen, Rosenberg.
60. Natanson, M. "Philosophy and Psychiatry." In: *Psychiatry and Philosophy,* W.E. Straus, M. Natanson, H. Ey, eds. New York: Springer Verlag, 1969: 85-110.
61. Sinha.
62. Department of Philosophy of Medicine and Science, Institute of History of Medicine.
63. Fleck, L. *Genesis and Development of Scientific Fact.* Chicago: University of Chicago Press, 1979.
64. Foucault, M. *The Birth of the Clinic: An Archaeology of Medical Perception.* New York: Pantheon Books, 1979.
65. Blane, G. *Elements of Medical Logick.* London: Underwood, 1819.
66. Oesterlen, F. *Medical Logic.* G. Whitney, ed. and trans. Sydenham Society, 1855.
67. Murphy, E. The Logic of Medicine. Baltimore: Johns Hopkins University Press, 1976.

68. Beauchamp, T.L. and J.F. Childress. *Principles of Biomedical Ethics*, 4th ed. New York: Oxford University Press, 1994.
69. Clouser, K.D., and B. Gert. "A Critique of Principlism." *Journal of Medicine and Philosophy* 15(2) (1990): 219-236.
70. Pellegrino. E.D. "The Four Principles and the Doctor-Patient Relationship: The Need for a Better Understanding." In: *Principles of Health Care Ethics*, R. Gillon, ed. Chichester, England: John Wiley & Sons, 1994: 353-366.
71. Osler, W. *Aequanimitas with Other Addresses to Medical Students, Nurses, and Practitioners of Medicine*. Philadelphia: P. Blakiston's Son and Company, 1905.
72. Peabody, F. *Doctor and Patient: Papers on the Relationship of the Physician to Men and Institutions*. New York: Macmillan, 1930.
73. Cabot, R.C. *Introduction, Differential Diagnosis*, vol. I, 3rd ed. Philadelphia and London: W.B. Saunders Company, 1916: 17-23.
74. Cabot, R.C. *What Men Live By: Work, Play, Love, Worship*. Boston and New York: Houghton Mifflin Company, 1914.
75. Thomas, L. *The Youngest Science: Notes of a Medicine Watcher*. New York: Viking Press, 1983.
76. Plato. "Gorgias." In: *The Collected Dialogues of Plato*. Bolligen Series LXXI. E. Hamilton and H. Cairns, eds. New Jersey: Princeton University Press, 1982; 501A: 283-284.
77. Plato. "Phaedrus." In: In: *The Collected Dialogues of Plato*. Bolligen Series LXXI. E. Hamilton and H. Cairns, eds. New Jersey: Princeton University Press, 1982; 268b-d and 270b-c: 513-516.
78. Castiglione, A. *A History of Medicine*. New York: Alfred Knopf and Company, 1941.
79. Garrison, F.H. *An Introduction to the History of Medicine*, 4th ed. Philadelphia: W.B. Saunders, 1966: 310-319.
80. King. *The Philosophy of Medicine: The Early Eighteenth Century*.
81. French, R., and A. Wear, eds. *The Medical Revolution of the Seventeenth Century*. Cambridge: Cambridge University Press, 1989.
82. Castiglione, 582-593.
83. Garrison.
84. Descartes, R. "Discourse on Method," in oeuvres vol. III, p. 78, 1. 8-13 as cited in Carter, R.B., *Descartes' Medical Philosophy: The Original Solution of the Mind-Body Problem*. Baltimore: Johns Hopkins University Press, 1983: 4.
85. Golson, E. *The Unity of Philosophical Experience*. New York: Charles Scribner's Sons, 1937: 147-148.
86. Hippocrates, "The Art," 185-218.
87. Hippocrates, "Ancient Medicine," 1-64.
88. Lain-Entralgo, P. *Quaestiones Hippocraticae: Disputatae Tres in La Collection Hippocratique et Son Role Dans L'Histoire de la Medicine*. Colloque de Strasbourg. Leiden: E.J. Brill, 1975: 23-27.
89. King. *The Philosophy of Medicine: The Early Eighteenth Century*.
90. Pellegrino, E.D. "Toward a Reconstruction of Medical Morality: The Primacy of the Act of Profession and the Fact of Illness." *Medicine and Philosophy* 4(1) (March 1979): 32-56.
91. Pellegrino, E.D. "The Healing Relationship: The Architectonics of Clinical Medicine." In: *The Clinical Encounter: The Moral Fabric of the Patient-Physician Relationship*. Philosophy and Medicine Series, 4. Dordrecht: D. Reidel Publishing Company, 1983: 153-172.
92. Wallace, W.A. *Causality and Scientific Explanation*, Volume II: Classical and Contemporary Science. Ann Arbor: University of Michigan Press, 1974: 141-154.
93. Pellegrino, Thomasma, *For the Patient's Good*.
94. Pellegrino, Thomasma, *The Virtues in Medical Practice*.

95. Ladd, J. "The Contract Model of the Doctor-Patient Relationship: A Critique and an Alternative Ethics of Responsibility." *Mount Sinai Medicine* 60(1) (Jan. 1993): 6-10.
96. Pellegrino, Thomasma, *For the Patient's Good.*
97. Pellegrino, Thomasma, *A Philosophical Basis of Medical Practice.*
98. Pellegrino, Thomasma, *The Virtues in Medical Practice.*
99. Pellegrino, E.D., and D.C. Thomasma. *Helping and Healing.* Washington: Georgetown University Press, 1996.
100. Pellegrino, E.D. and D.C. Thomasma. *The Christian Virtues in Medical Practice.* Washington: Georgetown University Press, 1996.
101. Gorovitz, S., and A. MacIntyre. "Toward a Philosophy of Medical Fallibility." *Medicine and Philosophy* 1 (1976): 51-71.
102. Caplan, A.L. "Does the Philosophy of Medicine Exist?" *Theoretical Medicine* 13 (1992): 70.
103. Pellegrino, E.D., and D.C. Thomasma. *A Moral Philosophy of Medicine* (forthcoming).

CHAPTER TWO

1. Edelstein, L. "The Professional Ethics of the Greek Physician." In *Ancient Medicine,* O. Temkin and C.L. Temkin, eds. Baltimore: Johns Hopkins Press, 1967: 336, 345, 346n.
2. Edelstein, L. *The Hippocratic Oath: Test, Translation and Interpretation.* Baltimore: Johns Hopkins Press, 1943.
3. Jones, W.H.S. *Philosophy and Medicine in Ancient Greece.* Baltimore: Johns Hopkins Press, 1946.
4. Hippocrates. "Epidemica." *Hippocrates,* W.H.S. Jones, trans. Loeb Classical Library. Cambridge, MA: Harvard University Press, 1923.
5. Hippocrates. "On Diseases." *Hippocrates,* W.H.S. Jones, trans. Loeb Classical Library. Cambridge, MA: Harvard University Press, 1923.
6. Hippocrates. "On Decorum." *Hippocrates,* W.H.S. Jones, trans. Loeb Classical Library. Cambridge, MA: Harvard University Press, 1923, xiv.
7. Edelstein, L. "The Professional Ethics of the Greek Physician."
8. Hippocrates. "On Decorum," xvi.
9. Ibid.
10. Hippocrates. "The Physician." *Hippocrates,* W.H.S. Jones, trans. Loeb Classical Library. Cambridge, MA: Harvard University Press, 1923.
11. Hippocrates. "On Joints." *Hippocrates,* W.H.S. Jones, trans. Loeb Classical Library. Cambridge, MA: Harvard University Press, 1923.
12. Edelstein, L. "The Professional Ethics of the Greek Physician."
13. Edelstein, L. *The Hippocratic Oath.*
14. Jonsen, A.E., and A.E. Hellegers. In: *Conceptual Foundations for an Ethics of Medical Care,* L. Tancredi, ed. Washington, 1974: 3-20.
15. Owens, J. "Aristotelian Ethics, Medicine and the Changing Nature of Man." In: *Philosophical Medical Ethics: Its Nature and Significance,* vol. 3, S. Spicker and H.T. Engelhardt, Jr., eds. Dordrecht: D. Reidel, 1977.
16. Spicker, S. "Medicine's Influence on Ethics: Reflections on the Putative Moral Role of Medicine." In: *Philosophical Medical Ethics: Its Nature and Significance,* vol. 3, S. Spicker and H.T. Engelhardt, Jr., eds. Dordrecht: D. Reidel, 1977.
17. Burns, C. "American Medical Ethics: Some Historical Roots." In: *Philosophical Medical Ethics: Its Nature and Significance,* vol. 3, S. Spicker and H.T. Engelhardt, Jr., eds. Dordrecht: D. Reidel, 1977.
18. Largus, Scribonius. *Compositions,* G. Helmreich, ed. Lepsiae, 1877.
19. Edelstein, L. "The Professional Ethics of the Greek Physician."

20. *Cicero on Moral Obligation: A New Translation of Cicero's "De Oficiis."* Bks. 1 and 2. Introduction and notes by J. Higginbotham. Berkeley: University of California Press, 1967.
21. Largus, Scribonius. *Compositions,* G. Helmreich, ed. Stuttgart: B.G. Teubner, 1887.
22. Deichgraber, K. *Professio medici zum Vorwort des Schibonius Largus.* Wiesbaden: Franz Steiner Verlag, 1950.
23. Edelstein, L. "The Professional Ethics of the Greek Physician."
24. Ibid.
25. Marcus Aurelius. *Meditations.* G. Long, trans. Garden City, NY: Doubleday & Co., 1960.
26. Edelstein, L. "The Professional Ethics of the Greek Physician."
27. Levey, M. "Medical Ontology in Ninth Century Islam." In: *Legacies in Ethics and Medicine,* C. Burns, ed. New York: Science History Publications, 1977.
28. Nortel, B. "AMA Judicial Activities." *Journal of the American Medical Association* 239 (April 1978): 1396-1397.
29. Pellegrino, E.D. "The Anatomy of Clinical Judgments: Some Notes on Right Reason and Right Action." Paper presented at the Fifth Trans-Disciplinary Symposium on Philosophy and Medicine: Clinical Judgment, University of California School of Medicine, Los Angeles, April 14-16, 1977.
30. Cassell, E. "Autonomy and Ethics in Action." *New England Journal of Medicine* 6 (Aug. 1977): 333-334.
31. Benarde, M., and E.W. Mayerson. "Patient-Physician Negotiation." *Journal of the American Medical Association* 239 (April 1978): 14-15.
32. Cabot, R. "The Use of Truth and Falsehood in Medicine, an Experimental Study." In: *Ethics in Medicine,* S. Reiser et al, eds. Cambridge, MA: M.I.T. Press, 1977.
33. Gert, B. *The Moral Rules.* New York: Harper Torchbooks, 1973.

Other references:

Ba-Sela, A., and H.E. Hoff. "Isaac Israeli's Fifty Admonitions to the Physician." In: *Legacies in Ethics and Medicine.* New York: Science History Publications, 1977.

Hooker, W. *Physician and Patient, a Practical View of Medical Ethics.* New York: Arno Press, 1849.

CHAPTER THREE

1. Plato. "Phaedrus." In: *The Dialogues of Plato,* vol. 1, B. Jowett, trans. New York: Random House, 1937.
2. Jaeger, W. *Paideia: The Ideals of Greek Culture,* vol. III, G. Highet, trans. New York: Oxford University Press, 1944: 3-45.
3. Versenyi, L. *Socratic Humanism.* New Haven, CT: Yale University Press, 1963: 33-35.
4. Plato. "Symposium 186." In: *The Dialogues of Plato,* vol. 1, B. Jowett, trans. New York: Random House, 1937: 313.
5. Rosen, S. *Plato's Symposium.* New Haven, CT: Yale University Press, 1969: 90-119, 273-277.
6. Plato. "Phaedo 67." In: *The Dialogues of Plato,* vol. 1, B. Jowett, trans. New York: Random House, 1937: 450.
7. Riese, Walther. "Philosophical Presuppositions of Present-Day Medicine." *Bulletin of the History of Medicine* 30, no. 2 (March-April 1956): 163-174.
8. Buchanan, S. *The Doctrine of Signature: A Defense of Theory in Medicine.* London: Kegan Paul, Trench, Trubner & Co., 1938. x, 194.
9. Wartofsky, M.W. "Roundtable Discussion." In: *Evaluation and Explanation in the Biomedical Sciences,* H.T. Engelhardt, Jr. and S.F. Spicker, eds. Philosophy and Medicine, vol. 1. Dordrecht: D. Reidel Publishing Co., 1975: b. 228.

10. Pellegrino, E.D. "Medicine and Philosophy: Some Notes on the Flirtations of Minerva and Aesculapius." *Annual Oration of the Society for Health and Human Values*, Nov. 1973. Philadelphia: Society for Health and Human Values, 1974.
11. Edelstein, L. "Hippocrates of Cos." In: *The Encyclopedia of Philosophy*, vol. 3, P. Edwards, ed. New York: Macmillan Co., 1967.
12. Jaeger.
13. Hippocrates. "De la Bein Séance." In: *Hippocrates oeuvres completes*, E. Littré, ed. Paris: J.B. Balliere, 1839-1861: 9: 232.
14. Aristotle. *De Sensu, In the Works of Aristotle*, J.I. Beare, trans., W.E. Ross, ed. New York: Oxford University Press, 1931: 1:436a.
15. Kuehn, C., ed. *Claudii Galeni, Opera Omnia*. Leipzig, 1820-1833. Cited in J.S. Kroffer, *Galen's Institutio Logica*. Baltimore: Johns Hopkins Press, 1964: 1:53-63.
16. Jaeger.
17. Galdston, I. "The Romantic Period in Medicine." *Bulletin of the New York Academy of Medicine* 32, no. 5 (May 1956): 346-362.
18. Risse, G.B. "The Quest for Certainty in Medicine: John Brown's System of Medicine in France." *Bulletin of the History of Medicine* 45, no. 1 (Jan.-Feb. 1971): 1-10.
19. Risse, G.B. "Kant, Schelling and the Early Search for a Philosophical Science of Medicine in Germany." *Journal of the History of Medicine* 27, no. 2 (April 1972): 145-158.
20. McMullin, E. "Two Faces of Science." *Review of Metaphysics* 27, no. 4 (June 1974): 655-676.
21. Edwards, P., editor-in-chief. *The Encyclopedia of Philosophy*. New York: Macmillan and Co. and Free Press, 1972.
22. Szumowski, W. "La Philosophie de la Médicine: Son Histoire, Son Essence, Sa Dénomination, et Sa Définition." *Archives Internationale d'Histoire des Sciences*. 2-9 (October 1949): 1097-1139.
23. de Waelhens, A. "The Ontological Encounter of Human Science and Philosophy." In: *Begegnung; Rencontre; Encounter*, F.B. Sullivan, trans. Utrecht: Vitgeverij The Spectrum, 1957.
24. Marcel, G. "Incarnate Being as the Central Datum of Metaphysical Reflection." In: *Creative Fidelity*, R. Rosthal, trans. New York: Noonday Press, 1964.
25. Merleau-Ponty, M. "The Spatiality of the Lived Body and Motility." C. Smith, trans. In: The *Philosophy of the Body*, S. Spicker, ed. Chicago: Quadrangle Books, 1970.
26. Spicker, S. "The Lived Body as Catalytic Agent: Reaction at the Interface of Medicine and Philosophy." In: *Evaluation and Explanation in the Biomedical Sciences*, H.T. Engelhardt, Jr., and S.F. Spicker, eds. Philosophy and Medicine, vol. 1. Dordrecht: D. Reidel Publishing Co., 1975: 181-204.
27. Straus, E. *Phenomenological Psychology, Selected Papers*. Translated in part by E. Eng. New York: Basic Books, 1966.
28. Straus, E., M. Natanson, and H. Ey. *Psychiatry and Philosophy*. M. Natanson, ed. New York: Springer-Verlag, Inc., 1969.
29. Grene, M. "People and Other Animals." *Philosophia Naturalis* 14 (1973): 25-38.
30. Engelhardt, H.T., Jr. "The Philosophy of Medicine: A New Endeavor." *Texas Reports on Biology and Medicine* 31, no. 3 (Fall 1973): 443-452.
31. Engelhardt, H.T., Jr. "The Concepts of Health and Disease." In: *Evaluation and Explanation in the Biomedical Sciences*, H.T. Engelhardt, Jr. and S.F. Spicker, eds. Philosophy and Medicine, vol. 1. Dordrecht: D. Reidel Publishing Co., 1975.
32. Buytendijck, F.D.A. *Prolegomena to an Anthropological Physiology*. Pittsburgh: Duquesne University Press, 1974.
33. Lain-Entralgo, P. "The Health and Perfection of Man." *Diogenes* 31 (Fall 1960): 1-19.
34. Lain-Entralgo, P. *La relacion medico-enfermo*. Madrid: Revista de Occidente, 1964.

35. Lain-Entralgo, P. *The Therapy of the Word in Classical Antiquity.* L.J. Rather and J.M. Sharp, trans. New Haven, CT: Yale University Press, 1970.
36. Wartofsky, M.W. "Organs, Organisms and Disease: Human Ontology and Medical Practice." In: *Evaluation and Explanation in the Biomedical Sciences,* H.T. Engelhardt, Jr. and S.F. Spicker, eds. Philosophy and Medicine, vol. 1. Dordrecht: D. Reidel Publishing Co., 1975.
37. Zaner, R. "The Radical Reality of the Human Body." *Humanitas 2,* no. 1 (1966): 73-87.
38. Zaner, R. "The Unanchored Leaf: Humanities and the Discipline of Care." *Texas Reports on Biology and Medicine* 32, no. 1 (Spring 1974): 1-18.
39. Zaner, R. "Context and Reflexivity: The Genealogy of Self." In: *Evaluation and Explanation in the Biomedical Sciences,* H.T. Engelhardt, Jr. and S.F. Spicker, eds. Philosophy and Medicine, vol. 1. Dordrecht: D. Reidel Publishing Co., 1975.
40. Engelhardt, H.T., Jr., and S.F. Spicker, eds. *Evaluation and Explanation in the Biomedical Sciences.* Philosophy and Medicine, vol. 1. Dordrecht: D. Reidel Publishing Co., 1975.
41. Shaffer, J. "Roundtable Discussion." In: *Evaluation and Explanation in the Biomedical Sciences,* H.T. Engelhardt, Jr. and S.F. Spicker, eds. Philosophy and Medicine, vol. 1. Dordrecht: D. Reidel Publishing Co., 1975.
42. Toulmin, S. "Concepts of Function and Mechanism in Medicine and Medical Science (Hommage á Claude Bernard)." In: *Evaluation and Explanation in the Biomedical Sciences,* H.T. Engelhardt, Jr. and S.F. Spicker, eds. Philosophy and Medicine, vol. 1. Dordrecht: D. Reidel Publishing Co., 1975: 54.
43. Szumowski.
44. Ortega y Gasset, J. *What Is Philosophy?* M. Adams, trans. New York: W.W. Norton Co., 1960.
45. Heidegger, M. *An Introduction to Metaphysics.* R. Manheim, trans. New York: Doubleday & Co., Anchor Books, 1961.
46. Merleau-Ponty, M. *In Praise of Philosophy.* Chicago: Northwestern University Press, 1963.
47. Husserl, E. "Philosophy as Rigorous Science." In: E. Husserl, *Phenomenology and the Crisis of Philosophy,* Q. Lauer, trans. New York: Harper & Row, Torchbooks, 1965.
48. Toulmin.
49. Jonas, H. "Technology and Responsibility." *Social Research* 40 (1973): 31-54.
50. Temkin, O. "On the Interrelationship of the History and Philosophy of Medicine." *Bulletin of the History of Medicine* 30, no. 3 (May/June 1956): 241-251.
51. Osler, W. *A Way of Life and Selected Writings.* New York: Dover Publications, 1951.
52. Clouser, K.D. "Medical Ethics: Some Uses, Abuses and Limitations." *New England Journal of Medicine* 293, no. 8 (Aug. 1975): 384-387.
53. Straus, R. "The Nature and Status of Medical Sociology." *American Sociological Review* 22, no. 2 (1957): 203.
54. Heidegger, M. *What Is Called Thinking?* F.D. Wieck and J.G. Gray, trans. New York: Harper & Row, Torchbooks, 1968: 33.
55. Dreyfus, H. "The Critique of Artificial Reason." In: *Interpretations of Life and Mind: Essays Around the Problem of Reduction,* M. Grene, ed. London: Routledge & Kegan Paul, 1974.
56. Scheler, M. *Man's Place in Nature.* New York: Noonday Press, 1961.
57. Cassirer, E. *An Essay on Man.* New York: Bantam Books, 1970.
58. Buber, M. *Between Man and Man,* R. Smith, trans. New York: Macmillan Co., 1972.
59. Stent, G.S. "Limits to the Scientific Understanding of Man." *Science* 187 (March 21, 1975): 1052-1057.
60. Pellegrino, E.D. "Physicians, Patients and Society: Some New Tensions in Medical Ethics." In: *Human Aspects of Biomedical Innovation,* E. Mendelsohn, J. Swazey, and I. Taviss, eds. Cambridge, MA: Harvard University Press, 1971: 77-97, 210-220.

61. Gorovitz, S. "Bioethics and Social Responsibility." *Monist* 60, no. 1 (Jan. 1976).
62. Bronowski, J. *Science and Human Value.* Baltimore: Penguin Books, 1964: 63-64.
63. Holton, G. "Modern Science and the Intellectual Tradition." *Science* 131 (April 22, 1960): 1187-1193.
64. Jonas, H. "The Scientific and Technological Revolutions, Their History and Meaning." *Philosophy Today* 15, no. 2-4 (Summer 1971): 76-101.
65. Price, D.K. *The Scientific Estate.* Cambridge, MA: Harvard University Press, 1967: 105.
66. Pellegrino, E.D. "The Most Humane Science: Some Notes on Liberal Education in Medicine and the University." *Bulletin of the Medical College of Virginia* 2, no. 4 (Summer 1970): 11-39.
67. Foucault, M. *The Birth of the Clinic: An Archaeology of Medical Perception.* New York: Random House, 1973.
68. Pellegrino, E.D. "Medicine, Philosophy and Man's Infirmity." In: Conditio Humana: Festschrift for Professor Erwin Straus on His 75th Birthday, W. von Beyer and R.H. Griffith, eds. New York: Springer-Verlag, Inc., 1966.
69. MacIntyre, A. "Moral Philosophy and Medical Perplexit: Comments on 'How Virtues Becomes Vices.'" In: *Philosophical Medical Ethics: Its Nature and Significance,* H.T. Engelhardt, Jr., and S. Spicker, eds. Philosophy and Medicine, vol. 3. Dordrecht: D. Reidel Publishing Co., 1975: 97-111.
70. Wartofsky. "Organs, Organisms and Disease: Human Ontology and Medical Practice."
71. Institute on Human Values in Medicine. "Human Values Teaching Programs for Health Professionals." Philadelphia: Society for Health and Human Values, 1974.
72. Fried, C. Medical Experimentation: Personal Integrity and Social Policy. Amsterdam: North-Holland Publishers, 1974.
73. Buchanan.

CHAPTER FOUR

1. Wittgenstein, L. *Philosophical Investigations,* 3rd ed., G.F.M. Anscombe, trans. New York: Macmillan, 1968: 16.
2. Ibid.
3. Ibid., 6.
4. *Quill v. Vacco,* 80FBd 716; 2nd Cir., 1996.
5. *Compassion in Dying v. State of Washington* 49FBd 790; 9th Cir., 1996.
6. Engelhardt, H.T., Jr. *The Foundations of Bioethics,* 2nd ed. New York: Oxford University Press, 1996, 189-238.
7. Berger, P.L., and T. Luckmann. *The Social Construction of Reality: A Treatise in the Sociology of Knowledge.* Garden City, NY: Doubleday, 1996.
8. Lobkowicz, N. *Theory and Practice: History of a Concept from Aristotle to Marx.* Notre Dame, IN: Notre Dame University Press, 1967.
9. Schutz, A. "Collected Papers." In: *The Problem of Social Reality,* 2nd ed., M. Natanson, ed. The Hague: Martinus Nijhoff, 1967.
10. Hippocrates. "Ancient Medicine." *Hippocrates I,* W.H.W. Jones, trans. Loeb Classical Library 148. Cambridge, MA: Harvard University Press, 1972: 21.
11. Hippocrates. "The Art." *Hippocrates II,* W.H.W. Jones, trans. Loeb Classical Library 148. Cambridge, MA: Harvard University Press, 1981: 193.
12. Ibid., 205.
13. Hippocrates. "On Joints." *Hippocrates,* W.H.S. Jones, trans. Loeb Classical Library. Cambridge, MA: Harvard University Press, 1923: 339.
14. Brown, J. *Horae Subsecivae.* London: A. and C. Black, 1907: 407.

15. Jaeger, W. *Paideia: The Ideals of Greek Culture*, vol. III, G. Highet, trans. New York: Oxford University Press, 1944: 3-45.
16. See W. Jaeger, "Commentary on Plato's Gorgias," 465a, 464a, in *Paideia: The Ideals of Greek Culture*, vol. II, G. Highet, trans. New York: Oxford University Press, 1944.
17. Pellegrino, E.D., and D.C. Thomasma. *For the Patient's Good: The Restoration of Beneficence in Health Care.* New York: Oxford University Press, 1988.
18. Pellegrino, E.D., and D.C. Thomasma. *A Philosophical Basis of Medical Practice: Toward a Philosophy and Ethic of the Healing Professions.* New York: Oxford University Press, 1981.
19. Callahan, D. *What Kind of Life: The Limits of Medical Progress.* New York: Simon & Schuster, 1990.
20. Callahan, D. *The Trouble Dream of Life: Living with Mortality.* New York: Simon & Schuster, 1993.
21. Schutz, A. xxxvi.

CHAPTER FIVE

1. Burleigh, M. *Death and Deliverance: "Euthanasia" in Germany.* c. 1900-1945. Cambridge: Cambridge University Press, 1994.
2. Frey, R.G. "Moral Standing, the Value of Lives, and Speciesism." *Between the Species* 4 (1988): 191-201.
3. Leavitt, F. "Let's Keep Metaphysics Out of Medical Ethics: Critique of Poplawski and Gillet." *Journal of Medical Ethics* 18 (1992): 206-209.
4. Parkin, C. "Metaphysics and Medical Ethics." Journal of Medical Ethics 21 (1995): 106-111.
5. Rorty, A.O. "Socrates and Sophia Perform the Philosophic Turn." In: A. Cohen and M. Dascal, eds., *The Institution of Philosophy: A Discipline in Crisis.* La Salle, IL: Open Court, 1989: 273.
6. Pellegrino, E.D. "Toward a Reconstruction of Medical Morality: The Primacy of the Act of Profession and the Fact of Illness." Journal of Medicine and Philosophy 4 (1979): 32-56.
7. Pellegrino, E.D. "The Healing Relationship: The Architectonics of Clinical Medicine." In: *The Clinical Encounter: The Moral Fabric of the Patient-Physician Relationship.* Philosophy and Medicine Series, 4. Dordrecht: D. Reidel Publishing Company, 1983: 153-172.
8. Pellegrino, E.D., and D.C. Thomasma. "Filosofia della Medicina." In: G. Russo (a cura di), *Bioetica fondamentale e generale.* Torino: SEI, 1995: 169-178.
9. Pellegrino, E.D., and D.C. Thomasma. *For the Patient's Good: The Restoration of Beneficence in Health Care.* New York: Oxford University Press, 1988.
10. King, L.S. *The Philosophy of Medicine.* Cambridge, MA: Harvard University Press, 1978.
11. Galen. Galen: *On the Therapeutic Method, Books I and II,* R.J. Harkinson, trans. Oxford: Clarendon Press, 1991.
12. Scarborough, J. "Review of Galen: On the Therapeutic Method, Books I and II." *Bulletin of the History of Medicine* 69 (1991): 628-629.
13. Hippocrates. "Ancient Medicine." *Hippocrates I,* W.H.S. Jones, trans. Loeb Classical Library 148. Cambridge, MA: Harvard University Press, 1972: 13-64.
14. Pellegrino, E.D. "Medical Ethics: Entering the Post-Hippocratic Era." *Journal of the American Board of Family Practice* 1 (1988): 230-237.
15. Pellegrino, E.D., and D.C. Thomasma. *A Philosophical Basis of Medical Practice: Toward a Philosophy and Ethic of the Healing Professions.* New York: Oxford University Press, 1981.
16. Pellegrino, E.D., and D.C. Thomasma. *For the Patient's Good: The Restoration of Beneficence in Health Care.* New York: Oxford University Press, 1988.
17. Pellegrino, E.D., and D.C. Thomasma. *The Virtues in Medical Practice.* New York: Oxford University Press, 1993.

18. Toulmin, S. "The Primacy of Practice: Medicine and Postmodernism." In: *A Twenty-Year Retrospective.* Carson, Burns, eds. 41-54.
19. Marx, W. *The Meaning of Aristotle's "Ontology."* The Hague: Martinus Nijhoff, 1954: 25.
20. Aristotle. "Metaphysics." In: *The Basic Works of Aristotle*, R. McKlon, ed. New York: Random House, 1941: 1027a, 19-22, 782.
21. Marx.
22. Dinan, S.A. "The Particularity of Moral Knowledge, Practical Reasoning." *Proceedings of the American Catholic Association* LVIII (1983): 65-72.
23. Gadamer, H.G. *Reason in the Age of Science.* Cambridge, MA: Massachusetts Institute of Technology Press, 1981: 69.
24. Marx, 15.
25. Aristotle, "Metaphysics," 691.
26. Ibid., 689-692.
27. Ibid., 689.
28. Gadamer, H.G. *The Idea of Good in Platonic and Aristotelian Philosophy.* New Haven, CT: Yale University Press, 1986.
29. Jaeger, W. "Aristotle's Use of Medicine as a Model of Method in Ethics." *Journal of Hellenic Studies* 77 (1957): 54.

CHAPTER SIX

1. Ortega y Gasset, J. *Meditations on Quixote.* E. Rugg and D. Marin, trans. New York: Norton, 1963: 45; see also nn. 7, 36.
2. Dixon, J.W., Jr. "Ortega and the Redefinition of Metaphysics." *Cross Currents* 39 (Fall 1979): 281-299. The implications of this view of the philosophical foundations of medical morality are more extensively discussed in E.D. Pellegrino, *Humanism and the Physician* (Knoxville: University of Tennessee Press, 1979) and in E.D. Pellegrino and D.C. Thomasma, *A Philosophical Basis of Medical Practice* (New York: Oxford University Press, 1981).
3. Pellegrino, E.D. "Plus la Change: The Changeless, the Changing, and the Unchangeable in the Healing Relationship." *2004-Medicine in the 21st Century.* Kingston, Ontario: Queens University, 1980: 54-68.
4. Pellegrino, E.D., and L. Newton, eds. "Collective Responsibility in Medicine." *Journal of Medicine and Philosophy* 7:1 (Feb. 1982).

CHAPTER SEVEN

1. de Unamuno y Jugo, M. *Selected Works of Muguel de Unamuno*, vol. 6. A. Kerrigan and M. Nozick, eds. Novela/Nivola Series LXXXV 6. Princeton: Princeton University Press, 1976: 366.
2. Kass, L. "Regarding the End of Medicine and the Pursuit of Health." *The Public Interest* 40 (Summer 1975): 11-42.
3. Burnham, J. "American Medicine's Golden Age: What Happened to It?" *Science* 215 (1982): 1474-1479.
4. Seldin, D. "The Medical Model: Biomedical Science as the Basis for Medicine." In: *Beyond Tomorrow.* New York: The Rockefeller University Press, 1977: 40.
5. Constitution of the World Health Organization. "Preamble: The First Ten Years of the World Health Organization." Geneva, 1958.
6. Caplan, A.J., et al., eds. *Concepts of Health and Disease.* Reading, MA: Addison Wesley, 1981.
7. Seldin, D.
8. Seldin, D. "The Boundaries of Medicine." Presidential address. *Transactions of the Association of American Physicians* 94 (1981): 75-86.

9. Kenty, S. "From Rationalization to Reason." *American Journal of Psychiatry* 131 (1974): 957-963.
10. Nozick, R. *Philosophical Explanations.* Cambridge, MA: Belknap-Harvard University Press, 1981.
11. Jacob, F. *The Possible and the Actual.* Seattle and London: University of Washington Press, 1982: 44.
12. Engel, G. "The Clinical Application of the Biopsychosocial Model." *The American Journal of Psychiatry* 137 (May 1980): 535-544.
13. Engel, G. "The Need for a New Medical Model: A Challenge for Biomedicine." *Science* 196 (1977): 129-136.
14. Ibid.
15. Allen, D., et al. *Whole Person Medicine.* Downers Grove, IL: Inter-Varsity Press, 1980.
16. Engel, G. "The Clinical Application of the Biopsychosocial Model."
17. Pellegrino, E.D. "Biology and Public Administration: Some Touchstones Scrutinized." *Proceedings,* Colloquium Series. C.W. Post Center, Long Island University, Greenvale, NY: nd.
18. Kass.
19. Ibid.
20. Ibid.
21. Pellegrino, E.D., and D.C. Thomasma. *A Philosophical Basis of Medical Practice: Toward a Philosophy and Ethic of the Healing Professions.* New York: Oxford University Press, 1981.
22. Siegler, M. "The Doctor-Patient Encounter and Its Relationship to Health and Disease." In: *Concepts of Health and Disease,* A. Caplan et al., eds. Reading, MA: Addison-Wesley: 627-644.
23. Ibid.
24. Ibid.
25. Pellegrino, E. "Philosophy and Medicine: Problematic and Potential." *Journal of Medicine and Philosophy* 1 (March 1976): 5-31.
26. Whitbeck, C. "A Theory of Health." In: *Concepts of Health and Disease,* A. Caplan et al., eds. Reading, MA: Addison-Wesley: 611-626.
27. Fabrega, H. "Concepts of Disease: Logical Features and Social Implications." *Perspectives in Biology and Medicine* 1 (Summer 1973): 538-617.
28. Pellegrino, E.D. *Humanism and the Physician.* Knoxville, TN: The University of Tennessee Press, 1979.
29. Sade, R. "Medical Care as a Right: A Refutation." *New England Journal of Medicine* 285 (Dec. 2, 1971): 1288-1292.
30. Bayles, M. "Physicians as Body Mechanics." In: *Contemporary Issues in Biomedical Ethics,* J. Davis et al., eds. Clifton, NJ: Humana Press, 1979.
31. Pellegrino and Thomasma. *A Philosophical Basis of Medical Practice.*
32. Edwards, P., ed. "The Good." *The Encyclopedia of Philosophy,* vol. 3. New York: Free Press, 1967: 367-270.
33. Frankena, W.K. *Ethics.* Englewood Cliffs, NJ: Prentice-Hall, 1963.
34. Gorovitz, S., and A. MacIntyre. "Toward a Theory of Medical Fallibility." *Journal of Medicine and Philosophy* 1 (March, 1976): 51-71.
35. Edwards.
36. Pellegrino, E.D. "The Anatomy of Clinical Judgments: Some Notes on Right Reason and Right Action." In: *Clinical Judgment: A Critical Appraisal,* H.T. Engelhardt, Jr., et al., eds. Dordrecht: D. Reidel, 1979: 169-194.
37. Engel, "The Need for a New Medical Model."
38. Engel, "The Clinical Application of the Biopsychosocial Model."

39. Pellegrino, "The Anatomy of Clinical Judgments."
40. Fabrega.
41. Pellegrino, *Humanism and the Physician.*
42. Pellegrino, E.D. "Toward a Reconstruction of Medical Morality: The Primacy of the Act of Profession and the Fact of Illness." *Journal of Medicine and Philosophy* 4 (March 1979): 32-56.
43. Pellegrino, E.D. "Optimizing the Uses of Medical Knowledge." Academy of Independent Scholars Symposium, nd.
44. Frankena.
45. Burnham.
46. Gorovitz and MacIntyre.

CHAPTER EIGHT

1. Santayana, G. Dominations and Powers: *Reflections of Liberty, Society and Government.* New York: Charles Scribner's Sons, 1951: 3.
2. MacIntyre, A. *After Virtue.* Notre Dame, IN: University of Notre Dame Press, 1981.
3. Oates, W., ed. *The Stoic and Epicurean Philosophers.* New York: Modern Library, 1957.
4. Foot, P. *Virtues and Vices.* Berkeley and Los Angeles: University of California Press, 1978.
5. Geach, P. *The Virtues.* Cambridge: Cambridge University Press, 1977.
6. Guthrie, W. *Socrates.* Cambridge: Cambridge University Press, 1971.
7. Kenny, A. *The Aristotelian Ethics.* Oxford: Clarendon Press, 1978.
8. May, W. Personal communication. "Virtues in a Professional Setting." Unpublished.
9. Pieper, J. *The Four Cardinal Virtues.* Notre Dame, IN: University of Notre Dame Press, 1966.
10. Shelp, E., ed. *Beneficence and Health Care.* Dordrecht: D. Reidel, 1982.
11. Shelp, E., ed. *Justice and Health Care.* Dordrecht: D. Reidel, 1981.
12. Sokolowski, R. *The Good Faith and Reason.* Notre Dame, IN: University of Notre Dame Press, 1982.
13. Von Wright, G. *The Varieties of Goodness.* New York: The Humanities Press, 1965: 139-141.
14. Wallace, J. *Virtues and Vices.* Berkeley and Los Angeles: University of California Press, 1978.
15. MacIntyre.
16. Pellegrino, E.D. "The Anatomy of Clinical Judgments: Some Notes on Right Reason and Right Action." In: *Clinical Judgment: A Critical Appraisal,* H.T. Engelhardt, Jr., et al., eds. Dordrecht: D. Reidel, 1979: 169-194.
17. Pellegrino, E.D. "Toward a Reconstruction of Medical Morality: The Primacy of the Act of Profession and the Fact of Illness." *Journal of Medicine and Philosophy* 4 (March 1979): 32-56.
18. Jhingran, S. *Aspects of Hindu Morality.* Delhi: Barnaasidass Publishers, 1989.
19. Pinckaers, S. *Les Sources de la Moral Chretienne.* Fribourg: Editions Universitaires, 1985.
20. Wilson, E.O. *Sociobiology.* Cambridge, MA: Belknap Press of Harvard University Press, 1980.
21. MacIntyre, A. *Whose Justice? Which Rationality?* Notre Dame, IN: University of Notre Dame Press, 1988.
22. Gould, J. *The Development of Plato's Ethics.* New York: Russell and Russell, 1972.
23. Ross, W. Aristotle: *A Complete Exposition of His Works and Thoughts.* New York: Meridian Books, 1959.
24. Ibid.
25. MacIntyre.
26. Copleston, F. *Aquinas.* New York: Penguin Books, 1959.
27. Ibid.
28. Aquinas, T. *Summa Theologica,* vol. 23. Cambridge: Blackfriars, 1964.
29. Cornford, F. *Before and After Socrates.* Cambridge: Cambridge University Press, 1932.

30. Aquinas, T. "De Virtutibus in Communi." In: *Opera Omnia*, vol. 14, S. Fretté, ed. Paris: Louis Virés, 1875; 178-229.
31. Maritain, J. *Art and Scholasticism With Other Essays.* New York: Charles Scribner's Sons, 1962: 166, 178, 245.
32. Pieper.
33. Ibid.
34. Geach.
35. Kenny.
36. MacIntyre.
37. May.
38. Oates.
39. Pieper.
40. MacIntyre.
41. Hauerwas, S. *A Community of Character.* Notre Dame, IN: University of Notre Dame Press, 1981.
42. Lewis, C.S. *Mere Christianity.* New York: Macmillan Company, 1952.
43. Pellegrino, E.D. "The Healing Relationship: The Architectonics of Clinical Medicine." In: *The Clinical Encounter: The Moral Fabric of the Patient-Physician Relationship.* Philosophy and Medicine Series, 4. Dordrecht: D. Reidel Publishing Company, 1983: 153-172.
44. Pellegrino, E.D. "Moral Choice, The Good of the Patient and the Patient Good." In: *Moral Choice and Medical Crisis,* J. Moskop and L. Kopelman, eds. Dordrecht: D. Reidel, 1983.
45. Engel, G. "The Clinical Application of the Biopsychosocial Model." *American Journal of Psychiatry* 137:2; 535-544.
46. Von Wright.
47. Ibid.
48. MacIntyre.
49. Pellegrino, "The Anatomy of Clinical Judgments."
50. Pellegrino, "Toward a Reconstruction of Medical Morality."
51. May.
52. Frankena, W. "Beneficence in an Ethics of Virtue." In: *Beneficence and Health Care,* E. Shelp, ed. Dordrecht: D. Reidel, 1982: 63-81.
53. Pellegrino, E.D. "Optimizing the Uses of Medical Knowledge." Academy of Independent Scholars Symposium, nd.
54. Pellegrino, E.D. "Value Desiderata in Logical Structuring of Clinical Diagnosis." In: *Ethics of Diagnosis,* J.L. Peset et al., eds. Dordrecht: D. Reidel.
55. Sade, R. "Medical Care as a Right: A Refutation." *New England Journal of Medicine* 285 (Dec. 2, 1971): 1288-1292.
56. Cicero. *Moral Obligations.* J. Higginbotham, trans. Berkeley: University of California Press, 1967.
57. Pellegrino, E.D. "Scribonius Largus and the Origins of Medical Humanism." Address to the American Osler Society, 1983.
58. Reader, J. "Beneficence, Supererogation, and Role Duty." In: *Beneficence and Health Care,* E. Shelp, ed. Dordrecht: D. Reidel, 1982: 83-108.
59. Josen, A. "Watching the Doctor." New England Journal of Medicine 308: 25 (1983); 1531-1535.
60. Cushing, H. *Consecratio Medici and Other Papers.* Boston: Little, Brown and Co., 1929.
61. Edelstein, L. "The Professional Ethics of the Greek Physician." In: *Ancient Medicine: Selected Papers of Ludwig Edelstein,* O. Temkin, ed. Baltimore: Johns Hopkins University Press, 1967.

CHAPTER NINE

1. MacIntyre, A. *After Virtue: A Study in Moral Theory*, 2nd ed. South Bend, IN: University of Notre Dame Press, 1984: 187.
2. Cua, A.S. *Dimensions of Moral Creativity.* University Park and London: Pennsylvania State University Press, 1978.
3. Waley, A. *Three Ways of Thought in Ancient China.* New York: Doubleday-Anchor, 1956.
4. Yearly, L.H. *Mencius and Aquinas.* Albany: State University of New York Press, 1990.
5. Jhingran, S. *Aspects of Hindu Morality.* Delhi: Barnaasidass Publishers, 1989.
6. Wiredu, K. "The Moral Foundations of African American Culture and the African Concept of Personhood." In: *African American Perspectives on Biomedical Ethics.* Eds. H. Flack and E.D. Pellegrino, pp. 80-93 and 104-117 respectively. Washington: Georgetown University Press, 1992.
7. Reale, G. *The Systems of the Hellenistic Age*, J. Catan, trans. Albany: State University of New York Press, 1985.
8. Rist, J.M. *Stoic Philosophy.* Cambridge: Cambridge University Press, 1980.
9. MacIntyre.
10. Gomez-Lobo, A. *The Foundations of Socratic Ethics.* Indianapolis: Hackett Publishing Company, 1995.
11. Plato. *The Collected Dialogues Including the Letters*, E. Hamilton and H. Cairns, eds. Princeton: Bollinger Series, 1961.
12. Aristotle. *The Complete Works of Aristotle*, J. Barnes, ed. Princeton: Bollinger Series, 1984.
13. Ibid.
14. Ibid.
15. Ibid.
16. Ibid.
17. Ibid.
18. Ibid.
19. Ibid.
20. Ibid.
21. Ibid.
22. Ibid.
23. Prior, W.J. *Virtue and Knowledge: An Introduction to Ancient Greek Ethics.* London and New York: Signet Books, 1991: 159-160.
24. Aquinas, T. *Summa Theologiae*, vol. 1-60. New York and London: Blackfriars/McGraw-Hill Book Company, 1963.
25. Aristotle.
26. Ibid.
27. Ibid.
28. Pinckaers, S. *Les Sources de la Moral Chretienne.* Fribourg: Editions Universitaires, 1985.
29. Pieper, J. *The Four Cardinal Virtues.* Notre Dame, IN: University of Notre Dame Press, 1966.
30. Maritain, J. *Art and Scholasticism.* New York: Charles Scribner's Sons, 1949: 116.
31. Hume, D. *Enquiries Concerning Human Understanding and the Principles of Morals*, 3rd ed., L.A. Selby-Bigge, ed. Oxford: Clarendon Press, 1975: 211.
32. Sidgwick, H. *Outlines of the History of Ethics.* Indianapolis: Hackett Publishing Company, 1988.
33. Becker, L.C., and C.B. Becker, eds. *A History of Western Ethics.* New York and London: Garland Publishing, 1992.
34. Machiavelli, N. *The Prince*, G. Bull, trans. London: The Folio Society, 1970.

35. Mandeville, B. *The Fable of the Bees, Or Private Vices, Publick Benefits.* New York: Capricorn Books, 1962.
36. Nietzsche, F. *Thus Spoke Zarathustra,* A. Tille, trans. New York: Macmillan Publishing Co., 1954.
37. Nietsche, F. *On the Genealogy of Morals and Ecce Homo,* W. Kaufmann, trans. New York: Vintage Books, 1967.
38. Rand, A. *The Virtue of Selfishness.* New York: Signet Books, 1964.
39. Hume.
40. Kant, I. *Ethical Philosophy,* J.W. Ellington, trans. Indianapolis: Hackett Publishing Company, 1986: 394-396.
41. Bentham, J. A Bentham Reader, M.P. Mack, ed. New York: Pegasus Books, 1969.
42. Kuperman, J. *Character.* New York: Oxford University Press, 1991.
43. MacIntyre.
44. Foot, P. *Virtues and Vices.* New York: Oxford University Press, 1978: 8.
45. Frankena, W. "Beneficence in an Ethics of Virtue." In: *Beneficence and Health Care.* Notre Dame: University of Notre Dame Press, 1982.
46. French, P.A., T.E. Uehling, Jr., and H.K. Wettstein, eds. *Midwest Studies in Philosophy, Volume XIII: Ethical Theory, Character and Virtue.* Notre Dame: University of Notre Dame Press, 1988.
47. Hauerwas, S. *A Community of Character.* Notre Dame, IN: University of Notre Dame Press, 1981.
48. MacIntyre, A. *Three Rival Versions of Moral Enquiry.* Notre Dame: University of Notre Dame Press, 1990.
49. Baynes, K., J. Bohman, and T. McCarthy. "Introduction." In: *After Philosophy,* K. Baynes, J. Bohman, and T. McCarthy, eds. Cambridge, MA: Massachusetts Institute of Technology Press, 1987; 1-18.
50. Rockmore, T., and B.J. Singer. *Antifoundationalism Old and New.* Philadelphia: Temple University Press, 1992.
51. Foot.
52. Warnock, G. *The Object of Morality.* London: Methuen and Company, 1971.
53. Casey, J. *Pagan Virtue.* New York: Oxford University Press, 1990.
54. Wilson, E.O. *Sociobiology.* Cambridge, MA: Belknap Press of Harvard University Press, 1980.
55. MacIntyre, *Whose Justice? Which Rationality?*
56. MacIntyre, *After Virtue.*
57. MacIntyre, *Whose Justice? Which Rationality?*
58. MacIntyre, *Three Rival Versions of Moral Enquiry.*
59. Murdoch, I. *Metaphysics as a Guide to Morals.* New York: Penguin Press, 1992: 481-484.
60. Ibid.
61. Pincoffs, E.L. *Quandaries and Virtue: Against Reductivism in Ethics.* Lawrence, KS: University Press of Kansas, 1986: 85.
62. Moore, G.E. *Principia Ethica.* Cambridge: Cambridge University Press, 1903.
63. Casey.
64. Wilson.
65. Veatch, R.M. "The Hippocratic Ethic Is Dead." *The New Physician* Sept. 1984: 41-42, 48.
66. Pellegrino, E.D. "Rationing Health Care: The Ethics of Medical Gatekeeping." *The Journal of Contemporary Health Law and Policy* 2 (1986): 23-45.
67. Veatch.
68. Pellegrino, E.D. "Medical Ethics: Entering the Post-Hippocratic Era." *The Journal of the American Board of Family Practice* 1 (1988): 20-37.

69. Clouser, K.D., and G. Bernard. "A Critique of Principlism." *Journal of Medicine and Philosophy* 15 (1990): 219-236.
70. Carse, A.L. "The 'Voice of Care': Implications for Bioethical Education." *Journal of Medicine and Philosophy* 16 (1991): 5-28.
71. Pellegrino, E.D., and D.C. Thomasma. *For the Patient's Good: The Restoration of Beneficence in Health Care.* New York: Oxford University Press, 1988.
72. Pellegrino, "Medical Ethics: Entering the Post-Hippocratic Era."
73. Pellegrino, E.D., and D.C. Thomasma. *The Virtues in Medical Practice.* New York: Oxford University Press, 1993.
74. Pellegrino, E.D. "The Four Principles and the Doctor-Patient Relationship: The Need for a Better Understanding." In: *Principles of Health Care Ethics*, R. Gillon, ed. Chichester: John Wiley & Sons, 1994: 353-366.
75. Pellegrino, E.D. "The Caring Ethic: The Relationship of Physician to Patient." In: *Caring, Curing, Coping: Nursing-Physician Relationships*, A.H. Bishop and J.R. Scudder, Jr., eds. Alabama: University of Alabama Press, 1985.
76. Pellegrino, "Rationing Health Care."

CHAPTER TEN

1. Cabot, R. *Differential Diagnosis*, vol. 1. Philadelphia: W.B. Saunders Co., 1916: 19.
2. Black, D.A.K. *The Logic of Medicine.* Edinburgh: Oliver & Boyd, 1968: 17-19.
3. Feinstein, A.R. "The Haze of Bayes, the Aerial Palaces of Decision Analysis, and the Computerized Ouija Board." *Clinical Bio-statistics* 39.
4. Jacquez, J.A., ed. *The Diagnostic Process.* Ann Arbor: University of Michigan Press, 1964.
5. Ledley, R.S., and L.B. Lusted. "Reasoning Foundation of Medical Diagnosis." *Science* 130 (1959): 9-21.
6. Murphy, E.A. *The Logic of Medicine.* Baltimore: Johns Hopkins University Press, 1976.
7. Wulff, H.R. *Rational Diagnosis and Treatment.* Oxford: Blackwell Scientific Publications, 1976.
8. Jaeger, W. *Paideia: The Ideals of Greek Culture*, vol. III, G. Highet, trans. New York: Oxford University Press, 1944: 17-19.
9. Elstein, A.S. "Clinical Judgment: Psychological Research and Medical Practice." *Science* 194 (1976): 696-700.
10. Pellegrino, E.D. "Philosophy of Medicine: Problematic and Potential." *Journal of Medicine and Philosophy* 1-1 (1976): 5-31.
11. MacIntyre, A. "Patients as Agents." In: *Philosophical Medical Ethics*, S. Spicker and H. Engelhardt, eds. Dordrecht: D. Reidel, 1977: 197-212.
12. Pellegrino, E.D. "Moral Agency and Professional Ethics: Some Notes on Transformation of the Physician-Patient Encounter," commentary on A. MacIntyre, "Patients as Agents," in *Philosophical Medical Ethics*, S. Spicker and H. Engelhardt, eds. Dordrecht: D. Reidel, 1977: 213-220.
13. Koran, L.J. "The Reliability of Clinical Methods, Data and Judgments, first of two parts." *New England Journal of Medicine* 293:13 (1975): 642-646.
14. Koran, L.J. "The Reliability of Clinical Methods, Data and Judgments, first of two parts." *New England Journal of Medicine* 293:13 (1975): 695-701.
15. McNeill, B.J., E. Keeler, and S.J. Adelstein. "Primer on Certain Elements of Medical Decision-Making." *New England Journal of Medicine* 293:5 (1975): 211-215.
16. Feinstein, A.R. *Clinical Judgment.* Baltimore: Williams & Wilkins, 1967: 214.
17. Sober, E. "Learning Theory and Clinical Practice." np. nd. 29-44.

18. Raiffa, H. *Decision Analysis: Introductory Lectures on Choices Under Uncertainty, Clinical Judgment.* Reading, PA: Addison-Wesley, 1968.
19. Feinstein, "The Haze of Bayes…"
20. Weaver, R. *The Ethics of Rhetoric.* Chicago: Henry Regnery Co., 1968; 27-28, 101-117.
21. Adler, M.J. *Dialectic.* New York: Harcourt, Brace & Co., 1927; 31, 243, 247 n. 1.
22. Sober.
23. Feinstein, A.R., and C.K. Wells. "Randomized Trials vs. Historical Controls: The Scientific Plagues of Both Houses." Association of American Physicians, nd.
24. Chambers, E.E., J.A. Inciardi, and H.A. Siegal. *Chemical Coping: A Report on Legal Drug Use in the U.S.A.* New York: Spectrum Publications, 1975: 141.
25. Warnock, G. *The Object of Morality.* London: Methuen and Company, 1971.
26. Abercrombie, M.L.J. *The Anatomy of Judgment.* London: Penguin Books, 1974.
27. Bernard, C. *An Introduction to the Study of Experimental Medicine.* New York: Macmillan, 1927; 203.
28. Sokal, R.R. "Numerical Taxonomy and Disease Classification." In: *The Diagnostic Process,* J.A. Jacquez, ed. Ann Arbor: University of Michigan Press, 1964: 51-68.
29. Elstein.
30. Kroger, J. "Polanyi and Lonergan on Scientific Method." *Philosophy Today* Spring 1977: 2-20.
31. Schwartz, W.B., G.A. Gorry, J.P. Kassier, and A. Essig. "Decision Analysis and Clinical Judgment." *The American Journal of Medicine* 55 (1973): 459-472.
32. McNeill et al.
33. Sober.
34. Einstein, A. *Out of My Later Years.* Secaucus, NJ: Citadel Press, 1974: 24.
35. Aristotle. *Metaphysics,* W.D. Ross, trans. Oxford: Clarendon Press, 1940.
36. Maritain, J. *Art and Scholasticism With Other Essays.* New York: Charles Scribner's Sons, 1949; 7 n4, n5.
37. Schwartz et al.
38. Aristotle.
39. Aquinas, T. *Summa Theologiae,* vol. 1-60, W.P Hughes, trans. Leonine text, la2ae, Question 57, art, 3-4.
40. Pellegrino, E.D. "Educating the Humanist Physician: An Ancient Ideal Reconsidered." *Journal of the American Medical Association* 227:11 (1974): 1288-1294.
41. Pellegrino, E.D. "Preface." In: *Human Values Teaching Programs for Health Professionals,* T.K. McElhinney, ed. Philadelphia: Society for Health and Human Values, 1976: ix-x.
42. Buchanan, S. *The Doctrine of Signatures: A Defense of Theory in Medicine.* London: Kegan Paul, 1938: 174.

CHAPTER ELEVEN

1. *The Caraka Samhita,* vol. 1. S. Gulabkunverba, trans. Jamnagar, India: Ayurvedic Society, 1949: 469.
2. Aulus Gellius, cited by R.S. Crane. *The Idea of the Humanities and Other Essays Critical and Historical.* Chicago: University of Chicago Press, 1968: 23.
3. Pellegrino, E.D. "The Non-Renaissance Man." *Pharas of Alpha Omega Alpha* 32:1 (1969): 16-17.
4. Jung, C. *Psychological Reflections,* J. Jacobi, ed. Princeton, NJ: Bollington Series XXI, 1970: 90.
5. Merton, T. *New Seeds of Contemplation.* New York: New Directions, 1961: 38.
6. Hesse, H. *Demian.* New York: Bantam Books, Inc., 1970: prologue.
7. Jung, 90.

8. Hammarskjöld, D. *Markings.* New York: Alfred A. Knopf, Inc., 1965: 105.
9. Rogers, C. "Bringing Together Ideas and Feeling in Learning." *Learning Today* 5:2 (1972): 32-43.
10. Entralgo, P.L. *La Relacion Medico-Enfermo Historia y Teoria.* Madrid: Revista de Occidente, 1964.
11. Kristeller, P.O. *Renaissance Thought: The Classic and Scholastic and Humanist Strains.* New York: Harper Torchbooks, 1961: 8-23.
12. Edel, A. "Where Is the Crisis in Humanism?" *Revue Internationale de Philosophie* fasc 3-4 (1968): 284-295.
13. Murray, G., quoted by H. Cushing: *Introduction to Sir William Osler: The Old Humanities and the New Science.* Boston: Houghton-Mifflin Co., 1920: x.
14. Else, G. "The Old and the New Humanities." *Daedalus* 98 (1969): 803-804.
15. Berenson, B. *Italian Painters of the Renaissance: Florentine and Central Italian Schools,* vol. 2. New York: Phaidon, 1968: 1.
16. *Proceedings of the Institute on Human Values in Medicine.* Philadelphia: Society for Health and Human Values, 1972, vol. 2, pp BP 1-BP 83.
17. Booth, W. "Is There Any Knowledge a Man Must Have?" In: *The Knowledge Most Worth Having,* W.C. Booth, ed. Chicago: University of Chicago Press, 1967: i-28.
18. Pellegrino, E.D. "The Most Humane Science: Some Notes on Liberal Education in Medicine and the University, the Sixth Sanger Lecture." *Bulletin of the Medical College of Virginia* 2 (1970): 11-39.
19. Pellegrino, E.D. "Reflections, Refractions, and Perspectives." *Proceedings of the Institute on Human Values in Medicine.* Philadelphia: Society for Health and Human Values, 1972: vol. 1, 99-115.
20. Pellegrino, E.D. "Physicians, Patients, and Society: Some New Tensions in Medical Ethics." In: *Human Aspects of Biomedical Innovation,* E. Mendelsohn, J.P. Swazey, and I. Traviss, eds. Cambridge, MA: Harvard University Press, 1971: 77, 97, 219-220.
21. Ciardi, J. "Esthetic Wisdom." *Saturday Review* April 8, 1972: 22.

CHAPTER FIFTEEN

1. Engelhardt, H.T., and M.A. Rie. "Morality for the Medical-Industrial Complex: A Code of Ethics for the Mass Marketing of Health Care." New England Journal of Medicine 319 (1989): 1086.
2. Pellegrino, E.D., and D.C. Thomasma. *For the Patient's Good: The Restoration of Beneficence in Health Care.* New York: Oxford University Press, 1987.
3. Edelstein, L. Ancient Medicine: Selected Papers of Ludwig Edelstein, O. Temkin and C.L. Temkin, eds. Baltimore: Johns Hopkins University Press, 1967: 40-57.
4. Jones, W.H.S. *The Doctor's Oath: An Essay in the History of Medicine.* Cambridge: Cambridge University Press, 1924: 42-45.
5. Carrick, P. *Medical Ethics in Antiquity: Philosophical Perspectives on Abortion.* Dordrecht: Kluwer Academic Publishers, 1985: 76-77.
6. Pellegrino, E.D. "Toward an Expanded Medical Ethics: The Hippocratic Ethic Revisited." In: *In Search of the Modern Hippocrates,* R.J. Bulgar, ed. Iowa City: University of Iowa Press, 1987: 45-64.
7. Reale, G. *The Systems of the Hellenic Age: A History of Ancient Philosophy,* J. Catan, ed. and trans. Albany: State University of New York Press, 1985: 282-283.
8. Pellegrino, E.D. "Toward a Reconstruction of Medical Morality: The Primacy of the Act of Profession and the Fact of Illness." *Journal of Medicine and Philosophy* 4 (March 1979): 32-56.

9. Percival, T. *Medical Ethics.* Birmingham: Classics of Medicine Library, 1985.
10. Reck, A.J. "Nature, Law and the Constitution." *Review of Metaphysics* 1989: 482-511.
11. Dicey, A.V. "Lectures on the Relation Between Law and Public Opinion in England During the Nineteenth Century." Cited in A. Vincent, "Can Groups Be Persons?" *Review of Metaphysics* 1989: 687-715.
12. French, P.A. *Collective and Corporate Responsibility.* New York: Columbia University Press, 1984.
13. May, L. *The Morality of Groups: Collective Responsibility, Group Based Harm, and Corporate Rights.* Notre Dame, IN: University of Notre Dame Press, 1987.
14. Pellegrino and Thomasma.
15. Lifton, R.J. *The Nazi Doctors: Medical Killing and the Psychology of Genocide.* New York: Basic Books, 1986.
16. Gallagher, H. *By Trust Betrayed: Patients, Physicians and the License to Kill.* New York: Holt, nd.
17. Lundbert, G.D. "Fifty Hours for the Poor." Editorial. *Journal of the American Medical Association* 258: 1987.
18. Jacobi, J. Inaugural Address. In: *Collected Essays, Addresses, Scientific Papers and Miscellaneous Writings*, vol. VII, Collectanea Jacobi, W.J. Robinson, ed. New York: Critic and Guide Company, 1909.

CHAPTER SEVENTEEN

Note: Chapter XVII references a bibliography rather than footnotes.

1. *Academic Plan,* Campus Academic and Development Plan, Health Sciences Center, State University of New York at Stony Brook. February 1968.
2. Muir Committee Report, Education for the Health Professions: A Comprehensive Plan for Comprehensive Care to Meet New York's Needs in an Age of Change. Malcolm Muir, chairman. June 1963.
3. Pellegrino, E.D. "The Crisis in Medical Education: The School Years, Changing Concepts in the Delivery of Health Service." American Society of Internal Medicine, 13th Annual Meeting, pp. 6-11. April 1969.
4. Pellegrino, E.D. (a) "A Health Sciences Consortium," (b) "Historical Sketch-The State University of New York at Stony Brook: Health Sciences Center-Medical School." *Notes and Tips*, Harper and Row, vol. 1, no. 9, p. 164, and p. 180. March 1971.
5. Pellegrino, E.D. "Human Values and the Medical Curriculum." *Journal of the American Medical Association*, vol. 209, p. 1349. September 1969.
6. Pellegrino, E.D. "Medical Practice and the New Curricula." *Journal of the American Medical Association*, vol. 213, p. 748. August 1970.
7. Pellegrino, E.D. "Planning the Health Science Center at Stony Brook-Academic Commitments and Architectural Constraints." Presentation at the 1968 Conference on Architecture and the College, Department of Architecture, University of Illinois. April 1968.
8. Pellegrino, E.D. "Planning the Health Sciences within a University Context: The Health Sciences Center at Stony Brook." Annals of the New York Academy of Sciences, vol. 166, no. 3, p. 874. December 1969.

CHAPTER EIGHTEEN

1. Morrill, R.L. "A Conceptual Basis for Values Education in the University." *Soundings*, LXT (1978): 421-438.
2. The Role of the University in the Search for International Value Consensus, A Bellagio Conference, July 1980. The Rockefeller Foundation, 1982.
3. MacIntyre, A. "The Nature of the Virtues." *The Hastings Center Report* April 1981: 32.

4. Calabresi, G., and P. Bobbitt. *Tragic Choices.* New York: W.W. Norton and Co., 1978.
5. Ginzberg, E. "Health Institutions and Market Incentives." *Bulletin of the New York Academy of Medicine* 58:6 (Sept. 1982): 545-555.
6. Abelson, P. "Differing Values in Academia and Industry." Editorial. *Science* 217:456 (Sept. 17, 1982).
7. Relman, A.S. "The New Medical-Industrial Complex." *New England Journal of Medicine* 303 (1980): 963-970.
8. Stockman, D. "Premises for a Medical Marketplace." *Health Affairs* Winter 1981: 5-18.
9. Bayles, M. "Physicians as Body Mechanics." In: *Concepts of Health and Disease,* A.L. Caplan, H.T. Engelhardt, Jr., and J.J. McCartney, eds. Reading, MA: Addison-Wesley Publishing co., 1981: 665-675.
10. Sade, R. "Medical Care as a Right: A Refutation." *New England Journal of Medicine* 285 (Dec. 2, 1971): 1288-1292.
11. Havighurst, C.C. "Competition in Health Services: Overview, Issues and Answers." *Vanderbilt Law Review* 34:4 (May 1981): 1117-1158.
12. Marmor, T.R., R. Boyer, and J. Greenberg. "Medical Care and Procompetitive Reform." *Vanderbilt Law Review* 34:4 (May 1981), 1003-1028.
13. Gephardt, R.A. "Do We Need Legislation to Achieve Competition? The View of an Advocate." *Health Affairs* Spring 1982: 53-68.
14. *A.M.A. v. Federal Trade Commission Respondent, Connecticut State Medical Society and New Haven County Medical Association Petitioners v. Federal Trade Commission Respondent.* Nos. 995, 1050 docket 79-4214, 79-4226, U.S. Court of Appeals, 2nd Circuit, Oct. 1980.
15. Howell, J.T. "The Profession of Medicine in the New Competitive Marketplace." *Alabama Journal of Medical Sciences* 19:3 (1982).
16. Pellegrino, E.D. "Toward a Reconstruction of Medical Morality: The Primacy of the Act of Profession and the Fact of Illness." *Journal of Medicine and Philosophy* 4 (March 1979): 32-56.
17. Toynbee, A. *A Study of History.* Oxford.

CHAPTER NINETEEN

1. Enthoven, A. "The History and Principles of Managed Competition." *Health Affairs* 12: 24-48.
2. Shearer, G. *Hidden from View: The Growing Burden of Health Care Costs.* Washington: Consumers Union, 1998.
3. Ware, J.E. "Differences in Health Outcomes for Elderly and Poor Chronically Ill Patients: Results from Outcome Studies." *Journal of the American Medical Association* 216:1039-1047.
4. Worland, S.T. "Adam Smith, Economic Justice and the Founding Fathers." In: *New Directions in Economic Justice,* R. Skurski, ed. Notre Dame: University of Notre Dame Press 1983: 1-12.
5. Daniels, N. *Just Health Care.* Cambridge: Cambridge University Press, 1985.
6. Daniels, N., D. Light, and R. Caplan. *Benchmarks of Fairness for Health Care Reform.* New York: Oxford University Press, 1996.
7. Light, D.W. "The Sociological Character of Health Care." In: *Health Care Markets, Handbook of Social Studies in Health,* G.L. Albrecht, R. Fitzpatrick, and S.C. Scrimshaw, eds. London: Sage Publications, 2000.
8. Rice, T. "Can Market Forces Give Us the Health Care System We Want?" *Journal of Health Politics, Policy and Law* 22 (1987): 383-426.
9. Pellegrino, E.D., and D.C. Thomasma. *For the Patient's Good: The Restoration of Beneficence in Health Care.* New York: Oxford University Press, 1987.
10. Lewis, I.T., and C.G. Sheps. *The Sick Citadel: American Academic Health Centers and the Public Interest.* Cambridge, MA: Oelgeselager, Gunn, and Hain, 1983.

11. Pellegrino, E.D. "Academic Health Centers and the Medical Marketplace: A Faustian Compact Examined." In: *Dr. Partridge's Dilemma-The Academic Health Center: Keeping It All Together Is Not Easy.* (Proceedings of the 1982 Association of Academic Health Centers Annual Meeting.) Washington: Association of Academic Health Centers, 1983: 19-39.

Also noted:

Novak, M. The Spirit of Democratic Capitalism. Lanham, MD: Madison Books, 1982.

Pellegrino, E.D. "The Commodification of Medical and Health Care: The Moral Consequences of a Paradigm Shift from a Professional to a Market Ethic." *Journal of Medicine and Philosophy* 24 (1999): 243-266.